PERSPECTIVES IN HYPERTENSION
Volume 1

The Kidney in Hypertension

PERSPECTIVES IN HYPERTENSION SERIES

Series Editors
Barry M. Brenner, Norman M. Kaplan,
and John H. Laragh

Vol. 1 The Kidney in Hypertension, *edited by Norman M. Kaplan, Barry M. Brenner, and John H. Laragh,* 288 pp., 1987.

PERSPECTIVES IN HYPERTENSION
Volume 1

The Kidney in Hypertension

Editors

Norman M. Kaplan, M.D.
University of Texas
Health Science Center at Dallas
Dallas, Texas

Barry M. Brenner, M.D.
Department of Medicine
Harvard Medical School
Boston, Massachusetts

John H. Laragh, M.D.
Department of Medicine
The New York Hospital
Cornell Medical Center
New York, New York

Raven Press New York

Raven Press, 1185 Avenue of the Americas, New York, New York 10036

Made in the United States of America

Library of Congress Cataloging-in-Publication Data
The Kidney in hypertension.

(Perspectives in hypertension ; v. 1)
Includes index.

1. Renal hypertension. I. Kaplan, Norman M., 1931– II. Brenner, Barry M., 1937– III. Laragh, John H., 1924– . IV. Series.
[DNLM: 1. Hypertension. 2. Kidney—physiopathology. WG 340 K465]
RC918.R38K53 1987 616.1′32 874527
ISBN 0-88167-298-X

The material contained in this volume was submitted as previously unpublished material, except in the instances in which credit has been given to the source from which some of the illustrative material was derived.

Great care has been taken to maintain the accuracy of the information contained in the volume. However, Raven Press cannot be held responsible for errors or for any consequences arising from the use of the information contained herein.

9 8 7 6 5 4 3 2 1

Preface

Hypertension is now the single most common reason for visits to physicians and for the use of prescription drugs. This tremendous increase in clinical attention, occurring mainly over the past 10 years, reflects a similar increase in research and in both writing and teaching about hypertension.

Consider that in 1973, Sir George Pickering's book *High Blood Pressure* was virtually the only one available. In 1986, there must be 50.

Consider that in 1980, there were no journals exclusively covering hypertension. In 1986, there are at least six.

It should then be obvious that a virtual flood of material is now available, more than any one physician can assimilate. There is, then, a need for concise, timely reviews of the field, written by those who are both involved in the research and able to communicate effectively.

This series—*Perspectives in Hypertension*—hopes to provide such timely reviews that will be authoritative in their coverage and easily assimilated into clinical practice. This volume—the first in what is planned to be an annual series—covers an area wherein major diagnostic and therapeutic advances have been made but which remains a difficult and unsettled relationship: the kidney and hypertension. As covered in the first section of six chapters, the kidney is undoubtedly involved in the pathophysiology of all forms of hypertension. New insights as to this role provide the basis for the following two sections of 12 chapters detailing the clinical aspects and therapeutic strategies now available.

Since hypertension is the most common cause of renal failure and since renal dysfunction is involved in all hypertension, this subject seems appropriate for the first in our series. The editors and authors hope that this book—and those that follow—will clarify some of the major issues in hypertension and help clinicians deal with them to our patients' benefit.

The Editors

Contents

The Role of the Kidney in the Pathogenesis of Hypertension

The Kidney and Hypertension—Clinical Aspects

Therapeutic Strategies in Hypertension

Contributors

Sharon Anderson
Department of Medicine
Harvard Medical School
Boston, Massachusetts 02115

William M. Bennett
Oregon Health Sciences University School of Medicine
Portland, Oregon 97201

Barry M. Brenner
Department of Medicine
Harvard Medical School
Boston, MA 02115

Thomas G. Coleman
Department of Physiology and Biophysics
University of Mississippi Medical Center
Jackson, Mississippi 39216–4505

Gerald F. DiBona
Department of Internal Medicine
University of Iowa College of Medicine
Iowa City, Iowa 52242

Arthur C. Guyton
Department of Physiology and Biophysics
University of Mississippi Medical Center
Jackson, Mississippi 39216–4505

John E. Hall
Department of Physiology and Biophysics
University of Mississippi Medical Center
Jackson, Mississippi 39216–4505

Bruce J. Hillman
Department of Radiology
University of Arizona College of Medicine
Tucson, Arizona 85724

Norman M. Kaplan
University of Texas Health Science Center at Dallas
Dallas, Texas 75235

Michael Kashgarian
Department of Pathology
Yale University School of Medicine
New Haven, Connecticut 06510

John P. Koepke
Department of Internal Medicine
University of Iowa College of Medicine
Iowa City, Iowa 52242

Ulla C. Kopp
Department of Internal Medicine
University of Iowa College of Medicine
Iowa City, Iowa 52242

John H. Laragh
Department of Medicine
The New York Hospital
Cornell Medical Center
New York, New York 10021

H. Leland Mizelle
Department of Physiology and Biophysics
University of Mississippi Medical Center
Jackson, Mississippi 39216–4505

Richard S. Muther
Divisions of Nephrology/Hypertension
University of Missouri
Kansas City School of Medicine
Kansas City, Missouri 64108

Andrew C. Novick
Department of Urology
Cleveland Clinic Foundation
Cleveland, Ohio 44106

Thomas G. Pickering
Department of Medicine
The New York Hospital
Cornell University Medical Center
New York, New York 10021

C. Venkata S. Ram
Department of Internal Medicine
Southwestern Medical School
Dallas, Texas 75235–9030

Gerald M. Reid
Divisions of Nephrology/Hypertension
University of Missouri
Kansas City School of Medicine
Kansas City, Missouri 64108

Brian F. Robinson
Department of Medicine
St. George's Hospital Medical School
London, England SW17 ORE

Burton D. Rose
The Brigham and Women's Hospital
Boston, Massachusetts 02115

D. E. Schwarten
St. Vincent Hospital and Health Care Center
Indianapolis, Indiana 46260

Stephen C. Textor
Renal Physiology Laboratory
City of Hope National Medical Center
Duarte, California 91010

Lawrence A. Turka
The Brigham and Women's Hospital
Boston, Massachusetts 02115

E. D. Vaughan, Jr.
Department of Medicine
University of Virginia School of Medicine
Charlottesville, Virginia 22908

Lori L. Woods
Department of Physiology and Biophysics
University of Mississippi Medical Center
Jackson, Mississippi 39216–4505

Randall M. Zusman
Hypertension Division, Cardiac Unit
Harvard Medical School
Boston, Massachusetts 02115

The Kidney in Hypertension, edited by Norman M. Kaplan, Barry M. Brenner, and John H. Laragh. Raven Press, New York © 1987.

Renal Excretory Function and Hypertension

John E. Hall, Arthur C. Guyton, Thomas G. Coleman, Lori L. Woods, and H. Leland Mizelle

Department of Physiology and Biophysics, University of Mississippi Medical Center, Jackson, Mississippi 39216-4505

Most forms of experimental hypertension begin with some obvious insult to the kidney that alters renal hemodynamics and/or tubular reabsorption. For example, Goldblatt hypertension begins with stenosis of one or both of the renal arteries; mineralocorticoid hypertension begins with increased tubular sodium reabsorption; and hypertension caused by infusion of vasoconstrictors such as angiotensin II (ANGII) or norepinephrine may be associated with increased tubular reabsorption as well as renal vasoconstriction. As hypertension develops, many of these initial changes in renal function are obscured by various compensatory mechanisms that return sodium and water excretion to normal. Some of these compensations are mediated by intrinsic renal mechanisms, but when systemic changes such as increased arterial pressure are needed to maintain sodium balance, a cascade of secondary alterations in circulatory function may occur. In some instances, these secondary abnormalities may be even more striking than the initial disturbances of renal function after various compensatory changes have taken place, even though the original insult was to the kidney.

In searching for the mechanisms involved in the pathogenesis of human essential hypertension, it is tempting to focus on those changes that are readily observable after hypertension is established. However, this approach can lead to confusion regarding those abnormalities that are *causal* versus those that merely *result from* hypertension. Therefore, rather than providing a compilation of the changes in renal hemodynamics and tubular reabsorption that occur in different forms of experimental and human hypertension, we will briefly review the mechanisms by which the kidneys normally regulate blood pressure and the physiological bases for increased arterial pressure caused by various disturbances of renal function.

RENAL-BODY FLUID FEEDBACK CONTROL OF ARTERIAL PRESSURE

One of the most basic mechanisms by which the kidneys regulate arterial pressure is by altering renal excretion of salt and water, and therefore circulatory volume. Changes in arterial pressure, in turn, influence renal excretion (60,63) (the phenomena of pressure natriuresis and diuresis), providing a negative feedback mechanism for control of arterial pressure and extracellular fluid volume. The basic components of this mechanism, often referred to as the renal-body fluid feedback (26,27), are illustrated in Fig. 1. This feedback mechanism normally acts as a powerful stabilizer of arterial pressure, because increases in pressure above the normal set-point tend to raise sodium and water excretion and decrease extracellular fluid volume until arterial pressure returns to normal. Conversely, reductions in arterial pressure tend to cause sodium and water retention, thereby elevating extracellular fluid volume until arterial pressure increases to normal. An important feature of this feedback system is that there are many neurohumoral controls that act to amplify

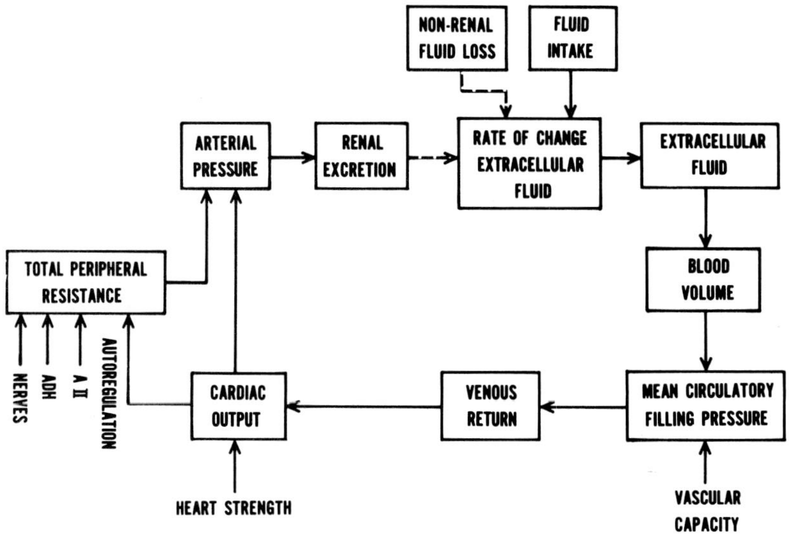

FIG. 1. Basic components of renal-body fluid feedback system for regulation of arterial pressure. *Solid lines* indicate positive effects and *dashed lines* indicate negative effects. (ADH) Antidiuretic hormone; (AII) angiotensin II.

its effectiveness in regulating arterial pressure. For example, increases in arterial pressure not only tend to raise renal excretion directly, but also inhibit formation of ANGII and aldosterone, which further elevates renal excretion and decreases extracellular fluid volume, promoting a more rapid recovery of arterial pressure.

The renal-body fluid feedback, acting in conjunction with various neurohumoral controls, is potentially very powerful in long-term regulation of arterial pressure because it continues to operate until pressure is restored to the normal set-point, providing an "infinite gain" control system (26). Thus, disturbances that tend to increase arterial pressure by raising cardiac output or total peripheral resistance but do not alter the set-point of the renal pressure natriuresis mechanism would cause only transient increases in arterial pressure, because natriuresis and diuresis would continue to decrease extracellular fluid volume until arterial pressure returned to normal (26,35).

Although the renal pressure natriuresis mechanism normally acts to prevent changes in arterial pressure, abnormalities of renal hemodynamics or tubular reabsorption can alter the set-point at which arterial pressure and sodium excretion are controlled. For example, excessive formation of a powerful antinatriuretic hormone such as ANGII, or a renal disease that reduces renal excretory capability, would tend to cause fluid retention and increase extracellular fluid volume if intake remained constant. Accumulation of fluid would continue until blood pressure increased sufficiently to restore renal excretion to normal, via the pressure natriuresis mechanism. In the steady state, renal excretion would be maintained equal to intake, but at the expense of hypertension.

The renal-body fluid feedback concept implies that long-term regulation of arterial pressure is dictated by renal excretory capability; functional or pathological changes that decrease renal excretory capability would necessitate increased arterial pressure to maintain sodium and water balance. However, factors that do not alter renal excretory capability would not cause chronic hypertension. Thus, changes in total peripheral resistance or cardiac output would not be considered as *causes* of hypertension, but merely a means of adjusting arterial pressure to the level dictated by renal excretory function.

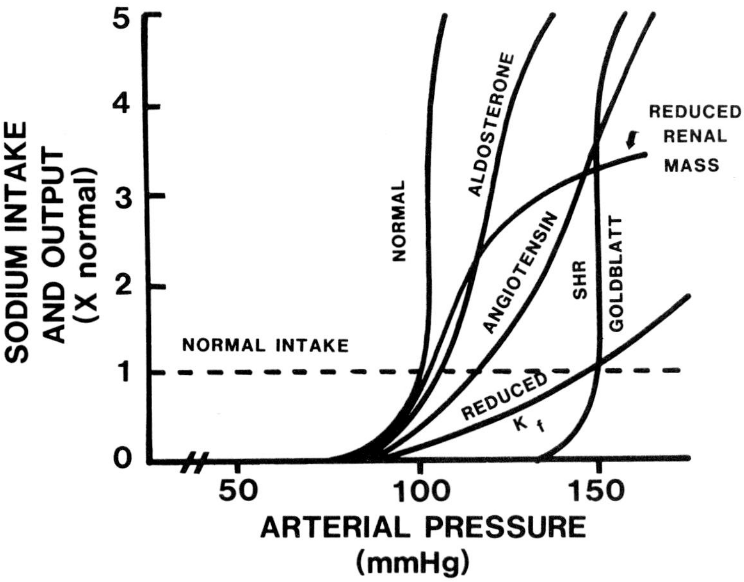

FIG. 2. Steady-state relationships between arterial pressure and urinary sodium excretion and sodium intake in various forms of hypertension. (K_f) Glomerular capillary filtration coefficient; (SHR) spontaneously hypertensive rats.

ABNORMAL PRESSURE NATRIURESIS AND DIURESIS: A CAUSE OR A CONSEQUENCE OF HYPERTENSION?

In all forms of chronic hypertension, the pressùre natriuresis mechanism is abnormal, since the steady-state level of sodium excretion is approximately the same as in normotension, assuming that sodium intake is normal. Figure 2 illustrates the approximate steady-state relationships between arterial pressure and sodium excretion in several types of experimental hypertension (26). In each of these examples, the pressure natriuresis curve is shifted so that sodium balance occurs at elevated blood pressures. Obviously, a shift of the pressure natriuresis curve to a higher pressure level must occur in all forms of chronic hypertension, otherwise sodium excretion would remain higher than sodium intake until it caused severe volume depletion, circulatory collapse and death.

One explanation for the shift of the pressure natriuresis curve in hypertension that is consistent with the renal-body fluid feedback concept is that a primary reduction in renal excretory capability initiates a compensatory increase in arterial pressure to maintain fluid balance. The reduction in renal excretory capability could be caused by decreased glomerular filtration rate (GFR) or increased tubular reabsorption, due to various functional or pathological changes in the kidney. In the steady state, normal sodium excretion is maintained at the expense of chronic hypertension. An opposing view of the abnormal pressure natriuresis mechanism in hypertension is that it occurs *secondarily* to increased arterial pressure (50,57,63). This concept predicts that hypertension can be initiated by elevations in cardiac output or total peripheral vascular resistance and that the kidneys secondarily adapt to the increased arterial pressure, through various intrinsic or neurohormonal mechanisms, to maintain sodium balance. Obviously, if the kidneys could *completely* reset their excretion of sodium after chronic changes in arterial pressure initiated by nonrenal abnormalities, the renal pressure natriuresis mechanism could not play a major role in long-term blood pressure regulation. Therefore, one of the most important issues concerning the role of the kidneys in the pathogenesis of hypertension is whether arterial pressure has a long-term effect on sodium and water excretion. To answer this question, it may be useful to consider the pressure natriuresis mechanism in a few examples of experimental hypertension in which the direct effects of increased arterial pressure can be separated from other factors that influence renal excretion.

Mineralocorticoid Hypertension

Excessive secretion of mineralocorticoids, or infusion of mineralocorticoids such as aldosterone, typically causes transient sodium and water retention and gradual elevation of arterial pressure (34,45). Sodium retention lasts for only a few days, depending on sodium intake and the severity of mineralocorticoid excess, and is followed by an "escape" in which sodium excretion returns to normal. Although the phenomenon of renal escape has been extensively studied, the mechanisms that enable the kidney to maintain sodium balance in the face of continued mineralocorticoid excess and the factors involved in causing hypertension have been very controversial.

According to the renal-body fluid feedback concept, mineralocorticoids reduce renal excretory capability by increasing tubular reabsorption, thereby initiating a sequence of events that culminates in hypertension. Increased arterial pressure, in turn, restores sodium and water excretion to normal via the pressure natriuresis mechanism. However, because mineralocorticoid excess is almost invariably associated with increased total peripheral vascular resistance, the increased arterial pressure has also been postulated to be caused by a direct or an indirect effect of mineralocorticoids to constrict the peripheral vasculature (3,43,54). Two ideas that have received considerable attention are that mineralocorticoids may activate the sympathetic nervous system or stimulate release of a oubain-like circulating inhibitor of sodium-potassium ATPase, which, in turn, might constrict the peripheral vasculature and elevate arterial pressure (22,28,29). The escape from sodium retention could also be independent of increased arterial pressure and be mediated by increased formation of various natriuretic factors, such as a oubain-like natriuretic hormone, atrial natriuretic factor, kinins, prostaglandins, or decreased renal sympathetic nerve activity (1,8,21,45,51,62).

To resolve these issues and to directly test the importance of the pressure natriuresis mechanism in regulating sodium balance in mineralocorticoid hypertension, we compared the chronic blood pressure and renal effects of aldosterone infusion in dogs in which renal perfusion pressure was either permitted to increase or servocontrolled at the normal level (34). In normal dogs, aldosterone infusion increased arterial pressure by only about 19 mm Hg after 7 days. Sodium excretion decreased transiently but returned toward control on the second day of infusion, and after 7 days cumulative sodium balance was only slightly elevated. In contrast, when renal perfusion pressure was servocontrolled during aldosterone infusion (Fig. 3), sodium excretion remained approximately 80 mEq/day below intake (263 mEq/day) throughout the 7 days of infusion. Therefore, cumulative sodium balance continued to increase, causing marked ascites and peripheral edema in several dogs. The systemic arterial hypertension was also much more severe when renal arterial pressure was prevented from increasing, with mean arterial pressure rising to approximately 60 mm Hg above control. When the servocontroller was stopped and renal perfusion pressure was allowed to increase to hypertensive levels, there was a prompt escape from sodium retention and cumulative sodium balance, and arterial pressure returned to about the same levels as measured in normal dogs during aldosterone infusion.

These observations indicate that the pressure natriuresis mechanism plays an essential role in maintaining sodium balance during mineralocorticoid hypertension. Because the increase in systemic arterial pressure had not plateaued even after 7 days of aldosterone infusion, it seems likely that arterial pressure would have continued to increase as long as renal perfusion pressure was servocontrolled, eventually causing circulatory collapse. If various natriuretic fac-

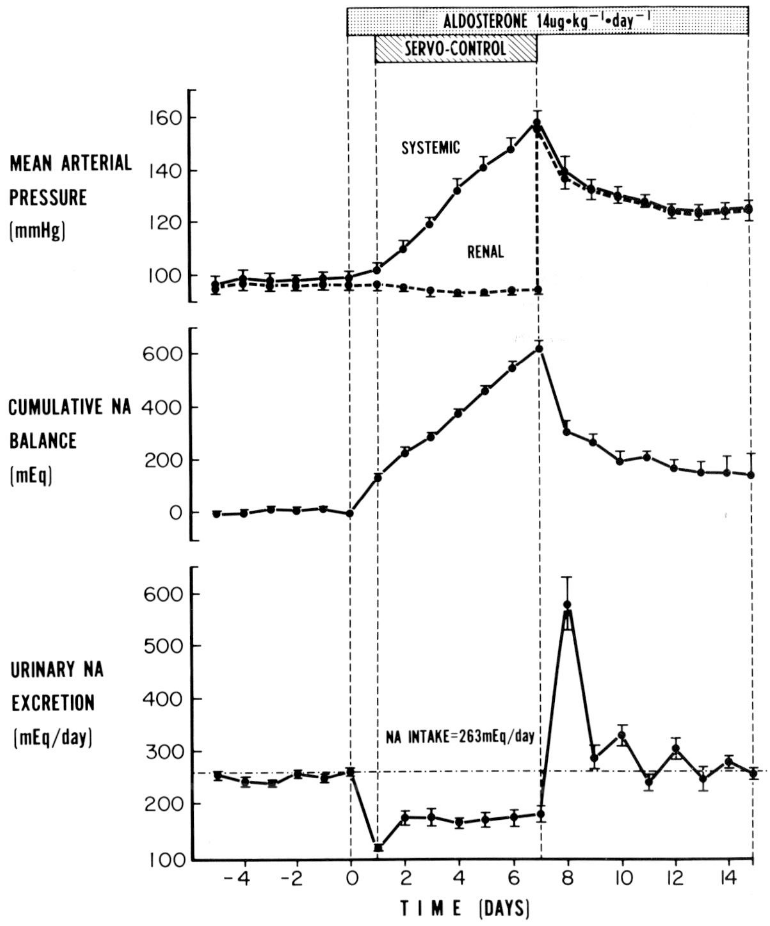

FIG. 3. Effects of aldosterone infusion when renal perfusion pressure was servocontrolled at the normal level in dogs maintained on high sodium intake. (From ref. 34.)

tors are released in aldosterone hypertension, they are apparently not sufficiently powerful to offset the antinatriuretic actions of mineralocorticoids in the absence of increased perfusion pressure. However, it is possible that natriuretic influences could play a role in minimizing the increase in arterial pressure needed to maintain sodium balance. We have previously demonstrated that suppression of ANGII formation is an important mechanism for minimizing the rise in arterial pressure needed to maintain sodium balance during chronic increases in sodium intake (37). Presumably, decreased ANGII formation could also play a role in attenuating the hypertensive effects of mineralocorticoids and in allowing escape from sodium retention during mild mineralocorticoid excess that is insufficient to cause hypertension. However, when mineralocorticoid excess is severe enough to cause hypertension, plasma renin activity is suppressed to undetectable levels and increased arterial pressure is apparently the remaining mechanism that is essential for maintaining sodium balance.

The intrarenal mechanisms by which increased arterial pressure allows escape from the antinatriuretic effects of aldosterone appear to be related to small increases in GFR and renal plasma flow and decreases in fractional sodium reabsorption (34). The observation that GFR and renal plasma flow are elevated in mineralocorticoid hypertension, even though renal excretory capability is reduced, illustrates an important point: evaluation of renal excretory capability cannot be based on steady-state measurements of renal hemodynamics, tubular reabsorption, or even urinary sodium excretion, since each of these variables is influenced by various compensatory mechanisms that are set into motion as hypertension develops. In the case of mineralocorticoid hypertension, increases in GFR and renal plasma flow, along with a reduction in proximal fractional reabsorption, appear to be important compensations for a primary increase in distal tubular sodium reabsorption. In the steady state, a reduction in renal excretory capability is apparent only when one considers the arterial pressure that is needed to maintain sodium excretion equal to intake.

Angiotensin II Hypertension

Excessive ANGII formation is an even more potent hypertensive stimulus than mineralocorticoid excess. ANGII hypertension may have an adrenal component, since ANGII stimulates aldosterone secretion (48), but ANGII also has important direct effects on the kidney that contribute to sodium retention and increased arterial pressure (31,32,38). Infusion of physiological doses of ANGII normally causes a transient decrease in sodium excretion followed by a return of sodium balance as arterial pressure increases (36). According to the renal-body fluid feedback concept, increased arterial pressure is a compensatory response essential for maintaining sodium balance in the face of the continued antinatriuretic effects of ANGII. However, ANGII is also believed to increase arterial pressure by raising total peripheral vascular resistance directly or indirectly by activating the sympathetic nervous system (22,58,69). Moreover, renal escape from sodium retention during chronic ANGII hypertension could be independent of increased arterial pressure and mediated by increased formation of various natriuretic factors that are stimulated by ANGII.

To quantitate the importance of the renal pressure natriuresis mechanism in ANGII hypertension, we examined the chronic effects of ANGII infusion when renal perfusion pressure was servocontrolled (33) (Fig. 4). As long as renal arterial pressure was maintained constant, escape from sodium retention did not occur and cumulative sodium balance and systemic arterial pressure in the upper part of the body continued to increase. Although the rate of ANGII infusion in these experiments (5 ng/kg/min) normally raises arterial pressure only 25 to 30 mm Hg, systemic arterial pressure increased to 50 to 70 mm Hg above control, in parallel with increased sodium balance, when renal artery pressure was servocontrolled. In some experiments, sodium retention was so severe and arterial pressure increased to such an extent that pulmonary edema developed after 4 to 6 days of ANGII infusion (33). When the servocontroller was stopped and renal artery pressure was allowed to increase to hypertensive levels while ANGII infusion was continued, cumulative sodium balance and arterial pressure decreased to approximately the same levels observed in normal dogs (i.e., renal artery pressure not servocontrolled) during ANGII infusion. These observations add further evidence that the renal-pressure natriuresis mechanism plays a dominant role in long-term control of sodium balance and that hypertension is a necessary "tradeoff" for decreased renal excretory capability.

Like aldosterone hypertension, ANGII hypertension is associated with very few detectable abnormalities of renal function after various compensations have taken place. GFR, tubular reabsorption, and sodium excretion are nearly normal, although renal plasma flow may be slightly reduced and filtration fraction is elevated in ANGII hypertension (33,36). However, before various compensatory mechanisms are activated and prior to increases in renal perfusion pressure, ANGII has several effects that tend to increase sodium reabsorption markedly (31,32). Increased arterial pressure offsets these antinatriuretic actions of ANGII by causing small increases in glomerular filtration and decreases in fractional sodium reabsorption in proximal and distal tubules (31–33). Thus, in analyzing

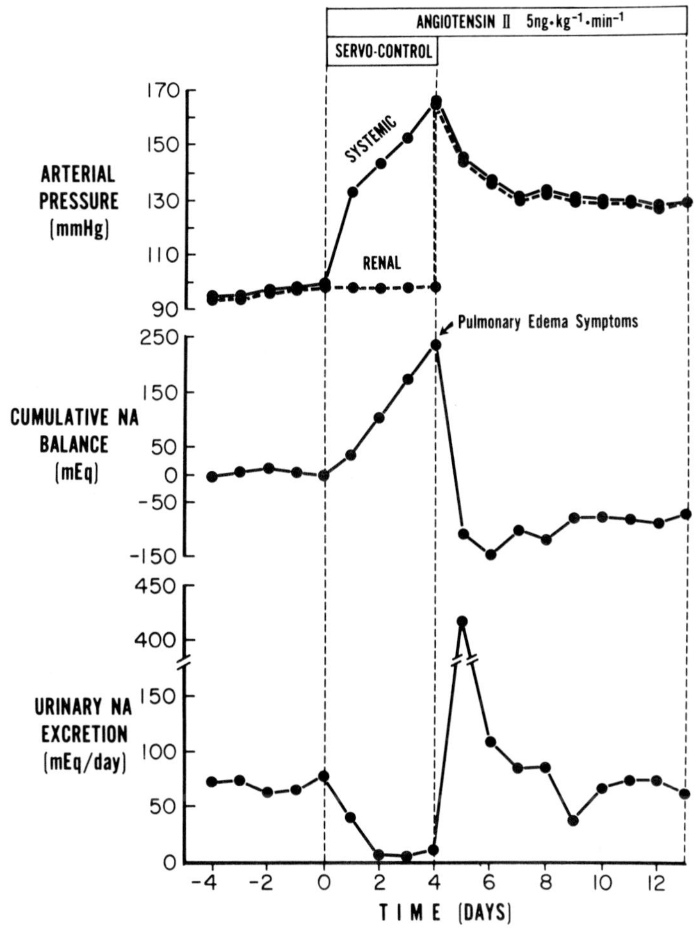

FIG. 4. Effects of angiotensin II infusion in a dog in which renal perfusion pressure was servocontrolled at the normal level. After 4 days, severe hypertension in sodium and water retention resulted in pulmonary edema. (From ref. 33.)

the effect of ANGII on renal excretory function, one must consider the effects of compensatory changes in arterial pressure. Normal sodium excretion associated with high ANGII levels and high arterial pressure represents reduced excretory capability, because increased arterial pressure would usually cause natriuresis. Likewise, when ANGII formation is blocked and arterial pressure decreases, normal sodium excretion is indicative of increased renal excretory capability.

Figure 5 shows a more complete analysis of the interrelationships between ANGII, arterial pressure, and sodium excretion during progressive changes in sodium intake in three groups of dogs with different levels of activity of the renin-angiotensin system (RAS) (37). In these experiments, sodium intake was raised in steps from 5 to 500 mEq/day and maintained at each level for 8 days until balance between intake and output of sodium was achieved. In normal dogs with an intact RAS, sodium balance was maintained with only minor changes (5–10 mm Hg) in arterial pressure over the entire range of sodium intakes, indicating a very effective pressure natriuresis mechanism. However, when ANGII was infused at a low rate (5 ng/kg/min) throughout the experiment so that circulating

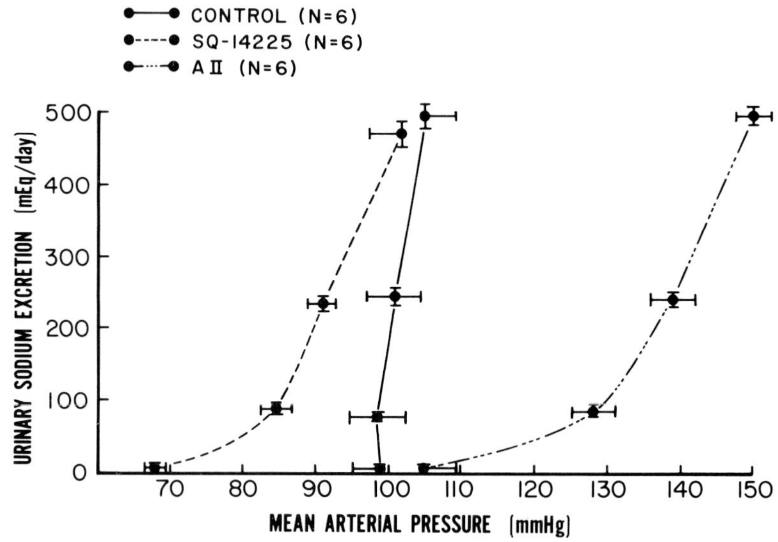

FIG. 5. Steady-state relationships between arterial pressure and sodium excretion in control dogs and in dogs infused with the converting enzyme inhibitor SQ-14225 or angiotensin II (5 ng/kg/min). (From ref. 37.)

levels of ANGII could not be suppressed, much larger increases in arterial pressure (40–50 mm Hg) were required to maintain sodium balance when intake was raised. This observation indicates that inappropriately high levels of ANGII, or an inability to suppress ANGII formation normally, greatly reduce the effectiveness of the renin-pressure natriuresis mechanism. An obvious implication of these observations is that hypertension could occur as a result of an inability to suppress ANGII normally during disturbances that tended to increase extracellular fluid volume and arterial pressure. After blockade of ANGII formation with the converting enzyme inhibitor SQ-14225, renal excretory capability was increased markedly, since sodium balance was maintained at lower than normal arterial pressures. This effect of converting enzyme inhibitors on renal excretory function provides the basis for their long-term antihypertensive action.

Vasopressin Hypertension

Although vasopressin is one of the most potent vasoconstrictors in the body, minimal increases in arterial pressure are observed in patients with inappropriate antidiuretic hormone (ADH) syndrome or during chronic vasopressin infusion in normal animals (13,61). Vasopressin may cause moderate increases in arterial pressure and extracellular fluid volume for a few days because of its antidiuretic effects, but the kidneys quickly escape the fluid retention and extracellular fluid volume and arterial pressure eventually returns toward normal (13,40,61). The fact that a vasoconstrictor as powerful as vasopressin does not cause sustained hypertension is difficult to explain if one considers increases in total peripheral resistance to be a primary determinant of hypertension. However, the failure of vasopressin to sustain hypertension is easy to explain considering its renal actions. Although vasopressin has a potent antidiuretic effect on the kidney, it does not have a major antinatriuretic action. Therefore, increases in arterial pressure would tend to cause natriuresis and offset the fluid retention initiated by vasopressin.

To directly test the role of the pressure natriuresis and diuresis mechanisms in mediating renal escape from fluid retention and in minimizing the hypertensive effects of vasopressin, we compared the chronic effects of arginine vasopressin (AVP) in dogs in which renal artery pressure was servocontrolled with the responses measured when pressure was allowed to increase (40). In normal dogs, AVP infusion at rates that produced maximal antidiuresis (0.2 mU/kg/min) increased arterial pressure to peak values of 25 to 30 mm Hg above control while causing fluid retention and increased urine osmolality for 3 days. However, after 3 to 4 days urine volume and osmolality returned toward normal and mean arterial pressure began to decline, averaging only 10 to 15 mm Hg above control after 9 days. This decline of arterial pressure was associated with a net loss of approximately 180 mEq of sodium. In contrast to the response of normal dogs, AVP caused sustained antidiuresis when renal perfusion pressure was servocontrolled, despite continuous expansion of body fluid volume (Fig. 6). Urine osmolality remained elevated and mean systemic arterial pressure continued to increase in parallel with the fluid retention. After 8 days of AVP infusion

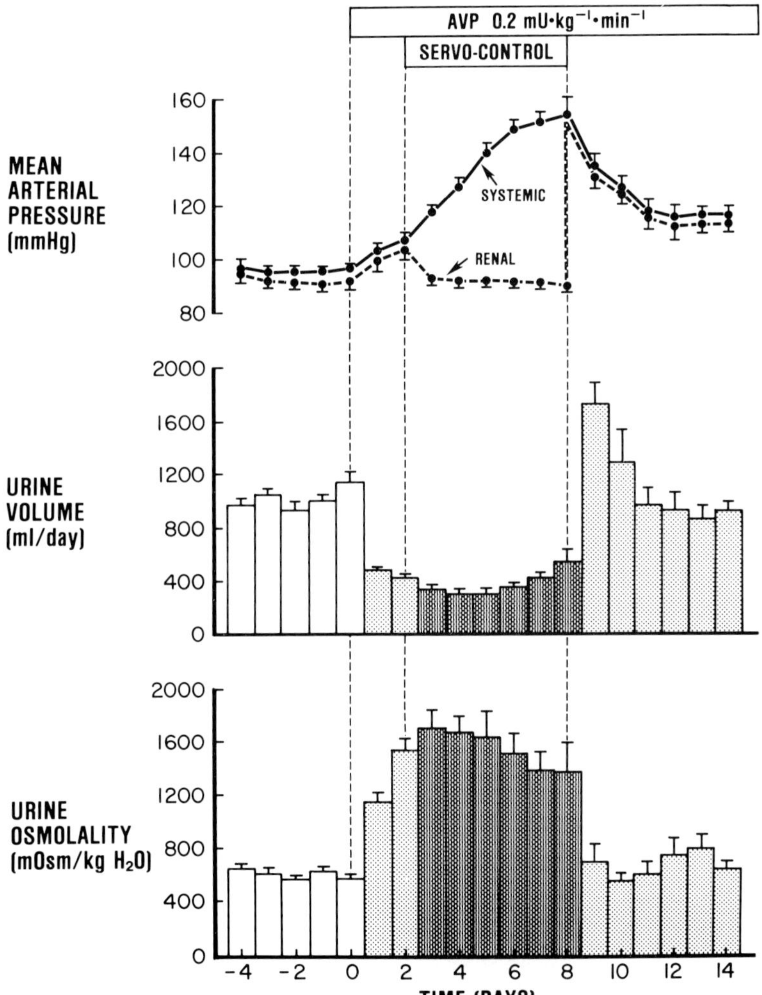

FIG. 6. Effects of arginine vasopressin (AVP) infusion when renal perfusion pressure was servocontrolled at the normal level. (From ref. 40.)

with renal artery pressure held constant, mean systemic arterial pressure increased to approximately 55 mm Hg above control. Servocontrolling renal artery pressure also prevented the large loss of sodium chloride normally seen with AVP infusion. When the servocontroller was stopped and AVP infusion was continued, there was a rapid escape from fluid retention with urine volume and sodium excretion increasing and urine osmolality decreasing toward normal. Mean arterial pressure also decreased to levels similar to those seen with AVP infusion when renal artery pressure was allowed to increase.

Thus, the pressure natriuresis and diuresis mechanisms play an essential role in offsetting the antidiuretic effect of AVP, thereby minimizing volume expansion and hypertension. These results support the view that the chronic hypertensive effects of AVP depend on fluid retention (14). Although AVP is a potent peripheral vasoconstrictor, this effect does not appear to cause chronic hypertension as long as the pressure natriuresis and diuresis mechanisms are functioning normally. However, when pressure natriuresis and diuresis are impaired (e.g., with renal disease or reduced renal mass), AVP may be capable of causing severe fluid retention and hypertension.

We have also seen similar results in other forms of experimental hypertension that we have studied, including norepinephrine and corticotropin (ACTH) hypertension (39). In each case, increased renal perfusion pressure is essential for maintaining sodium excretion in balance with intake. Thus, there is substantial experimental support for the major premise of the renal-body fluid feedback concept of blood pressure regulation that arterial pressure has a profound long-term effect on renal excretion. We have found no evidence that sodium balance is maintained independently of renal perfusion pressure in hypertension. And if one is willing to accept the conclusion that increased arterial pressure has important long-term effects on renal excretion, then it is clear that chronic hypertension can occur only when there is an abnormality of renal excretory capability.

Essential Hypertension

In human essential hypertension, no specific renal disease can be identified, at least in the early stages of hypertension, and there is little evidence for increased levels of antinatriuretic hormones such as ANGII or aldosterone. These observations have led many researchers to believe that renal function is entirely normal in human essential hypertension. However, it is clear that renal excretory function is not normal in essential hypertension, since the renal pressure natriuresis mechanism is shifted along the arterial pressure axis and normal sodium excretion is maintained only at elevated blood pressure (Fig. 7). This observation alone indicates that the kidneys' capability to excrete sodium is reduced. Omvik et al. (57) have also demonstrated that when arterial pressure in patients with essential hypertension was acutely reduced by infusion of nitroprusside, sodium excretion decreased below normal, indicating that the pressure natriuresis mechanism was attenuated in these patients. A similar abnormality of the renal-pressure natriuresis mechanism has also

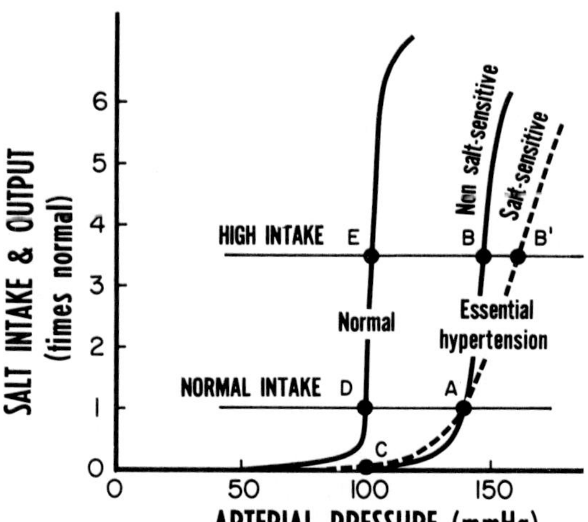

FIG. 7. Steady-state relationships between arterial pressure and sodium intake and output in normal subjects and essential hypertensives. The two types of curves for essential hypertensives represent the salt-sensitive and non-salt-sensitive type of hypertensive. (From ref. 26.)

been observed in all animal models of genetic hypertension that have been studied (12,56,65).

Evidence that abnormalities of renal function play a causal role in hypertension and are not merely secondary to increased arterial pressure comes from kidney cross-transplantation studies in experimental models of genetic hypertension. In Okamoto spontaneously hypertensive rats (SHR), Dahl salt-sensitive rats, and the Milan strain of SHR, transplantation of kidneys from hypertensive donors into normotensive controls increased arterial pressure in the recipient (4,5,9,12,16,17,44). One drawback of these studies is that it is possible that the kidneys from hypertensive rats may have been damaged as a result of increased arterial pressure before transplantation. However, more persuasive is the observation that transplantation of kidneys from normotensive controls into hypertensive rats normalized blood pressure in the recipient (4,5; see 9,12 for review). Thus, normotension or hypertension follows the kidneys and is not dictated by the various systemic abnormalities that have been reported in these models of genetic hypertension. These observations suggest that a genetic renal defect is involved in initiating and sustaining hypertension in these experimental models. That these observations in animals may be relevant to the pathogenesis of human essential hypertension is supported by the recent observations of Curtis et al. (15). These investigators reported that transplantation of kidneys from normotensive donors into patients with essential hypertension and renal failure due to nephrosclerosis led to a complete normalization of arterial pressure. If increased arterial pressure had been caused by some factor extrinsic to the kidneys, hypertension should have eventually reappeared after transplantation. However, blood pressure remained normal in all patients for an average follow-up period of 4.5 years. These observations support the view that essential hypertension may be caused by some type of intrinsic renal defect.

Unfortunately, the precise nature of the defect responsible for altering the renal-pressure natriuresis mechanism in human essential hypertension is still uncertain (11). It seems likely that essential hypertension is a very heterogeneous disease, beginning with different abnormalities of renal hemodynamics or tubular reabsorption in different patients. Unfortunately, measurements of various indices of renal function after hypertension is established, or even during the development of hypertension, may not give a great deal of insight into the pathophysiological processes that initiate the hypertension, because such measurements represent a summation of compensatory mechanisms and abnormalities involved in causing the hypertension. For example, renal vascular resistance is almost invariably increased in patients with essential hypertension (2,11,20,42). Yet, increased renal vascular resistance could be an autoregulatory response to increased arterial pressure in some instances, or it could play a causal role in hypertension if it is increased sufficiently to lower renal blood flow and GFR.

Some abnormalities of renal function are associated with reduced excretory capability and *increased* renal blood flow, as observed in mineralocorticoid hypertension (34). In an attempt to document abnormalities of renal hemodynamics in essential hypertension, various workers have reported increased, decreased, or no change in renal blood flow (20,42). Such variability is to be expected with different insults to the kidney and when factors known to influence renal blood flow and GFR, such as sodium or protein intake, are uncontrolled in clinical studies. Also, episodic measurements made during resting conditions may not reflect the average values of renal hemodynamics existing throughout the day, during periods of stress as well as inactivity. If patients with hypertension have a greater responsiveness to vasoconstrictors, as some studies suggest (42), then reductions in renal blood flow and GFR that would not be apparent under resting conditions could occur during periods of activity and could play a role in the pathogenesis of hypertension. Perhaps even more important, it is usually not possible to analyze the sequential changes in renal function that occur during the onset of hypertension in humans, or to conduct detailed and invasive experiments that allow separation of those abnormalities that could cause hypertension from those that merely occur as part of an overall compensatory response. Therefore, rather than listing the various alterations in renal function that have been reported, it may be more useful to consider the types of renal abnormalities that have been shown experimentally to cause hypertension and to determine which changes in renal function most closely resemble those observed in essential hypertension.

RENAL HEMODYNAMIC AND TUBULAR ABNORMALITIES THAT CAN CAUSE CHRONIC HYPERTENSION

As discussed above, chronic hypertension is an essential compensatory response to impaired renal sodium and water excretory capability. In theory, this impairment could be caused by factors that decrease GFR or increase tubular reabsorption. Since tubular reabsorption and GFR are both approximately 100-fold greater than urinary excretion, relatively small changes in either of these variables could have large effects on urinary excretion. Obviously, any long-term reduction in GFR must be perfectly compensated for by mechanisms that restore GFR or reduce tubular reabsorption if renal excretion is to be returned to normal so that fluid balance is maintained. Likewise, any chronic increase in tubular reabsorption must be completely compensated for by increased GFR or by restoration of tubular reabsorption to normal. Otherwise, fluid retention would continue, eventually causing complete circulatory collapse.

To the extent that compensations for abnormalities of kidney function can be achieved locally, through intrinsic renal mechanisms, systemic changes (e.g., hypertension) would not be required to maintain fluid balance. However, the fact that hypertension occurs so frequently suggests that intrinsic renal mechanisms are not powerful enough to completely prevent alterations in renal excretion in many circumstances in which there is a primary abnormality of GFR or tubular reabsorption. Apparently, systemic changes are often recruited to maintain perfect glomerulotubular balance. Unfortunately, the most powerful systemic hormonal mechanisms are geared mainly toward increasing, rather than decreasing, tubular reabsorption. Therefore, when renal excretory capability is reduced and arterial pressure increases, the primary antinatriuretic hormones (e.g., aldosterone and ANGII) can be suppressed to some extent and can help to minimize increases in blood pressure. However, once the lower limits of these hormonal controls have been reached, increases in arterial pressure serve as an essential mechanism for maintaining fluid balance when renal excretory capability is further reduced. Some of the renal abnormalities that can cause chronic hypertension by reducing renal excretory function include increased preglomerular resistance, decreased glomerular capillary filtration coefficient (K_f), increased tubular reabsorption, and decreased renal mass combined with other insults to the kidney.

Hypertension Caused by Increased Preglomerular Resistance

Perhaps one of the best examples of hypertension initiated by increased preglomerular resistance is that associated with constricting one of the renal arteries and removal of the contralateral kidney, i.e., the one-kidney, one-clip Goldblatt model of hypertension. Although Goldblatt hypertension is associated with many circulatory and neurohumoral abnormalities; it is important to keep in mind that the hypertension is *caused* by increased preglomerular resistance (due to the clip) and that blood pressure returns to normal when the clip is removed and preglomerular resistance returns to normal.

Immediately after partial constriction of one renal artery, renal blood flow is reduced and there is an increase in renin secretion and fluid retention (2,9,26,59). If the stenosis on the renal artery is not too severe, a steady state is reached in a few days, with most indices of renal function, including renal blood flow, GFR, tubular reabsorption, and plasma renin activity, returning nearly to normal in the clipped kidney

(2,9,19,26). The main abnormality that persists is increased total peripheral vascular resistance and hypertension (9,26). When the stenosis is severe, renal function cannot be restored and there is a continued increase in plasma renin activity that eventually leads to malignant hypertension (26).

Although the renal origin of Goldblatt hypertension is obvious, impairment of renal function is not readily apparent after various compensations have taken place. Without knowledge of the fact that a clip had been placed on the renal artery, one could easily conclude that hypertension may have been caused by other abnormalities, such as a primary increase in total peripheral resistance, that are more striking.

Functional or pathological increases in preglomerular resistance at other sites besides the renal artery, (e.g., the afferent arterioles) would increase arterial pressure through the same mechanisms that are activated when a clip is placed on the main renal artery. For example, widespread structural increases in afferent arteriolar resistance (e.g., nephrosclerosis) would tend to decrease GFR and renal blood flow, thereby reducing renal excretory capability and requiring increases in arterial pressure to restore renal function to normal and to maintain fluid balance. Similarly, functional increases in preglomerular resistance caused by excessive activation of the sympathetic nervous system or increased circulating levels of catecholamines (e.g., pheochromocytoma) could also cause hypertension. Whether or not a primary increase in preglomerular resistance plays a role in initiating human essential hypertension is still unclear. However, it is interesting to note that most patients with essential hypertension demonstrate many of the same characteristics seen in one-kidney, one-clip Goldblatt hypertension, including nearly normal renal blood flow, GFR, and plasma renin activity. Moreover, the steady-state relationship between urinary output and arterial pressure in patients with essential hypertension is shifted along the arterial pressure axis in parallel to the normal pressure natriuresis curve, similar to the shift seen in one-kidney, one-clip Goldblatt hypertension and the SHR (see Figs. 2 and 7). A parallel shift of the pressure natriuresis curve occurs with increased preglomerular resistance, because arterial pressure must be increased by an amount proportional to the pressure drop along the preglomerular vessels, caused by the clamp or by vasoconstriction, in order to return glomerular hydrostatic pressure to normal. Experimental models of hypertension caused by a primary increase in tubular reabsorption (e.g., mineralocorticoid hypertension) are generally associated with a decreased slope of the pressure natriuresis curve, rather than a parallel shift. Thus, it is possible that "essential" hypertension in some patients could be initiated by a functional or pathological increase in preglomerular resistance.

The two-kidney, one-clip model of Goldblatt hypertension presents a slightly more complicated picture than described above. Although this model also begins with increased preglomerular resistance, caused by placement of a clip on one renal artery, the contralateral untouched kidney initially acts to blunt the hypertension. However, the excretory function of the "normal" untouched kidney is also attenuated, partly because of functional changes such as increased secretion of renin by the clipped kidney and the subsequent antinatriuretic effects of ANGII (52). In the early stages of hypertension, removal of the clipped kidney restores blood pressure to normal, whereas removing the contralateral kidney exacerbates the hypertension (49). However, with prolonged hypertension, pathological changes in the vasculature of the contralateral kidney begin to appear and add to the impairment of renal excretory capability (66). At this stage, removal of the clipped kidney or unclipping only partially restores arterial pressure (64,66). However, removal of the contralateral "normal" kidney and unclipping normalizes arterial pressure (24). This observation suggests that chronic exposure to high blood pressure in the untouched kidney may cause structural changes that contribute to the progression of hypertension in this model. Thus, the two-kidney, one-clip model of Goldblatt hypertension, while initiated by increased preglomerular resistance in part of the renal tissue, is characterized by functional and pathological changes in the remaining "normal" renal tissue that contribute to the maintenance of increased arterial pressure. A similar situation may occur with patchy areas of renal ischemia (e.g., renal infarcts).

Hypertension Caused by Decreased Glomerular Capillary Filtration Coefficient

Various disorders associated with decreased K_f would also tend to reduce GFR and renal excretory capability, and increase arterial pressure. Initially, reducing K_f should lower GFR and sodium excretion while increasing renin secretion, via a macula densa mechanism (18,26). However, as arterial pressure increases, GFR and renin release could be restored toward normal so that the only persistent abnormalities of renal function would be reduced filtration fraction, increased glomerular hydrostatic pressure, and perhaps small increases in renal blood flow. Increases in renal blood flow and glomerular hydrostatic pressure could occur, in part, through a local tubuloglomerular feedback (30,55) as well as through increases in arterial pressure. Unfortunately, a compensatory increase in glomerular hydrostatic pressure could lead to additional renal dysfunction over a period of years by causing glomerulosclerosis, thereby reducing K_f even further and requiring additional increases in arterial pressure and glomerular hydrostatic pressure to maintain GFR constant. Obviously, such a sequence could initiate a vicious cycle leading to progressive renal damage and eventually renal failure. The clinical counterpart to the sequence described above may be found in hypertension caused by glomerulonephritis.

In contrast to hypertension caused by increased preglomerular resistance, hypertension due to reduced K_f is associated with a decreased slope of the renal pressure natriuresis curve (Fig. 2). The reason for this is that reduced K_f decreases the amount of glomerular filtrate formed for each millimeter of mercury of glomerular hydrostatic pressure and therefore lowers urinary output for any given level of arterial pressure; however, decreased K_f should not alter the initial pressure level at which glomerular filtrate begins to be formed. The significance of a reduced slope of the pressure natriuresis curve is that it causes arterial pressure to be very salt sensitive.

Hypertension Caused by Increased Tubular Reabsorption

An example of hypertension caused by increased tubular reabsorption is that initiated by mineralocorticoids which stimulate sodium reabsorption in the late distal and cortical collecting tubules. When renal function is normal, mineralocorticoids have only a weak hypertensive effect (9,26). However, when renal function is impaired or when sodium intake is high, the hypertensive potency of mineralocorticoids is greatly enhanced (9,26). Although mineralocorticoids have little or no direct effect on renal hemodynamics or arterial pressure, there is a gradual increase in GFR, renal plasma flow, and arterial pressure during prolonged mineralocorticoid excess (34). Other abnormalities of various systems also begin to appear, such as inhibition of sodium-potassium ATPase activity, increased levels of various natriuretic hormones, renal hypercalcuria, and changes in vascular reactivity, and each of these disturbances has been postulated to play a causal role in elevating arterial pressure (3,29,28,53). However, it seems likely that many of these abnormalities may be secondary to increased arterial pressure.

Increased ANGII levels can also cause hypertension by increasing tubular reabsorption directly and indirectly by stimulating aldosterone secretion (32,48). The precise mechanisms by which ANGII increases tubular reabsorption are still unclear, but may be related to direct effects on tubular transport, or constriction of efferent arterioles and subsequent changes in peritubular capillary dynamics (31,32). One difference between ANGII and aldosterone hypertension is that increases in tubular reabsorption are not counterbalanced by increased renal blood flow or large increases in GFR, as occur with mineralocorticoid excess. The renal vasoconstrictor action of ANGII, coupled with its effects on renal tubular reabsorption, may be one reason that ANGII hypertension is usually more severe than with mineralocorticoid excess (Fig. 2).

One feature of hypertension caused by increased tubular reabsorption is that it is usually very salt sensitive, so that increasing sodium intake exacerbates the hypertension and low salt ameliorates the increase in blood pressure (Fig. 2). Also, hypertension caused by primary increases in distal tubular reabsorption is often associated with secondary suppression of plasma renin activity and ANGII formation and a tendency toward expansion of the extracellular fluid volume. However, when increased tubular reabsorption is coupled with peripheral vasoconstriction (e.g., ANGII hypertension), the degree of volume expansion depends on the relative effects of the vasoconstrictor on the peripheral vasculature and on the kidney. With severe peripheral vasoconstriction and decreased vascular capacitance, much less volume is needed to raise arterial pressure sufficiently to offset the increase in tubular reabsorption and maintain fluid balance.

Each of the renal abnormalities discussed above causes chronic hypertension with different characteristics of renal and circulatory dynamics. The common feature of these abnormalities is that they all reduce renal excretory capability by increasing the ratio of tubular reabsorption to glomerular filtration, and it is important to recognize that the severity of hypertension depends on the *relative* changes in these two variables. Compensatory changes in renal hemodynamics and tubular reabsorption, as well as circulatory dynamics, can differ markedly depending on the initial insult to the kidney. Also, as discussed below, the various renal abnormalities that cause hypertension may have different consequences with regard to the progression of renal disease. For example, those abnormalities associated with increased preglomerular resistance that tend to decrease glomerular hydrostatic pressure should not cause injury to the glomerular membrane and sclerosis of renal vessels distal to the site of increased resistance. However, hypertension initiated by patchy areas of increased preglomerular resistance could eventually cause damage to the remaining normal renal tissues. Disturbances that decrease K_f or increase renal tubular reabsorption may be compensated for by renal vasodilation and increased glomerular hydrostatic pressure which, over a period of years, could lead to further injury to the kidney. Another important point to remember is that the abnormalities described above are not mutually exclusive; some forms of hypertension may result from a combination of disorders that influence GFR as well as tubular reabsorption.

Reduced Renal Mass

Considering the discussion above, one might predict that reductions in renal mass should impair renal excretory capability and cause hypertension. Yet, experimental studies have demonstrated that removal of large portions of the kidney, to the point that uremia occurs, rarely causes severe hypertension as long as sodium intake is normal (9,26). However, the failure of decreased renal mass to cause severe hypertension is easier to understand when one considers that it is the *difference* between glomerular filtration and tubular reabsorption that determines whether hypertension is necessary to maintain sodium balance. When entire nephrons are lost, glomerular filtration and tubular reabsorption capability are simultaneously reduced, so that balance between filtration and reabsorption can be maintained without major adaptive changes in arterial pressure.

Although kidneys with reduced numbers of nephrons can effectively maintain sodium balance under normal conditions, they are very susceptible to additional insults that impair renal excretory function. Thus, hypertension associated with mineralocorticoid administration is much more severe after reducing renal mass (9).

Also, the ability to increase sodium excretion in response to the additional challenge of high sodium intake requires a greater arterial pressure after decreasing renal mass (10,47) (Fig. 2). Apparently, the remaining nephrons of remnant kidneys have already undergone hypertrophy and functional changes (e.g., decreased fractional reabsorption and vasodilation), and further reductions in reabsorption or increases in GFR and sodium excretion cannot occur unless blood pressure is elevated. Thus, with high sodium intake, hypertension may be the primary remaining mechanism for maintaining sodium balance.

CHANGES IN RENAL FUNCTION THAT OCCUR SECONDARILY TO CHRONIC HYPERTENSION

In addition to its role in the pathogenesis of hypertension, the kidney is also a target organ of increased arterial pressure and responds to various intrinsic and extrinsic compensatory mechanisms. Depending on the initial disturbance that raises arterial pressure, renal abnormalities may differ. For example, a primary increase in distal tubular reabsorption, such as occurs with mineralocorticoid excess, would be compensated for by increased arterial pressure, which, in turn, would tend to raise intrarenal vascular pressures as well as glomerular hydrostatic pressure. Initially, these changes would tend to increase renal blood flow and GFR and restore distal tubular delivery to normal, thereby helping to maintain sodium and water balance. However, sustained increases in intrarenal vascular pressures and glomerular hydrostatic pressure could initiate structural changes that could lead to further impairment of renal function over a period of months or years. Brenner and his colleagues (6,7) have amassed considerable evidence that chronic increases in glomerular hydrostatic pressure may cause hemodynamic injury to the glomerular membranes and eventually complete loss of glomeruli.

Chronic increases in intrarenal pressures would also be expected to cause structural changes of the renal vasculature, including wall hypertrophy, that could tend to raise renal vascular resistance (25). Although the structural changes may be an appropriate tissue response to increased load, they could also contribute to renal dysfunction and progression of hypertension. As long as the initial disturbance of increased tubular reabsorption is maintained, reductions in K_f or increases in preglomerular resistance would necessitate further increases in arterial pressure to restore renal excretory function to normal, eventually causing a vicious cycle characterized by progressive decreases in renal function and severe hypertension.

Rats treated with desoxycorticosterone acetate (DOCA) and salt eventually show diffuse glomerular sclerosis associated with increased glomerular hydrostatic pressure and systemic hypertension. If these animals are returned to normal or low sodium diet in the early stages of hypertension, arterial pressure may be restored to nearly normal (see 9 for review). However, in the later stages of hypertension, decreasing sodium intake does not normalize arterial pressure. Similar mechanisms for irreversible hypertension and renal damage may occur in patients with longstanding primary aldosteronism in which removal of the hyperplastic adrenal gland may not return arterial pressure to normal (23). Thus, although mineralocorticoid excess may initially cause only a mild hypertension, over a long period of time various compensatory changes in renal function, necessary to maintain sodium balance, may worsen the hypertension.

A similar sequence of pathological changes of the renal circulation could be involved in causing the hypertension associated with Cushing's disease due to excess glucocorticoid secretion. Previous studies in our laboratory have suggested that the functional effect of glucocorticoids may be to increase renal excretory capability and lower blood pressure, due to increased GFR (41). However, despite these observations, there is still widespread belief among many investigators that glucocorticoid excess can cause chronic hypertension, partly because a large fraction of patients with Cushing's disease have hypertension (46). One possible explanation for the apparent discrepancy between the results obtained when glucocorticoids are infused over a period of several days and the observations in patients with longstanding glucocorticoid excess is that chronic high levels of glucocorticoids may cause gradual pathological changes in the kidney that could lead to hypertension. Glucocorticoids are known to cause glomerular hyperfiltration (41), which may be due to hyperglycemia and glucosuria, as well as catabolism of proteins and a rise in plasma amino acids. Increased blood levels of glucose or amino acids may cause renal vasodilation and marked increases in GFR and renal blood flow (67,68). The renal vasodilation and glomerular hypertension associated with glucocorticoid excess could, over a period of years, damage renal arterioles and glomerular membranes and reduce renal excretory capability, eventually causing systemic arterial hypertension.

Thus, functional or pathological changes in the kidneys that are compensated for by increased arterial pressure, increased intrarenal pressures, or increased glomerular hydrostatic pressure may initiate a series of renal changes that could not only obscure the initial disturbance, but also lead to progressive worsening of the hypertension. At different stages of the hypertension, the changes in renal hemodynamics and tubular reabsorption would reflect the effects of various compensatory changes as well as any initial disturbances that tended to influence these variables.

SUMMARY

Our major goals in this chapter have been to describe the most basic and powerful feedback control system for blood pressure regulation—the renal-body fluid feedback—and to discuss how abnormalities of this mechanism can cause hypertension. A key component of this feedback is the pressure natriuresis mechanism that stabilizes arterial pressure as long as renal excretory capability is not impaired. However, abnormalities that reduce renal excretory capability often require increased arterial pressure to restore renal excretion to normal so that balance between intake and output of salt and water can be maintained. Recent studies indicate that when the renal pressure natriuresis mechanism is prevented from operating in various forms of experimental hypertension, by servocontrolling renal perfusion pressure, sodium and water excretion remain below intake, resulting in severe increases in body fluid volumes and complete cardiovascular failure within a few days. Thus, chronic hypertension appears to be an *essential* compensatory response for an inability of the kidney to excrete the required amounts of sodium and water at normal arterial pressure.

A common feature of renal abnormalities that cause hypertension is that they increase the ratio of tubular reabsorption to GFR. This can occur as a result of primary reductions in GFR, due to increased preglomerular resistance (e.g., Goldblatt hypertension) or decreased K_f (e.g., glomerulonephritis), or a primary increase in tubular reabsorption (e.g., excessive formation of antinatriuretic hormones). After various compensations have taken place, due to increased arterial pressure or intrarenal and extrarenal feedbacks, the initial insult to renal hemodynamics or tubular reabsorption is often obscured, but other circulatory abnormalities that occur secondarily to increased arterial pressure begin to appear. The renal abnormalities responsible for essential hypertension are still unclear, probably because the onset of hypertension is usually very insidious and compensatory changes mask many of the initial insults to the kidneys that lead to the increased arterial pressure. However, it is clear that renal excretory capability is reduced in all forms of hypertension, including essential hypertension, since normal excretion of sodium and water is maintained only at the expense of chronic increases in arterial pressure.

ACKNOWLEDGMENTS

We thank Ivadelle Heidke, Gwendolyn Robbins, and Susan Pace for expert secretarial assistance. The authors' research was supported by National Institutes of Health Grants HL 23502 and HL 11678.

REFERENCES

1. Ballerman, B. J., Block, K. D., Seidman, J. G., and Brenner, B. M. (1986): Atrial natriuretic peptide (ANP) secretion, biosynthesis and glomerular receptor activity during mineralocorticoid escape (Abstr.). *Kidney Int.*, 29:329.
2. Baylis, C. (1981): Renal hemodynamics in experimental hypertension. In: *Hypertension (Contemporary Issues in Nephrology, Vol. 8)*, edited by B. M. Brenner and J. H. Stein, pp. 39–64. Churchill Livingston, New York.
3. Berecek, K. H., and Bohr, D. F. (1978): Whole body vascular reactivity during the development of deoxycorticosterone acetate hypertension in the pig. *Circ. Res.*, 42:764–771.
4. Bianchi, G., Fox, U., DiFrancesco, G. F., Bardi, U., and Radice, M. (1973): The hypertensive role of the kidney in spontaneously hypertensive rats. *Clin. Sci. Mol. Med.* 45(*Suppl.*):135s–139s.
5. Bianchi, G., Fox, U., DiFrancesco, G. F., Giovanetti, P. M., and Pagetti, D. (1978): Blood pressure changes produced by kidney cross transplantation between spontaneously hypertensive rats and normotensive rats. *Clin. Sci. Mol. Med.*, 47:435–448.
6. Brenner, B. M. (1983): Hemodynamically mediated glomerular injury and the progressive nature of kidney disease. *Kidney Int.*, 23:647–655.
7. Brenner, B. M., Meyer, T. W., and Hostetter, T. H. (1982): Dietary protein intake and the progressive nature of kidney disease: The role of hemodynamically mediated injury in the pathogenesis of progressive glomerular sclerosis in aging, renal ablation, and intrinsic renal disease. *N. Engl. J. Med.*, 307:652–659.
8. Buckalew, V. M., and Dimond, K. A. (1976): Effect of vasopressin on sodium excretion and plasma antinatriferic activity in the dog. *Am. J. Physiol.*, 231:28–33.
9. Coleman, T. G. (1980): *Blood Pressure Control, Vol. I.* Eden Press, St. Albans, VT.
10. Coleman, T. G., and Guyton, A. C. (1969): Hypertension caused by salt loading in the dog. III. Onset transients of cardiac output and other circulatory variables. *Circ. Res.*, 25:153–160.
11. Coleman, T. G., Guyton, A. C., Young, D. B., DeClue, J. W., Norman, R. A., Jr. and Manning, R. D., Jr. (1975): The role of the kidney in essential hypertension. *Clin. Exp. Pharmacol. Physiol.*, 2:571–581.
12. Coleman, T. G., Manning, R. D., Jr., Norman, R. A., Jr., and DeClue, J. W. (1975): The role of the kidney in spontaneous hypertension. *Am. Heart J.*, 89:94–98.
13. Cowley, A. W., Jr. (1982): Vasopressin and cardiovascular regulation. In: *International Review of Physiology, Cardiovascular Physiology IV*, edited by A. C. Guyton and J. E. Hall, pp. 189–242. University Park Press, Baltimore.
14. Cowley, A. W., Jr., Merrill, D. C., Quillen, E., Jr., and Skelton, M. M. (1984): Long-term blood pressure and metabolic effects of vasopressin with servo-controlled fluid volume. *Am. J. Physiol.*, 247:R537–R545.
15. Curtis, J. J., Luke, R. G., Dustan, H. P., Kashgarian, M., Whelchel, J. D., Jones, P., and Diethelm, A. (1983): Remission of hypertension after renal transplantation. *N. Engl. J. Med.*, 309:1009–1015.
16. Dahl, L. K., and Heine, M. (1975): Primary role of renal homografts in setting chronic blood pressure level in rats. *Circ. Res.*, 36:692–696.
17. Dahl, L. K., Heine, M., and Thompson, K. (1974): Genetic influences of the kidneys on blood pressure. *Circ. Res.*, 34:94–101.
18. Davis, J. O., and Freeman, R. H. (1976): Mechanisms regulating renin release. *Physiol. Rev.*, 56:1–56.
19. Deforrest, J. M., Davis, J. O., Freeman, R. H., Watkins, B. E., and Stephens, G. A. (1978): Separate renal function studies in conscious dogs with renovascular hypertension. *Am. J. Physiol.*, 235:F310–F316.
20. deLeew, P. W., and Birkenhager, W. H. (1983): The renal circulation in essential hypertension. *J. Hypertension*, 1:321–331.
21. DeWardener, H. E., and Clarkson, E. M. (1985): Concept of natriuretic hormone. *Physiol. Rev.*, 65:658–659.
22. Dickinson, C. J. (1981): Neurogenic hypertension revisited. *Clin. Sci.*, 60:471–477.
23. Ferris, J. B., Brown, J. J., Fraser, R., Haywood, E., Davis, D. L., Kay, A. W., Lever, A. F., Robertson, J. I. S., Owen, K., and Peart, W. S. (1975): Results of adrenal surgery in patients with hypertension, aldosterone excess, and low plasma renin activity. *Br. Med. J.*, 1:135.
24. Floyer, M. A. (1951): The effects of nephrectomy and adrenalectomy upon the blood pressure in hypertensive and normotensive rats. *Clin. Sci.*, 10:405–421.
25. Folkow, B. (1982): Physiological aspects of primary hypertension. *Physiol. Rev.*, 62:347–504.
26. Guyton, A. C. (1980): *Arterial Pressure and Hypertension.* W. B. Saunders Co., Philadelphia.
27. Guyton, A. C., Cowley, A. W., Jr., Young, D. B., Coleman, T. G., Hall, J. E., and DeClue, J. W. (1976): Integration and control of circulatory function. In: *International Review of Physiology, Cardiovascular Physiology II*, edited by A. C. Guyton and A. W. Cowley, Jr., pp. 341–385. University Park Press, Baltimore.
28. Haddy, F. J. (1983): Abnormalities of membrane transport in hypertension. *Hypertension*, 5(*Suppl. V*):V66–V72.
29. Haddy, F. J., and Pamani, M. B. (1984): The vascular Na^+-K^+ pump in low renin hypertension. *J. Cardiovasc. Pharmacol.*, 6:S61–S74.
30. Hall, J. E. (1982): Regulation of renal hemodynamics. In: *International Review of Physiology, Vol. 26: Cardiovascular Physiology IV*, edited by A. C. Guyton and J. E. Hall, pp. 243–322. University Park Press, Baltimore.
31. Hall, J. E. (1986): Regulation of glomerular filtration rate and sodium excretion by angiotensin II. *Fed. Proc.*, 45:1431–1437.

32. Hall, J. E. (1986): Control of sodium excretion by angiotensin: Intrarenal mechanisms and their role in blood pressure regulation. *Am. J. Physiol.*, 250:R960–R972.
33. Hall, J. E., Granger, J. P., Hester, R. L., Coleman, T. G., Smith, M. J., Jr., and Cross, R. B. (1984): Mechanisms of escape from sodium retention during angiotensin II hypertension. *Am. J. Physiol.*, 246:F627–F634.
34. Hall, J. E., Granger, J. P., Smith, M. J., Jr., and Premen, A. J. (1984): Role of renal hemodynamics and arterial pressure in aldosterone "escape." *Hypertension*, 6(*Suppl.* I):I183–I192.
35. Hall, J. E., Guyton, A. C., Granger, J. P., and Coleman, T. G. (1984): The kidney and experimental hypertension. In: *The Kidney in Essential Hypertension*, edited by F. H. Messerli, pp. 87–103. Martinus Nijhoff, Boston.
36. Hall, J. E., Guyton, A. C., Salgado, H. C., McCaa, R. E., and Balfe, J. W. (1978): Renal hemodynamics in acute and chronic angiotensin II hypertension. *Am. J. Physiol.*, 235:F174–F179.
37. Hall, J. E., Guyton, A. C., Smith, M. J., Jr., and Coleman, T. G. (1980): Blood pressure and renal function during chronic changes in sodium intake: Role of angiotensin. *Am. J. Physiol.*, 239:F271–F280.
38. Hall, J. E., Guyton, A. C., Trippodo, N. C., Lohmeier, T. E., McCaa, R. E., and Cowley, A. W., Jr. (1977): Intrarenal control of electrolyte excretion by angiotensin II. *Am. J. Physiol.*, 232:F538–F544.
39. Hall, J. E., and Montani, J. P. (1985): Role of the kidney in adrenocortical hypertension. In: *The Adrenal Gland and Hypertension*, edited by F. Mantero, E. G. Biglieri, J. W. Funder, and B. A. Scoggins, pp. 185–208. Raven Press, New York.
40. Hall, J. E., Montani, J. P., Woods, L. L., and Mizelle, H. L. (1986): Renal escape from vasopressin: Role of pressure natriuresis. *Am. J. Physiol.*, 250:F907–F916.
41. Hall, J. E., Morse, C. L., Smith, M. J., Jr., Young, D. B., and Guyton, A. C. (1980): Control of arterial pressure and renal function during glucocorticoid excess in dogs. *Hypertension*, 2:139–148.
42. Hollenberg, N. K., and Adams, D. F. (1976): The renal circulation in hypertensive disease. *Am. J. Med.*, 60:773–784.
43. Jones, A. W., and Hart, R. G. (1975): Altered ion transport in aortic smooth muscle during DOCA hypertension in the rat. *Circ. Res.*, 37:333–342.
44. Kawabe, K., Watanbe, T. X., Shiono, K., and Sokabe, H. (1978): Influences on blood pressure of renal isografts between spontaneously hypertensive and normotensive rats. *Jpn. Heart J.*, 19:886–899.
45. Knox, F. G., Burnett, J. C., Jr., Kohan, D. E., Spielman, W. S., and Strand, J. C. (1980): Escape from the sodium-retaining effects of mineralocorticoids. *Kidney Int.*, 17:263–276.
46. Krakoff, L., Nicolis, G., and Amsel, B. (1975): Pathogenesis of hypertension in Cushing's syndrome. *Am. J. Med.*, 58:216–220.
47. Langston, J. B., Guyton, A. C., Douglas, B. H., and Dorsett, P. E. (1963): Effect of changes in salt intake on arterial pressure and renal function in partially nephrectomized dogs. *Circ. Res.*, 12:508.
48. Laragh, J. H., and Sealey, J. E. (1973): The renin-angiotensin-aldosterone hormonal system and regulation of sodium, potassium, and blood pressure homeostasis. In: *Handbook of Physiology, Section 8: Renal Physiology*, edited by J. Orloff and R. W. Berliner, pp. 791–814. American Physiological Society, Washington, DC.
49. Liard, J. F. (1969): Effet de l'ablation partielle ou totale du tissu renal sur l'hypertension renovasculaire chez le rat. *Experientia*, 25:934–935.
50. Liard, J. F. (1979): Cardiogenic hypertension. In: *International Review of Physiology, Vol. 18: Cardiovascular Physiology III*, edited by A. C. Guyton and D. B. Young, pp. 317–355. University Park Press, Baltimore.
51. Marin-Grez, M., Oza, N. B., and Carretero, O. A. (1973): The involvement of urinary kallikrein in the renal escape from the sodium retaining effect of mineralocorticoids. *Henry Ford Hosp. Med. J.*, 21:85–90.
52. Masaki, Z., Ferrario, C. M., and Bumpus, F. M. (1980): Effects of SQ-20,881 on the intact kidney of dogs with two-kidney, one clip hypertension. *Hypertension*, 2:649–656.
53. McCarron, D. A. (1985): Is calcium more important than sodium in the pathogenesis of essential hypertension? *Hypertension*, 7:607–627.
54. Miller, A. W., Bohr, D. F., Schork, A. M., and Terris, J. M. (1979): Hemodynamic responses to DOCA in young pigs. *Hypertension*, 1:591–597.
55. Navar, L. G. (1978): Renal autoregulation: Perspectives from whole kidney and single nephron studies. *Am. J. Physiol.*, 234:F357–F370.
56. Norman, R. A., Jr., Enobakhare, J. A., DeClue, J. W., Douglas, B. H., and Guyton, A. C. (1978): Arterial pressure-urinary output relationships in hypertensive rats. *Am. J. Physiol.*, 234:R98–R103.
57. Omvik, P., Tarazi, R. C., and Bravo, E. L. (1980): Regulation of sodium balance in hypertension. *Hypertension*, 2:515–523.
58. Reid, I. A., Brooks, V. L., Rudolph, C. D., and Keil, L. C. (1982): Analysis of the actions of angiotensin on the central nervous system of conscious dogs. *Am. J. Physiol.*, 243:R82–R91.
59. Romero, J. C., Fiksen-Olsen, M., and Schryver, S. (1981): Pathophysiology of hypertension: The use of experimental models to understand the clinical features of the hypertension disease. In: *Clinical Medicine*, edited by J. A. Spittell, pp. 1–51. Harper & Row, Philadelphia.
60. Selkurt, E. E., Hall, P. W., and Spencer, M. P. (1949): Effect of graded arterial pressure decrement on renal clearance of creatinine, *p*-amino hippurate and sodium. *Am. J. Physiol.*, 159:369–384.
61. Smith, M. J., Jr., Cowley, A. W., Jr., Guyton, A. C., and Manning, R. D., Jr. (1979): Acute and chronic effects of vasopressin on blood pressure, electrolytes, and fluid volumes. *Am. J. Physiol.*, 237:F232–F240.
62. Sonnenberg, H., Chong, C. K., and Veress, A. T. (1981): Cardiac atrial factor—An endogenous diuretic? *Can. J. Physiol. Pharmacol.*, 59:1278–1279.

63. Thompson, J. M. A., and Dickinson, C. J. (1976): The relation between the excretion of sodium and water and the perfusion pressure in the isolated, blood-perfused, rabbit kidney, with special reference to changes occurring in clip-hypertension. *Clin. Sci. Mol. Med.*, 50:223–236.
64. Thurston, H., Bing, R. F., and Swales, J. P. (1980): Reversal of two-kidney one clip renovascular hypertension in the rat. *Hypertension,* 2:256–265.
65. Tobian, L., Lange, J., Azar, S., Iwai, J., Koop, D., Coffee, K., and Johnson, M. A. (1978): Reduction of natriuretic capacity and renin release in isolated, blood perfused kidneys of Dahl hypertension-prone rats. *Circ. Res.*, 43(*Suppl.* I):92–98.
66. Wilson, C., and Byrom, F. B. (1941): Vicious cycle in chronic Bright's disease: Experimental evidence from the hypertensive rat. *Q. J. Med.,* 10:65–93.
67. Woods, L. L., Mizelle, H. L., and Hall, J. E. (1987): Control of renal hemodynamics in hyperglycemia: Possible role of tubuloglomerular feedback. *Am. J. Physiol.*,252:F65–F73.
68. Woods, L. L., Mizelle, H. L., Montani, J.-P., and Hall, J. E. (1986): Mechanisms controlling renal hemodynamics and electrolyte excretion during amino acids. *Am. J. Physiol.,* 251:F303–F312.
69. Zimmerman, B. G., Sybertz, E. J., and Wong, P. C. (1984): Interaction between sympathetic and renin-angiotensin system. *J. Hypertension,* 2:581–588.

The Kidney in Hypertension, edited by Norman M. Kaplan, Barry M. Brenner, and John H. Laragh. Raven Press, New York © 1987.

Sodium and Calcium Handling

Brian F. Robinson

Department of Medicine, St. George's Hospital Medical School, London, England SW17 ORE

The human body contains in total some 4,500 mmol of sodium, not all of which is readily exchangeable, and 30,000 mmol or more of calcium, nearly all of which is stored in the bones. The preservation of the necessary total of these essential cations depends on the maintenance of an appropriate balance between absorption and urinary loss, and the homeostatic mechanisms concerned will be put under stress if the intake of either ion deviates widely from the optimum or if their handling by the kidney is abnormal.

For many years, the sodium ion has been widely regarded as of central importance in the hypertensive process, although there have always been those who were sceptics of this view or even frank disbelievers. More recently, evidence has accumulated that suggests that calcium may play a role in the development of hypertension. This chapter will review the data relating to abnormal handling of sodium and calcium in patients with primary hypertension and will also attempt the more difficult task of assessing the relative importance of the two ions in the causation and maintenance of the condition.

The diet of our remote ancestors cannot be known precisely, but archeological evidence suggests that it resembled that of primitive peoples alive today and may have contained approximately 30 mmol of sodium per day and 40 mmol of calcium (17). Modern urban diets typically contain from 120 to 300 mmol or more of sodium and 20 mmol or less of calcium. Our bodies are therefore faced with a much higher sodium intake than that to which they must be assumed to be adapted, and a somewhat lower calcium intake.

The mechanisms that are activated to compensate for deviations in the intake of sodium and calcium differ in some important respects between the two ions. The control of sodium metabolism is in principle simple, although the mechanisms involved are complex and still not fully understood. Since almost all ingested sodium is absorbed, the burden of dealing with an excessive intake falls entirely on the kidney. Humoral and other mechanisms induce the necessary increase in urinary sodium excretion at the cost, in normal subjects, of a small increase in extracellular fluid volume. Any impairment of the capacity of the kidney to eliminate sodium will necessarily augment the systemic effects of an abnormally high intake, but if disaster is to be avoided, renal sodium loss (together with the small extrarenal losses) must quickly come into strict balance with intake.

The control of calcium metabolism is more complex. Unlike sodium, the absorption of calcium from the gut is far from complete and is actively controlled by humoral mechanisms in accordance with need. The excretion of calcium by the kidney is also controlled by humoral mechanisms, but is, in addition, directly related to sodium excretion. As a consequence of this two-way control system, the coupling between intake and excretion is not as tight for calcium as it is for sodium and it is possible for small imbalances to persist for long periods. This can be tolerated without significant effect on the concentration of calcium ions in the extracellular fluid because of the buffering effect of the very large reserve of calcium within the bones.

SODIUM AND CALCIUM INTAKE IN RELATION TO ARTERIAL PRESSURE

Sodium

The epidemiological data showing a positive correlation between average sodium intake in different nations and groups and the prevalence of hypertension is well known and appears firmly based (see 40 for review). Almost equally well known is the criticism that a lower sodium content is only one of several ways in which the diets of populations with a low prevalence of hypertension differ from the North American/Western European norm: Diets that are naturally low in salt tend to be vegetarian with a high content of potassium and fiber and a low content of saturated fat. More damaging to the hypothesis of a causal link between sodium and hypertension has been the failure to demonstrate any consistent relationship between sodium intake and arterial pressure in individuals from within the same group (65). This is usually accounted for as the result of wide differences in genetically determined sensitivity to the blood-pressure-raising effect of salt. This explanation remains unproven, however, and received no support from a recent well-controlled study of two groups of young people, one group having both parents in the top third of the distribution for blood pressure and the other having both parents in the bottom third. Comparison of the effect of 4-week periods on a low-sodium (50 mmol/day) and a moderate sodium intake ($>$ 120 mmol/day) revealed no evidence at all of a blood-pressure-raising effect of sodium (71). It has been countered that it may take months or years for the blood-pressure-raising effect of a high-sodium intake to become apparent; if this is so it will be very difficult ever to demonstrate the link by controlled experiment.

Reduction of sodium intake in patients with established hypertension has yielded variable results. There is no doubt that severe restriction will lower arterial pressure, but a more modest reduction in intake induces, at the most, only a small fall in pressure. It has been pointed out, however, that the effect of salt restriction appears to be greater the higher the initial blood pressure, and the small reductions observed in most recent trials may reflect the selection of subjects with relatively mild hypertension (see 40 for review).

The evidence linking an excessive sodium intake to the development of hypertension is less overwhelming than is commonly supposed. It depends primarily on epidemiological studies comparing different populations, and a causal connection has not been firmly established. The effect on blood pressure of short-term alterations in sodium intake has been small or absent, but it may be that much longer periods are required for changes to be induced. The most that can be said with confidence is that sodium may have a permissive role in the development of hypertension and an intake of less than 60 to 70 mmol/day probably prevents initiation of the hypertensive process. There is no satisfactory evidence that dietary intakes above this level are associated with graded increases in arterial pressure until, perhaps, very high daily intakes are reached (24). It could be, however, that sodium intake in childhood or early adult life is critical in initiating the hypertensive process, but the relationship between intake and arterial pressure is lost when hypertension has become well established. The situation might then be similar to that in the salt-sensitive rat in which, once hypertension has been induced by the administration of an excess of salt, it cannot be reversed by a return to a normal salt intake.

Calcium

The collection of data on the relation between dietary calcium and hypertension is faced with the difficulty of assessing calcium intake. Sodium intake can be reliably estimated from the 24-hr urinary excretion, provided the subject can be assumed to be in balance. Calcium intake cannot be assessed in the same way, and it has therefore been necessary to resort to dietary histories. This approach may be of some value when applied to groups, but it is of little or no value when applied to individuals: Estimates of sodium intake based on dietary history show almost no correlation with the measured urinary sodium.

One epidemiological approach that avoids the pitfalls of the dietary history has been to examine the average level of blood pressure in different populations in relation to the calcium content of the water supply. In a few studies, a water supply with a high calcium content has been associated with lower levels of arterial pressure and vice versa (67). In other studies no such link was found, and it has been concluded that the evidence for a relationship is both weak and inconsistent (23). This is not very surprising, since calcium dissolved in water makes up only a small proportion of the total daily intake, and it is improbable that variations in water supply would have any major effect on the overall balance. If there is any effect of water supply, it may depend on altered absorption of trace metals rather than a direct effect of calcium itself.

A pioneer dietary study of students in Mississippi concluded that those with higher than average arterial pressures were eating less calcium than their siblings with lower pressure (36). Several subsequent studies have also reported an association between low calcium intake and raised blood pressure (18). In one of the best known of these studies, carried out by McCarron et al. (47), calcium intake estimated from a 24-hr dietary recall was reported to be approximately 25% lower in 46 subjects with essential hypertension than in 44 normotensive controls. Controversy continues over the interpretation of the United States National Health and Nutrition Examination Survey. Two analyses revealed an inverse relation between dietary calcium and blood pressure (27,48), but the analytical methods used in one of these studies have been heavily criticized (21). None of the individual studies relating low calcium intake to raised blood pressure are very convincing, but they all point with varying degrees of firmness in the same direction, and it seems likely that a weak relationship does exist within certain populations. There is little information relating calcium intake to blood pressure in different populations, but from what is known it seems unlikely that an inverse relationship exists. The situation regarding calcium is thus the reverse of that regarding sodium, for which a relationship to blood pressure can be demonstrated between populations, but not between individuals in the same population.

Additional evidence of a link between calcium intake and arterial pressure comes from studies of the epidemiology of pregnancy hypertension. For most communities, the major source of calcium in the diet comes from dairy products. In many impoverished countries where milk and milk products are in short supply, dietary calcium is low and the incidence of pregnancy hypertension is high. In Guatemala and Ethiopia, however, traditional foods provide an abundance of calcium and the incidence of pregnancy hypertension is reported to be low. In a number of countries for which figures are available, there is an inverse relation between calcium intake and the prevalence of pregnancy hypertension, and it has been suggested that a causal relationship may exist (5).

ALTERED SODIUM HANDLING BY KIDNEY

In an attempt to explain why a high sodium intake might lead to raised arterial pressure in some people and not in others, it has been postulated that the kidneys of patients with hypertension suffer a genetically determined impairment of their ability to excrete sodium (16). In support of this hypothesis, kidneys taken from Dahl salt-sensitive rats before the development of hypertension do show a reduced capacity to excrete sodium (70). It is difficult to obtain direct evidence for or against such a defect in patients. If the sodium excretory capacity of the kidneys is impaired, this must be compensated by changes in the regulatory mechanisms if balance is to be achieved. It would be predicted, therefore, that the end result would be a resetting of humoral and other factors controlling sodium handling rather than any observable change in the excretion of the ion. Evidence to support this hypothesis has recently appeared. The plasma concentration of atrial natriuretic factor is raised in some patients with hypertension (62), and there is in addition an excess of a circulating sodium pump inhibitor that is believed to be secreted in response to sodium loading (26). Suppression of renin secretion has, of course, been regarded as evidence of volume expansion, but there may be other explanations for this abnormality.

In addition to the regulatory effect of humoral and possible neural mechanisms, the excretion of sodium by the kidney is affected to an important extent by arterial pressure. This powerful mechanism acts to maintain long-term stability of arterial pressure, and, as Guyton has pointed out, it must be reset whenever permanent hypertension is present. It seems unlikely that there is a specific disorder of this mechanism in patients with hypertension. Impairment of sodium excretory capacity from whatever cause will, however, lead to diminished excretion of the ion at any given level of arterial pressure and so, in effect, reset the pressure natriuresis mechanism.

Although an impaired capacity for long-term renal excretion of sodium cannot be demonstrated directly in patients with primary hypertension, there is, paradoxically, evidence of an enhanced capacity for excretion in response to a sudden saline load. The enhanced excretory capacity can be demonstrated not only in patients with established hypertension, but also in the normotensive sons of hypertensive parents (72). The mechanism of this abnormal response is unknown, and it is not necessarily incompatible with an overall impairment of sodium excretion. It has been suggested that it reflects the presence of an abnormally high basal concentration of atrial natriuretic factor in the plasma (63).

ALTERED SODIUM HANDLING AT A CELLULAR LEVEL

If it is true that certain predisposed subjects may become hypertensive when faced with an inappropriately large intake of sodium in their diet, it is necessary to enquire what mechanism might link the two events. The most obvious link would be an increase in total body sodium with a consequent increase in blood volume and cardiac output. Such a mechanism appears to operate in patients with severe impairment of renal function, but in most patients with established primary hypertension, total body sodium is not increased (69), blood volume is, if anything, reduced, and cardiac output is normal or, in the later stages, reduced. It is therefore necessary to consider other ways in which disordered sodium handling might lead to a rise in arterial pressure. A number of alterations in the transport of sodium across cell membranes have now been identified in patients with hypertension, and the field has recently been subject to critical review (28). In brief, there is good evidence of an increase in intracellular sodium in leukocytes from patients with primary hypertension and possibly also in erythrocytes. The abnormality in the leukocytes results from diminished activity of the sodium pump. The depression of pump function is probably acquired and is thought to be caused by a circulating inhibitor, but some studies suggest it could be genetic in origin. The resistance vessels are almost certainly subject to a similar disorder of sodium handling. A recent study has shown that ouabain-sensitive sodium efflux from omental resistance vessels is quite closely correlated with that from leukocytes taken from the same patients (1). There is, furthermore, functional evidence of reduced sodium pump activity in the resistance vessels of patients with hypertension, as shown by a reduced dilator response to local infusion of potassium (50). Since the concentration of the circulating inhibitor of the sodium pump is believed to depend on sodium intake, it only remains to be demonstrated that inhibition of pump function can cause a sustained increase in peripheral resistance for a connection to be established between increased sodium intake and the development of hypertension. In support of the view that such a connection exists, a recent study has demonstrated a positive correlation between leukocyte sodium content and forearm vascular resistance and a negative correlation between sodium and venous compliance (54); venous compliance is, of course, inversely related to the degree of venoconstriction. An increased sodium content is not, however, the only factor inducing functional changes in the resistance vessels in patients with hypertension. Experimental inhibition of the sodium pump with ouabain in normal subjects reproduces the altered response to potassium that is seen in patients, but does not give rise to the same pattern of altered responsiveness to other dilator agents (62).

Increased activity of the sodium-lithium countertransport system is another abnormality of sodium handling that has been well documented in the erythrocytes of patients with hypertension; genetic factors may be important in determining this abnormality. Since, in its physiological mode, this system is assumed to work as a sodium-sodium exchanger, it is difficult to see how a change in activity could affect cell function. It is possible, however, that the system might be the same as the proton-sodium exchanger, in which case increased activity could modulate smooth muscle function by causing an increase in intracellular pH (41).

Alterations in sodium-potassium cotransport have also been reported in the erythrocytes of patients with hypertension, but the evidence is inconsistent and contradictory.

On present evidence, a link between increased sodium intake and hypertension would seem most likely to depend on increased production of the circulating inhibitor of the sodium pump with a resultant increase in peripheral resistance. Before this hypothesis can be accepted, however, it will be necessary to identify the circulating inhibitor and clearly demonstrate its dependence on sodium intake; it will also be necessary to show that inhibition of pump function by the circulating agent can in some way give rise to a sustained increase in peripheral resistance.

ALTERED CALCIUM HANDLING BY THE KIDNEY

There is convincing evidence of increased excretion of calcium by the kidney in patients with primary hypertension. McCarron et al. (49) measured the calcium and sodium content of 24-hr urine samples from 34 patients with hypertension and compared the results with those in timed urine samples from matched normal controls. The hourly rate of sodium excretion was similar in the two groups, but excretion of calcium was greater in patients than normal controls at any given rate of sodium loss. Strazzullo et al. (68) subsequently demonstrated that there is an absolute increase in calcium excretion in primary hypertension. They obtained full 24-hr urine samples from 55 patients with hypertension and a similar number of matched normal controls. Total calcium excretion was found to be nearly 30% higher in the patients than in the controls; the calcium/sodium ratio was also significantly raised, showing that the increased rate of calcium loss was not merely secondary to increased sodium excretion.

The increased urinary calcium excretion does not appear to be secondary to enhanced absorption from the gut, since the difference between the groups is even greater in the fasting state: In the study of Strazzullo et al. (68) the calcium excretion rate in the patients was approximately double that in the normal controls when two subgroups were reexamined after a 12-hr fast (Fig. 1). The increased excretion rate is not explained by an increase in serum calcium concentration: Total calcium was similar in the two groups in both studies cited (49,68), and serum ionized calcium was measured in one and was found not to differ between the groups (68). In both studies, the concentration of parathyroid hormone in the blood was shown to be slightly, but significantly, elevated. This combination of findings points to a disorder of renal function as the cause of the increased excretion of calcium in primary hypertension.

The renal calcium leak might reflect a specific defect in tubular reabsorption of the ion, and it is tempting to see a link with the altered function of the ATP-dependent calcium pump that has been observed in the vascular smooth muscle of the spontaneously hypertensive rat (SHR) and the platelets of humans (25,33–35,58). The tubular reabsorption of calcium is, however, directly linked to that of sodium (19), and the movement of calcium may depend to an important extent on a $Na^+ - Ca^{2+}$ exchange sys-

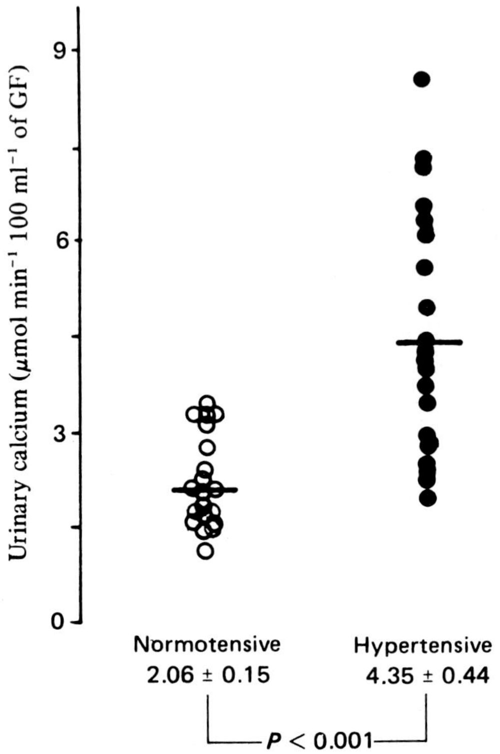

FIG. 1. Urinary calcium excretion rate after 12-hr fast in 20 normotensive and 20 hypertensive subjects. Values shown are mean ± SEM. (From ref. 68.)

tem in the outer surface of the tubular cells (39). It is therefore possible that the enhanced calcium loss in patients with hypertension is entirely secondary to an altered pattern of sodium handling. Such an alteration would seem likely to involve a reduction in the fractional reabsorption of sodium in the proximal tubule, since a rise in the urinary calcium/sodium ratio with an increase in total calcium loss is seen in dogs when fractional reabsorption of sodium in the distal tubule is increased by treatment with deoxycorticosterone acetate (DOCA) (42).

Whatever the cause of the renal calcium leak in primary hypertension, the increased urinary loss must put the mechanisms concerned with the maintenance of calcium balance in a state of constant mild stress in hypertensive patients. And if, as has been claimed, the increased urinary loss is accompanied in some patients by a suboptimal calcium intake, the stress on the homeostatic mechanisms will be correspondingly greater. The situation may be further complicated in the SHR by an impaired ability to absorb calcium from the gut (45), but this aspect is controversial and other workers have reported increased absorption (37).

The effect of the altered calcium metabolism on the plasma calcium concentration is no more than slight, and studies of the relation between plasma calcium and arterial pressure have yielded contradictory results. Two large epidemiological studies demonstrated a positive correlation between total plasma calcium concentration and arterial pressure (12,32). These studies related to normal populations, however, and they do not exclude the possibility of a different relationship between calcium and arterial pressure in patients with hypertension. In one study of patients with hypertension, the average total plasma calcium concentration did not differ from that in matched normotensive controls, but an inverse correlation was observed between calcium concentration and arterial pressure (49). In another study in which ionized calcium was measured, no difference was found between patients and controls (68); in a second report from the first laboratory, however, a significant reduction in ionized calcium was noted in a group of hypertensive patients as compared to normal controls (43). In yet another report, ionized calcium was claimed to be reduced in patients with suppressed renin activity, but not in those with normal or raised renin (57). When the results of all the studies are taken together, it appears that there is probably little or no difference overall in plasma ionized calcium concentration between patients with hypertension and normal subjects, but there may be a subgroup of patients in whom calcium is slightly reduced.

Two independent studies have agreed in finding a small, but significant, increase in the plasma concentration of parathyroid hormone in patients with hypertension (49,68). This can be seen as the compensatory mechanism by which ionized calcium is maintained at a normal, or near normal, level despite an inappropriately low intake in relation to urinary loss. It is to be expected that some increase in the plasma concentration of 1,25-dihydroxy vitamin D will also be present.

ALTERED CALCIUM HANDLING AT A CELLULAR LEVEL

It has been suggested that the disturbance of whole body calcium handling that has been demonstrated in patients with primary hypertension and in the SHR contributes in some way to the genesis or maintenance of the raised arterial pressure (44). If this is so, it seems likely that it would be as a result of alterations in calcium handling at a cellular level. There is convincing evidence of abnormal handling of the calcium ion by cells and cell membranes both in patients with hypertension and in the SHR. It is less clear, however, how these cellular mechanisms might be influenced by the calcium status of the organism as a whole.

Total and Free Calcium Within the Cell

The total calcium content of arteries from the SHR (22) and DOCA/salt hypertensive rat (31) has been shown to be elevated, but it is not clear where the excess calcium is located. Measurement of the kinetics of ^{45}Ca efflux from fat cells obtained from the SHR (51) and from patients with primary hypertension (53) revealed a substantial increase in exchangeable calcium within the cell, which was thought to be largely in the mitochondria. Recent studies have focused on the determination of free calcium within the cytosol, since this fraction alone is active in controlling other cellular functions. In one study, calcium activity was measured by an ion-sensitive electrode in a lysate of washed erythrocytes: Calcium activity was higher in preparations from patients with primary hypertension than in those from normotensive controls (73). The development of fluorescent probes, such as the dye quin 2, has provided a means for the estimation of free calcium within the cytosol of intact cells. The method is not without difficulty since the probe itself serves as a calcium sink and may thus alter the equilibrium concentration of the ion within the cell. Nonetheless, the demonstration by two groups (10,20) of a higher than normal concentration of free calcium within platelets derived from patients with primary hypertension provides strong evidence for an elevation of cytosolic Ca^{2+} in that condition. Not all workers are agreed, however, and free calcium showed no more than a small and statistically insignificant increase in two studies of mononuclear leukocytes from patients with hypertension (10,64) and was not raised at all in neutrophils (38). If the cells of the vascular smooth muscle are subject to the same disturbance of calcium handling as the platelets, it would account for the functional component of the rise in peripheral vascular resistance.

If the steady-state concentration of free calcium is increased in certain active cells in patients with hypertension, there must be either an increased delivery of calcium to the cytosol or impaired function of the systems responsible for the removal of calcium (or possibly a combination of the two). Evidence pointing to altered transport of calcium in patients and SHR will now be reviewed.

Calcium Influx

Measurement of calcium influx in platelets and lymphocytes of the SHR during inhibition of calcium pumping revealed influx to be 50 to 60% higher than normal (11). No direct measurements of calcium influx rates have been made in human cells. In studies of forearm resistance vessels of patients with hypertension, however, the dilator response to verapamil, which selectively inhibits potential-operated calcium channels, has been shown to be increased (29,60). There is no increase in the dilator response to nitroprusside, which induces relaxation by other mechanisms. The degree of enhancement of the responsiveness to verapamil is directly related to the severity of the hypertension (Fig. 2). These findings are consistent with an increased calcium flux through the potential-operated channels in the smooth muscle cells of hypertensive vessels.

No information is available concerning the

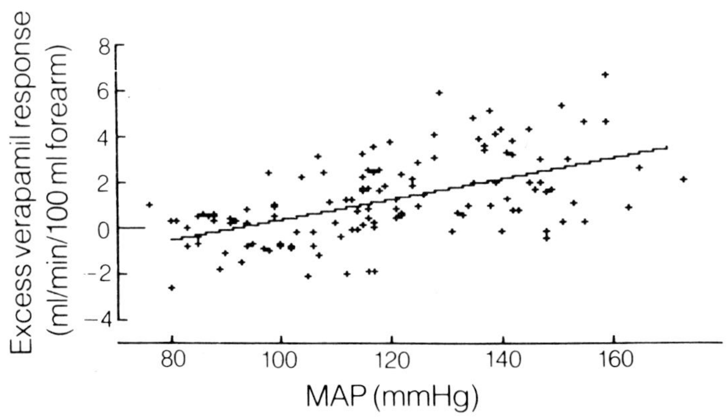

FIG. 2. Responsiveness of forearm resistance vessels to verapamil related to mean arterial pressure in 127 men. The "excess verapamil response" is the amount by which the sum of the responses to two infusions of verapamil at 5 μg/min exceeds that predicted from the response to nitroprusside using the regression line for normal subjects. There is a significant relation between response to verapamil and arterial pressure ($r = 0.55$; $p < 0.001$). (From ref. 59.)

release of calcium from the intracellular stores in the vascular smooth muscle.

Calcium Efflux

Two systems are known by which calcium can be pumped out of cells. They are the ATP-dependent calcium pump and the sodium-calcium exchange system, which makes use of the inwardly directed sodium gradient to drive calcium out of the cell (9,13). Sodium-calcium exchange is a low-affinity, high-capacity system and operates most effectively when the intracellular calcium concentration is relatively high; it is believed to be important in the rapid removal of calcium from myocardial cells at the end of systole. The ATP-dependent calcium pump is a high-affinity, low capacity system; it is believed to dominate the process of calcium extrusion when the concentration of the ion within the cell is relatively low, and this would normally be the case in the smooth muscle of the resistance vessels.

The intracellular sodium concentration is raised in the leukocytes of patients with primary hypertension (28). If, as is probable, a similar increase is present in other active cells, the rate of sodium-calcium exchange would be expected to be decreased, assuming no increase in the number of exchange sites. No measurements are available on the activity of this system in patients with hypertension, but from what is known of sodium-calcium exchange, an increase in intracellular sodium might be expected to have an important effect on calcium extrusion from the myocardium but not on the resistance vessels.

More information is available concerning ATP-dependent calcium pumping. Daniel et al. studied ATP-dependent calcium accumulation by inside-out vesicles derived from plasma membrane of rat mesenteric arteries. Accumulation was found to be below normal in preparations from rats with spontaneous hypertension (33), DOCA/salt hypertension (34), and two models of renovascular hypertension (35). This was thought to reflect defective functioning of the ATP-dependent calcium pump that operates in this model to move calcium inward across the inside-out membrane. The findings could, however, be accounted for by increased permeability to calcium, allowing a more rapid outward leak and so reducing accumulation. In a recent study of intact platelets and lymphocytes from the SHR by methods that enabled calcium influx to be distinguished from efflux, the rate of entry was found to be increased, whereas the rate of removal was as expected for the concentration of the ion in the cytosol (11). This finding suggests that the reduced ATP-dependent accumulation by inside-membrane vesicles may indeed reflect an increased leak rather than reduced pumping.

There is, however, evidence of abnormalities relating to the calcium pump in membrane preparations from the platelets of patients with primary hypertension. The molecular basis of the calcium pump is the calmodulin-sensitive fraction of the $(Ca^{2+} + Mg^{2+})-$ATPase of the plasma membrane. Total calcium-dependent ATPase activity in platelet plasma membrane is significantly increased in patients with hypertension (25,58). The enzyme is, however, functionally abnormal in that it shows reduced stimulation by calmodulin (58) and is less easily inactivated by lanthanum (25). These findings suggest that the $(Ca^{2+} + Mg^{2+})-$ATPase of hypertensive platelets may be less effective than usual in calcium pumping, but that the defect is compensated to a greater or lesser extent by an increase in total enzyme activity.

It remains an open question whether the elevation of cytosolic calcium believed to be present in the cells of patients with hypertension results solely from increased calcium influx, or is also dependent in part on impaired function of the calcium pump. Abnormalities can also be demonstrated in the $(Ca^{2+} + Mg^{2+})-$ATPase of endoplasmic reticulum in the platelets, and this raises the possibility that sequestration of calcium within the cell might also be disturbed.

Calcium Binding

Calcium binds to several molecular species in the plasma membrane, including anionic phospholipids and proteins. The internal surface of the membrane is exposed to ionic calcium concentrations that are typically below 1 μM, and high-affinity binding is involved. The outer surface is exposed to concentrations three or four orders of magnitude higher, and both high- and low-affinity binding are involved. Total calcium binding to the outer aspect of erythrocyte membranes is similar in hypertensive patients and normal controls as it is in SHR and appropriate controls (52). High-affinity binding of ^{45}Ca to the inner aspect of the membrane is, however, reduced both in patients with hypertension (52) and in the SHR (14,52). A similar reduction in binding has also been demonstrated with membrane preparations obtained from various other tissues of the SHR (15).

The significance of the reduced binding of calcium to the inner aspect of the plasma membrane is far from clear. Calcium exerts an important regulatory effect on various aspects of membrane function, and it is possible that the reduction in binding is a cause of some of the abnormalities of ion transport. It may be, however, that the reduction in binding is merely a marker of an alteration in membrane composition, which results in a reduced availability of binding sites.

RELATION BETWEEN WHOLE BODY CALCIUM METABOLISM AND EVENTS AT A CELLULAR LEVEL

If the abnormalities of calcium handling by cell membranes are in any way dependent on the disturbance of general calcium metabolism, some mechanism must exist by which the calcium balance of the body as a whole can influence events at a cellular level. The link could involve changes in the plasma ionized calcium concentration or changes in calcium-regulating substances such as parathyroid hormone or 1,23-dihydroxy vitamin D. A rising concentration of calcium in the extracellular fluid has been shown to inactivate certain potential-operated calcium channels in tenia coli (30), and a falling concentration must have contrary effects. It is probable that human resistance vessels respond in a similar way (61), although the manifest response to a rise in calcium concentration is contraction. The change in calcium concentration required to cause significant changes in vascular responsiveness is, however, large in relation to the small changes observed in patients with hypertension, and it seems unlikely that the small alterations in ionized calcium concentration reported in patients with primary hypertension could play a significant role in its causation. Parathyroid hormone probably acts on cells of many types apart from those of the renal tubules and bone, and an increase in its concentration may favor an increase in cytosolic calcium. At concentrations greatly in excess of those occurring physiologically, parathyroid hormone dilates resistance vessels (55), but the effect, if any, of the very small increases observed in patients with primary hypertension is unknown. Nothing is known of the direct effect on resistance vessels of 1,25-dihydroxy vitamin D. It must be concluded that no mechanism has yet been identified by which the changes in whole body calcium metabolism observed in hypertension could influence the changes at a cellular level. It is possible that a mechanism exists by which the free calcium in the cytosol can be modulated in response to changes in intake, but it seems likely that the disorder of calcium handling at a cellular level results predominantly from other causes.

EFFECT OF ALTERATION IN CALCIUM INTAKE

If a calcium intake that is suboptimal relative to need plays any part in the causation of primary hypertension, it would be expected that the administration of calcium supplements would lower pressure, at least in the early stages of the hypertensive process. In rats, the administration of large doses of calcium supplements ameliorates the hypertensive process (4), and severe calcium deprivation aggravates it (2). The changes in calcium intake were, however, very large in these experiments, and a more recent study in which more moderate changes in calcium balance were induced failed to demonstrate any effect on pressure (37).

Some studies on the effect of calcium supplementation in humans have suggested a small blood pressure lowering effect, but others have been essentially negative and the results overall are not very convincing. In one study of normotensive subjects, 30 volunteers were given an additional 25 mmol of calcium each day as "Calcium Sandoz"; diastolic (but not systolic) pressure showed a small but significant fall, which took many weeks to reach a maximum (6).

In a later study that was both better designed and better controlled, another group examined the effect of 8 weeks of treatment with a calcium supplement (calcium carbonate, 25 mmol/day) in 32 normal subjects and 48 patients with mild hypertension (46). In the normal subjects there was little effect, with no more than a small but statistically significant fall in supine diastolic pressure. In the patients treatment with calcium led after 8 weeks to significant reduction in systolic pressure in the supine position and both systolic and diastolic pressures standing. The fall in blood pressure was, however, no more than a few millimeters of mercury, and there was much variability in individual responses, with, for example, a third of the patients showing an increase in their standing systolic pressure. In another controlled study, 18 patients with mild to moderate hypertension were given an additional 40 mmol calcium daily as Sandocal for 4 weeks (66). Blood pressure was unaffected by calcium as compared to either placebo or pretreatment values. Both urinary calcium and total plasma calcium were significantly increased during the period of supplementation, but ionized calcium was unchanged. It should be noted, however, that no effect was seen in the previous trial after only 4 weeks of treatment. In a limited placebo-controlled and randomized study carried out in this department, eight subjects with mild to moderate hypertension were given 20 mmol calcium daily as Sandocal for 8-week periods: mean arterial pressure fell by less than 1 mmHg despite a significant increase in urinary calcium excretion (B.F. Robinson, R.J.W. Phillips, and Benjamin, N. *unpublished observations*).

It must be concluded that if administration of extra calcium does lower arterial pressure in patients with primary hypertension, the effect is small and inconsistent. It is possible, however, that a response to calcium occurs only in some subgroups of hypertensive patients, with no response at all in others. This possibility is supported by a study in which 10 patients with hypertension who had been classified by renin status were given 20 mmol of calcium carbonate daily for 5 days: diastolic pressure fell significantly in those with low plasma renin activity, but not in those with normal or raised renin (56). The results of the studies on calcium supplementation give little support to the view that relative deficiency of calcium is a common and important cause of primary hypertension. As with sodium, however, it would be rash to assume that short-term correction of an abnormality of intake will automatically correct secondary disorders that have taken years to develop.

In hypertension developing during pregnancy, altered calcium metabolism may play a more important role. Pregnancy and lactation impose a large demand for calcium on the mother, and the imbalance resulting from a suboptimal intake would be much greater than that in the nonpregnant state. It is of interest, therefore, that a controlled study of the effect of calcium supplementation during normal pregnancy (25 and 50 mmol/day) showed a significant reduction in diastolic pressure during the second trimester, and with the larger supplement, the normal increase in pressure in the third trimester was prevented (7). Pregnancy provides a unique opportunity to determine if calcium supplementation can prevent a rise in blood pressure and to investigate the possible relation between abnormalities of calcium balance and arterial pressure; it may be in this exceptional circumstance that a connection, if it exists, will be most easily demonstrated.

INTERRELATION OF SODIUM AND CALCIUM HANDLING

The abnormalities of handling of sodium and calcium have been considered separately, but there are many situations in which the handling of one ion may have important effects on the handling of the other. In the gut, high concentrations of sodium interfere with the absorption of calcium; an excessive sodium intake might therefore aggravate the effects of a suboptimal calcium intake. In the kidney, as has already been mentioned, calcium excretion is linked to sodium excretion (19), and an increased sodium load will augment the calcium leak that is characteristic of primary hypertension. A high sodium intake can thus reduce absorption of calcium while accelerating its excretion, and it may in this way increase the stress on the calcium homeostatic mechanisms. It would therefore seem important to consider the intake of sodium as well as calcium when trying to determine if there is a link between dietary calcium and the development of hypertension. Much of the epidemiological data would be more easily understood if it were postulated that a sodium intake of at least 100 to 120 mmol per day is necessary for the pressor effect of a low calcium intake to become apparent.

At a cellular level, too, sodium and calcium handling may interact. The effect of an increase in intracellular sodium in reducing sodium/calcium exchange and so raising cytosolic calcium has been stressed by Blaustein (8). It is now thought unlikely that the sodium/calcium exchange system is an important determinant of cytosolic calcium in vascular smooth muscle, but it is possible that sodium and calcium interact in other ways.

Finally, it should be noted that cytosolic calcium is the messenger controlling the secretion of the hormones involved in sodium and water handling. In nearly all endocrine cells, calcium is a stimulus for secretion, and an increase in cytosolic calcium might explain, for example, the small increase in plasma vasopressin concentration observed in hypertension. In the renin-secreting cells of the kidney, however, calcium is believed to serve an inhibitory function (3), and it is tempting to relate an increase in cytosolic calcium in patients with hypertension to the suppression of renin secretion that may develop.

CONCLUSIONS

Nearly everyone in the developed countries consumes more salt than is needed. Those who will develop hypertension are postulated to suffer in addition a diminished capacity for renal excretion of sodium. There is no direct evidence to support this view, but the recent demonstration of a raised concentration of atrial natriuretic factor in the plasma of some patients with primary hypertension offers indirect support. It is proposed that the sodium overload leads not to an increase in total body sodium, but to a compensatory increase in the plasma concentration of circulating natriuretic substances. These include not only the atrial factor, but a substance as yet unidentified that inhibits sodium pump activity; it is suggested that the pump inhibitor acts directly on the vascular smooth muscle to cause an increase in peripheral resistance. There is good evidence for depression of sodium pump activity in both leukocytes and resistance vessels of patients with hypertension, but it remains to be demonstrated that this can induce a sustained increase in peripheral resistance. The effect on raised blood pressure of restricting sodium intake is disappointingly small, but this may reflect the development of secondary changes that oppose a fall in pressure.

Calcium intake may be slightly lower than average in patients with hypertension, but the interpretation of the evidence is controversial and the deficit, if real, is small. There is convincing evidence of increased urinary calcium loss in patients with hypertension, and the homeostatic mechanisms regulating calcium balance appear to be under some stress with a small increase in the plasma concentration of parathyroid hormone. At a cellular level, there is evidence of increased calcium influx into platelets and vascular smooth muscle, and an increase in cytosolic calcium has been reported in platelets. A functional disorder affects the calcium pump, and the binding of calcium ions to the inner aspect of the plasma membrane is reduced. These changes could underly the increase in peripheral resistance. The disorder of calcium handling by the cells cannot be accounted for by altered sodium metabolism, and it is tempting to relate it to the altered whole body calcium metabolism. However, no mechanism has been identified by which the general disturbance might cause the cellular disorder. The effect on raised blood pressure of supplementing the diet with calcium is, at the most, small and inconsistent.

It is probable that abnormal whole body handling of sodium contributes to the hypertensive process and possible that abnormal handling of calcium is also involved, but neither ion has been shown to play a role of such dominance that a defect in its handling can reasonably be regarded as a primary cause of the condition.

At a cellular level, several abnormalities of transport of both sodium and calcium have been clearly defined and appear to result from immediate causes that are independent for the two ions; apart from the depression of sodium pump activity, the abnormalities of ion transport appear unconnected with altered whole body handling. It is probable that altered transport of both sodium and calcium contributes to the production of the raised peripheral resistance in established hypertension, and it may well be that several of the disorders that have been identified act in synergism to raise the concentration of free calcium in the cytosol.

REFERENCES

1. Aalkjaer, C., Heagerty, A. M., Parvin, S. D., Bell, P. R. F., Bing, R. F., and Swales, J. D. (1986): Cell membrane sodium transport: A correlation between human resistance vessels and leucocytes. *Lancet*, 1:649–651.
2. Anderson, S., Grady, J. R., Ellison, D. H., and McCarron, D. A. (1983): Calcium balance and parathyroid hormone mediated vasodilatation in the spontaneously hypertensive rat. *Hypertension*, 5(*Suppl.* 1):59–63.
3. Antonipillai, I., and Horton, R. (1985): Role of extra- and intracellular calcium and calmodulin in renin release from rat kidney. *Endocrinology*, 117:601–606.
4. Ayachi, S. (1979): Increased dietary calcium lowers blood pressure in the spontaneously hypertensive rat. *Metabolism*, 28:1234–1238.
5. Belizán, J. M., and Villar, J. (1980): The relationship between calcium intake and edema-, proteinuria-, and hypertension-gestosis: An hypothesis. *Am. J. Clin. Nutr.*, 33:2202–2210.
6. Belizán, J. M., Villar, J., Pineda, O., Gonzalez, A. E., Sainz, E., Garrera, G., and Sibrian, R. (1983): Reduction of blood pressure with calcium supplementation in young adults. *JAMA*, 249:1161–1165.
7. Belizán, J. M., Villar, J., Zalazar, A., Rojas, L., Chan, D., and Bryce, G. F. (1983): Preliminary evidence of the effect of calcium supplementation on blood pressure in normal pregnant women. *Am. J. Obstet. Gynecol.*, 146:175–180.
8. Blaustein, M. P. (1977): Sodium ions, calcium ions, blood pressure regulation, and hypertension: A reassessment and a hypothesis. *Am. J. Physiol.*, 232:C165–C173.
9. Brading, A. F., and Lategan, T. W. (1985): Na-Ca exchange in vascular smooth muscle. *J. Hypertension*, 3:109–116.
10. Bruschi, G., Bruschi, M. E., Caroppo, M., Orlandini, G., Spaggiari, M., and Cavatorta, A. (1985): Cytoplasmic free $[Ca^{2+}]$ is increased in the platelets of spontaneously hypertensive rats and essential hypertensive patients. *Clin. Sci.*, 68:179–184.
11. Bruschi, G., Bruschi, M. E., Orlandini, G., Cavatorta, A., Borghetti, A., Ferrandi, M., and Bianchi, G. (1985): Why is $[Ca^{2+}]_i$ increased in blood cells in

primary hypertension? *J. Hypertension,* 3(*Suppl.* 3):S45–S47.

12. Bulpitt, C. J., Hodes, C., and Everitt, M. G. (1976): The relationship between blood pressure and biochemical risk factors in a general population. *Br. J. Prevent. Soc. Med.,* 30:158–162.
13. Carafoli, E. (1984): How calcium crosses plasma membranes including the sarcolemma. In: *Calcium Antagonists and Cardiovascular Disease,* edited by L. H. Opie, pp. 29–41. Raven Press, New York.
14. Devynck, M. A., Pernollet, M. G., Nunez, A. M., and Meyer, P. (1981): Analysis of calcium handling in erythrocyte membranes of genetically hypertensive rats. *Hypertension,* 3:397–403.
15. Devynck, M. A., Pernollet, M. G., Nunez, A. M., and Meyer, P. (1981): Calcium binding alteration in plasma membrane from various tissues of spontaneously hypertensive rat. *Clin. Exp. Hypertension,* 3:797–807.
16. de Wardener, H. E., and MacGregor, G. A. (1980): Dahl's hypothesis that a saluretic substance may be responsible for a sustained rise in arterial pressure: Its possible role in essential hypertension. *Kidney Int.,* 18:1–9.
17. Eaton, S. B., and Konner, M. (1985): Paleolithic nutrition. *N. Engl. J. Med.,* 312:283–289.
18. Editorial (1986): Hypertension: Is there a place for calcium? *Lancet,* 1:359–361.
19. Edwards, B. R., Baer, P. G., Sutton, R. A. L., and Dirks, J. H. (1973): Micropuncture study of diuretic effects on sodium and calcium reabsorption in the dog nephron. *J. Clin. Invest.,* 52:2418–2427.
20. Erne, P., Bolli, P., Bürgisser, E., and Bühler, F. R. (1984): Correlation of platelet calcium with blood pressure. *N. Engl. J. Med.,* 310:1084–1088.
21. Feinleib, N., Lenfant, C., and Miller, S. A. (1984): Hypertension and calcium. *Science,* 226:384–386.
22. Fleckenstein, A. (1983): *Calcium Antagonism in Heart and Smooth Muscle.* John Wiley & Sons, New York.
23. Folsom, A. R., and Prineas, R. J. (1982): Drinking water composition and blood pressure: A review of the epidemiology. *Am. J. Epidemiol.,* 115:818–832.
24. Freis, E. D. (1981): Sodium deprivation as an approach to hypertension. In: *Frontiers in Hypertension Research,* edited by J. H. Laragh, F. R. Bühler, and D. W. Seldin, pp. 43–45. Springer-Verlag, New York.
25. Graham, J. M., Robinson, B. F., and Wilson, R. B. J. (1985): (Ca^{2+} + Mg^{2+}) ATPase activity of a platelet membrane fraction from normal subjects and patients with hypertension (Abstr.). *J. Hypertension,* 3:664.
26. Gray, H. H., Hilton, P. J., and Richardson, P. J. (1986): Effect of serum from patients with essential hypertension on sodium transport in normal leucocytes. *Clin. Sci.,* 70:583–586.
27. Harlan, W. R., Hull, A. L., Schmouder, R. L., Landis, J. R., Thompson, F. E., and Larkin, F. A. (1984): Blood pressure and nutrition in adults. The National Health and Nutrition Examination Survey. *Am. J. Epidemiol.,* 120:469–470.
28. Hilton, P. J. (1986): Cellular sodium transport in essential hypertension. *N. Engl. J. Med.,* 314:222–229.
29. Hulthén, U. L., Bolli, P., Amann, F. W., Kiowski, W., and Bühler, F. R. (1982): Enhanced vasodilatation in essential hypertension by calcium channel blockade with verapamil. *Hypertension,* 4(*Suppl.* II):26–31.
30. Hurwitz, L., McGuffee, L. J., Smith, P. M., and Little, S. A. (1982): Specific inhibition of calcium channels by calcium ions in smooth muscle. *J. Pharmacol. Exp. Ther.,* 220:382–388.
31. Jones, A. W., and Hart, R. G. (1975): Altered ion transport in aortic smooth muscle during deoxycorticosterone acetate hypertension in the rat. *Circ. Res.,* 37:333–341.
32. Kesteloot, H., and Geboers, J. (1982): Calcium and blood pressure. *Lancet,* 1:813–815.
33. Kwan, C. Y., Belbeck, L., and Daniel, E. E. (1979): Abnormal biochemistry of vascular smooth muscle plasma membrane as an important factor in the initiation and maintenance of hypertension in rats. *Blood Vessels,* 16:259–268.
34. Kwan, C. Y., Belbeck, L., and Daniel, E. E. (1980): Abnormal biochemistry of vascular smooth muscle plasma membrane isolated from hypertensive rats. *Mol. Pharmacol.,* 17:137–140.
35. Kwan, C. Y., Belbeck, L., and Daniel, E. E. (1980): Characteristics of arterial plasma membrane in renovascular hypertension in rats. *Blood Vessels,* 17:131–140.
36. Langford, H. G., and Watson, R. L. (1973): Electrolytes, environment and blood pressure. *Clin. Sci. Mol. Med.,* 45:111s–113s.
37. Lau, K., Gafter, U., Rydell, D., Eby, B., Pesigan, M., Tropp, I., Garno, J., and Zikos, D. (1986): Evidence against the role of calcium deficiency in genetic hypertension. *Hypertension,* 8:45–49.
38. Lew, P. D., Favre, L., Waldvogel, F. A., and Vallotton, M. B. (1985): Cytosolic free calcium and intracellular calcium stores in neutrophils from hypertensive subjects. *Clin. Sci.,* 69:227–230.
39. Lorenzen, M., Lee, C. O., and Windhager, E. E. (1984): Cytosolic Ca^{2+} and Na^{+} activities in perfused proximal tubules of *Necturus* kidney. *Am. J. Physiol.,* 247:F93–F102.
40. MacGregor, G. A. (1985): Sodium is more important than calcium in essential hypertension. *Hypertension,* 7:628–637.
41. Mahnensmith, R. L., and Aronson, P. S. (1985): The plasma membrane sodium-hydrogen exchanger and its role in physiological and pathophysiological processes. *Circ. Res.,* 56:773–788.
42. Massey, S. G., Corburn, J. W., Chapman, L. W., and Kleeman, C. R. (1968): The effect of long term deoxycorticosterone acetate administration on the renal excretion of calcium and magnesium. *J. Lab. Clin. Med.,* 71:212–219.
43. McCarron, D. A. (1982): Low serum concentration of ionized calcium in patients with hypertension. *N. Engl. J. Med.,* 307:226–228.
44. McCarron, D. A. (1985): Is calcium more important than sodium in the pathogenesis of essential hypertension? *Hypertension,* 7:607–627.
45. McCarron, D. A., Lucas, P. A., Shneidman, R. J., LaCour, B., and Drücke, T. (1985): Blood pressure development of the spontaneously hypertensive rat after concurrent manipulations of dietary Ca^{2+} and Na^{+}. *J. Clin. Invest.,* 76:1147–1154.
46. McCarron, D. A., and Morris, C. D. (1985): Blood pressure response to oral calcium in persons with mild

to moderate hypertension: A randomised double-blind placebo-controlled cross-over trial. *Ann. Intern. Med.*, 103:825–831.
47. McCarron, D. A., Morris, C. D., and Cole, C. (1982): Dietary calcium in human hypertension. *Science*, 217:267–269.
48. McCarron, D. A., Morris, C. D., Henry, H. J., and Stanton, J. L. (1984): Blood pressure and nutrient intake in the United States. *Science*, 224:1392–1398.
49. McCarron, D. A., Pingree, P. A., Rubin, R. J. Gaucher, S. M., Molitch, M., and Krutzik, S. (1980): Enhanced parathyroid function in essential hypertension: A homeostatic response to a urinary calcium leak. *Hypertension*, 2:162–168.
50. Phillips, R. J. W., and Robinson, B. F. (1984): The dilator response to K^+ is reduced in the forearm resistance vessels of men with primary hypertension. *Clin. Sci.*, 66:237–239.
51. Postnov, Yu. V., and Orlov, S. N. (1979): Features of intracellular calcium distribution in the adipose tissue of spontaneously hypertensive rats. *Experientia*, 35:1480–1481.
52. Postnov, Yu. V., Orlov, S. N., and Pokudin, N. I., (1979): Decrease of calcium binding by the red blood cell membrane in spontaneously hypertensive rats and in essential hypertension. *Pflügers Arch.*, 379:191–195.
53. Postnov, Yu. V., Orlov, S. N., and Pokudin, N. I. (1980): Alteration of intracellular calcium distribution in the adipose tissue of human patients with essential hypertension. *Pflügers Arch.*, 388:89–91.
54. Poston, L., Gray, H. H., Crowther, A., Dittrich, H. C., Hilton, P. J., Webb-Peploe, M. M., and MacGregor, G. A. (1984): Cellular sodium concentration and vasoconstrictor state in hypertension. *J. Cardiovasc. Pharmacol.*, 6:S16–S20.
55. Rambausek, M., Rascher, W., Mann, J., and Ritz, E. (1983): Action of parathyroid hormone on resistance vessels. *J. Hypertension*, 1(*Suppl.* 2):310–312.
56. Resnick, L. M., and Laragh, J. H. (1983): The hypotensive effect of short-term oral calcium loading in essential hypertension (Abstr.). *Clin. Res.*, 31:334A.
57. Resnick, L. M., Laragh, J. H., Sealey, J. E., and Alderman, M. H. (1983): Divalent cations in essential hypertension: Relations between serum ionised calcium, magnesium and plasma renin activity. *N. Engl. J. Med.*, 309:888–891.
58. Resink, T. J., Tkachuk, V. A., Erne, P., and Bühler, F. R. (1986): Platelet membrane calmodulin-stimulated calcium-adenosine triphosphatase. Altered activity in essential hypertension. *Hypertension*, 8:159–166.
59. Robinson, B. F. (1984): Altered calcium handling as a cause of primary hypertension. *J. Hypertension*, 2:453–460.
60. Robinson, B. F., Dobbs, R. J., and Bayley, S. (1982): Response of forearm resistance vessels to verapamil and sodium nitroprusside in normotensive and hypertensive men: Evidence for a functional abnormality of vascular smooth muscle in primary hypertension. *Clin. Sci.*, 63:33–42.
61. Robinson, B. F., and Phillips, R. J. W. (1984): Effect of small increments in plasma calcium concentration on the responsiveness of forearm resistance vessels to verapamil in normal subjects. *Clin. Sci.*, 67:613–618.
62. Robinson, B. F., Phillips, R. J. W., Wilson, P. N., and Chiodini, P. L. (1983): Effect of local infusion of ouabain on human forearm vascular resistance and on response to potassium, verapamil and sodium nitroprusside. *J. Hypertension*, 1:165–169.
63. Sagnella, G. A., Markandu, N. D., Shore, A. C., and MacGregor, G. A. (1986): Raised circulating levels of atrial natriuretic peptides in essential hypertension. *Lancet*, 1:179–181.
64. Shore, A. C., Beynon, G. W., Jones, J. C., Markandu, N. D., Sagnella, G. A., and MacGregor, G. A. (1985): Mononuclear leucocyte intracellular free calcium—Does it correlate with blood pressure? *J. Hypertension*, 3:183–187.
65. Simpson, F. O. (1979): Salt and hypertension: A skeptical review of the evidence. *Clin. Sci. Mol. Med.*, 57:463s–469s.
66. Singer, D. R. J., Markandu, N. D., Cappuccio, F. P., Beynon, G. W., Shore, A. C., Smith, S. J., and MacGregor, G. A. (1985): Does oral calcium lower blood pressure: A double-blind study (Abstr.). *J. Hypertension*, 3:661.
67. Stitt, F. W., Clayton, D. G., Crawford, M. D., and Morris, J. N. (1973): Clinical and biochemical indicators of cardiovascular disease among men living in hard and soft water areas. *Lancet*, 1:122–126.
68. Strazzullo, P., Nunziata, V., Cirillo, M., Giannatasio, R., Ferrara, L. A., Mattioli, P. L., and Mancini, M. (1983): Abnormalities of calcium metabolism in essential hypertension. *Clin. Sci.*, 65:137–141.
69. Swales, J. D. (1984): Ion transport in hypertension. *Biosci. Rep.*, 2:967–990.
70. Tobian, L., Lange, J., Azar, S., Iwai, J., Koop, D., Coffee, K., and Johnson, M. A. (1978): Reduction of natriuretic capacity and renin release in isolated, blood-perfused kidneys of Dahl hypertension-prone rats. *Circ. Res.*, 43(*Suppl.* I):I-92–I-97.
71. Watt, G. C. M., Foy, C. J. W., Hart, J. T., Bingham, G., Edwards, C., Hart, M., Thomas, E., and Walton, P. (1985): Dietary sodium and arterial pressure: Evidence against genetic susceptibility. *Br. Med. J.*, 291:1525–1528.
72. Wiggins, R. C., Basar, I., and Slater, J. D. H. (1978): Effect of arterial pressure and inheritance on the sodium excretory capacity of normal young men. *Clin. Sci. Mol. Med.*, 54:639–647.
73. Zidek, W., Vetter, H., Dorst, K.-G., Zumkley, H., and Losse, H. (1982): Intracellular Na^+ and Ca^{2+} activities in essential hypertension. *Clin. Sci.*, 63:41s–43s.

The Kidney in Hypertension, edited by
Norman M. Kaplan, Barry M. Brenner,
and John H. Laragh. Raven Press,
New York © 1987.

Role of the Renin-Angiotensin-Aldosterone Axis in Human Hypertensive Disorders

John H. Laragh

Cardiovascular Center, The New York Hospital-Cornell University Medical Center, New York, New York 10021

A glance at this book's table of contents should provide persuasive evidence that the phenomenon of high blood pressure reflects the participation of a great many endogenous and exogenous factors. There is no single pathogenesis for hypertension; it is not a single disease, despite the persistent clinical and nosological habit of treating it so. The column of mercury, in the sphygmomanometer as in the thermometer, rises in response to a number of disorders; it provides only a nonspecific finding, not a diagnosis.

Once the multiformity of the hypertensions is fully appreciated (1,2), there is a clearer basis for examining what they have in common. Etiology aside, they all have in common a state of increased peripheral vascular resistance and an obligatory disturbance, either reactive or causal, in the endocrinologic mechanism that is responsible for the ongoing regulation of blood pressure. Whatever the reason for the abnormality, internal or external, the central control system is bound to be affected.

This chapter will examine the ways in which the study of that central control, the renin-angiotensin-aldosterone axis, reveals differentiation among the hypertensions, refines analysis of the vasoconstrictive forces, suggests pathogenesis, and even guides specific therapies. A broad spectrum of cause and effect ranging between polar opposite vasoconstrictive mechanisms will be shown.

DISCOVERY OF THE RENIN SYSTEM

A kidney-based endocrine authority over blood pressure regulation was first proposed in 1898 by Tigerstedt and Bergman, who had produced hypertension in rabbits by injecting minced rabbit kidneys (3). They named their hypothetical substance renin. The proposal lost credence when most other workers failed to confirm the relationship, but interest revived when in 1934 Goldblatt (4) produced hypertension in dogs by clamping their renal arteries.

Renin was then identified and characterized in the laboratory. It was shown to be an enzyme with no pressor activity of its own (5,6). However, by its enzymatic action on a plasma substrate it releases the inactive decapeptide, angiotensin I (7), which then is converted (8) in the lungs (9) to the active octapeptide angiotensin II, the most powerful pressor agent known.

Shortly thereafter, renin, the kidney secretion, became linked to adrenal cortical activity by workers (10–12) investigating the newly discovered sodium-retaining corticosteroid, aldosterone, excesses of which were then identified in association with particular types of hypertension (13,14). In specific, the identification of a hypertensive syndrome, primary aldosteronism (15), associated with primary oversecretion of aldosterone and curable by removing a culpable adenoma, and then the discovery of massive oversecretions of aldosterone in patients with malignant hypertension (10,11,13) marked the first identifications of pathophysiologically significant endocrine abnormalities in any form of human hypertension.

It was especially intriguing that patients with malignant hypertension at laparotomy showed hyperplasia of both adrenal glands but no adrenal cortical tumors, as was the case in primary aldosteronism (14). Moreover, total adrenalectomy had no effect on the course of the malignant hypertension (14). Clearly, in malignant hypertension the adrenal cortex was receiving signals from elsewhere to stimulate its production of aldosterone. But this hyperaldosteronism was not the cause of malignant hypertension; rather the reverse seemed to be true. This became apparent when we found that even total adrenalectomy failed to reverse the inexorable course of the disease. Thus, it was logical to suspect the kidney as the source of the hyperaldosteronism because of the consistently severe renal damage associated with malignant hypertension. Pursuing this line, it was discovered that angiotensin, the pressor agent derived from renal renin secretion, was unique among pressor agents because it was found to be a potent and selective stimulator of adrenal cortical secretion of aldosterone in normal subjects (10).

Thus, the proposition emerged that malignant hypertension is, in fact the expression of a gross derangement of a newly identified renin-aldosterone-endocrine interplay with massive oversecretion of renin (as in the Goldblatt model) resulting in large excesses of angiotensin. This not only exerted a formidable pressor effect but it also stimulated the adrenal cortical secretion of aldosterone, which further complicated the situation by its volume-enhancing sodium-retaining and potassium-wasting actions. The combined onslaught of intense vasoconstriction with reduced flow and nutrition, plus stimulation of excess sodium-volume retention by aldosterone, leads to accelerating renal and vascular damage and thus fuels a vicious cycle, spiraling to fibrinoid and necrotizing lesions and to its inevitable fatal end. This concept of renin-mediated malignant vasculitis has been complemented by numerous animal studies in which injection of renin with aldosterone plus salt replicates the malignant syndrome with a uniform early fatal outcome (16).

Before long the existence of this renal-adrenal hormonal interplay between renin and aldosterone was abundantly verified and characterized in a range of human and animal studies involving normal as well as pathologic situations.

THE RENIN SYSTEM IN NORMAL OPERATION

The upshot of this effort was the charting of the biological characteristics of this renal-adrenal hormonal interaction and the demonstration that it served as a feedback control system that balances direct angiotensin-induced vasoconstriction and indirect sodium-induced vasoconstriction in the regulation of blood pressure. The thesis was put forward that the system's significance in disease lay in its fundamental physiologic assignment in health, which was no less than central authority over long-term blood pressure homeostasis and, concurrently, the regulation of sodium and potassium balance.

Figure 1 illustrates the normal operation of the renin system. The kidney secretes renin in response to changes in renal perfusion (e.g., shock, hemorrhage, heart failure, renal damage) or in renal distal tubular (i.e., sodium supply) flow. Renin's role is immediately realized by its invocation of angiotensin II, which quickly raises blood pressure by constricting the arterioles. At the same time angiotensin II stimulates the adrenal cortical production of aldosterone, which at a slower pace expands the extracellular fluid by means of sodium retention at the cost of potassium wastage. The sodium restores extracellular volume and also can act to induce its own vasoconstrictive effect by pathways not yet defined. The increased volume pays off in restored flow systemically and to the kidneys, thereby shutting off the initial signal for renin release.

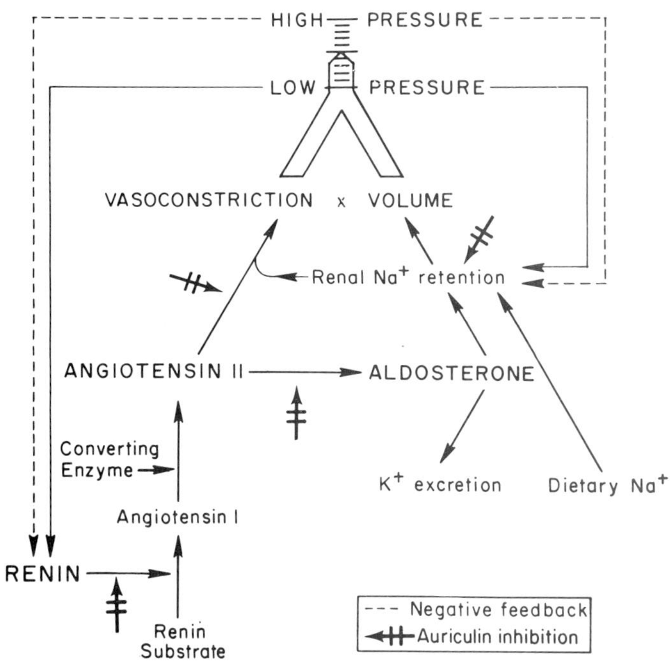

FIG. 1. The renin-angiotensin-aldosterone system and atrial natriuretic hormone. Renin, secreted in response to reduced renal arterial pressure or a reduction in the sodium supply in the renal distal tubule, acts to release angiotensin II. Angiotensin II raises blood pressure and stimulates aldosterone secretion, which leads to retention of sodium and water and to improved flow. These pressures and volume effects turn off the renin release. The atrial natriuretic peptide auriculin opposes the renin system at four points. Within the kidney, its natriuretic action opposes aldosterone action and stops renin secretion. The atrial hormone also opposes the vasoconstrictor action of angiotensin on blood vessels and, at the adrenal cortex, blocks angiotensin stimulation of aldosterone release. (From ref. 16a.) Broken lines denote negative feedback, crossed arrows auriculin inhibition.

In the 1960s clinical studies in normal volunteers demonstrated that prolonged continuous infusion of angiotensin for 10 days or more could produce sustained hypertension (17) with sodium retention. This hypertension could be maintained with progressively smaller doses. Moreover, neither sustained hypertension nor sodium retention could be produced by a similar continuous norepinephrine infusion. These studies established that angiotensin, effective at very low concentrations, was unique among pressor agents in that it could produce and sustain chronic hypertension, apparently indistinguishable from human essential hypertension.

A typical study that describes angiotensin's long-term hypertensionogenic effect in a normal subject is shown in Fig. 2. Here, an initial angiotensin-induced vasoconstriction is gradually replaced by increased aldosterone secretion and concomitant sodium retention. In the face of the resulting volume expansion and sodium-induced vasoconstriction, less and less angiotensin is required to maintain the hypertension.

RENIN SYSTEM BEHAVIOR IN HYPERTENSION DISORDERS: APPLICATIONS FOR RENIN PROFILING

If angiotensin is a vector for mediating chronic hypertension, plasma renin abnormalities, however subtle, should be detectable in all hypertensive patients in whom such a mechanism is operative. Previously, an appreciation of the renin system's role in hypertension was delayed by the inability of many investigators to find a consistent relationship between the serum renin level and the degree of the hypertension. This was likely in large part due to the popular assumption that essential hypertension is a single process. Thus, patients with low renin values can have very high blood pressures too, thereby leading to the possibly erroneous conclusion that renin has no relevance to any hypertensive process. However, if one assumes that there is heterogeneity in mechanisms, then the low-renin group can be presumed to reflect different pathophys-

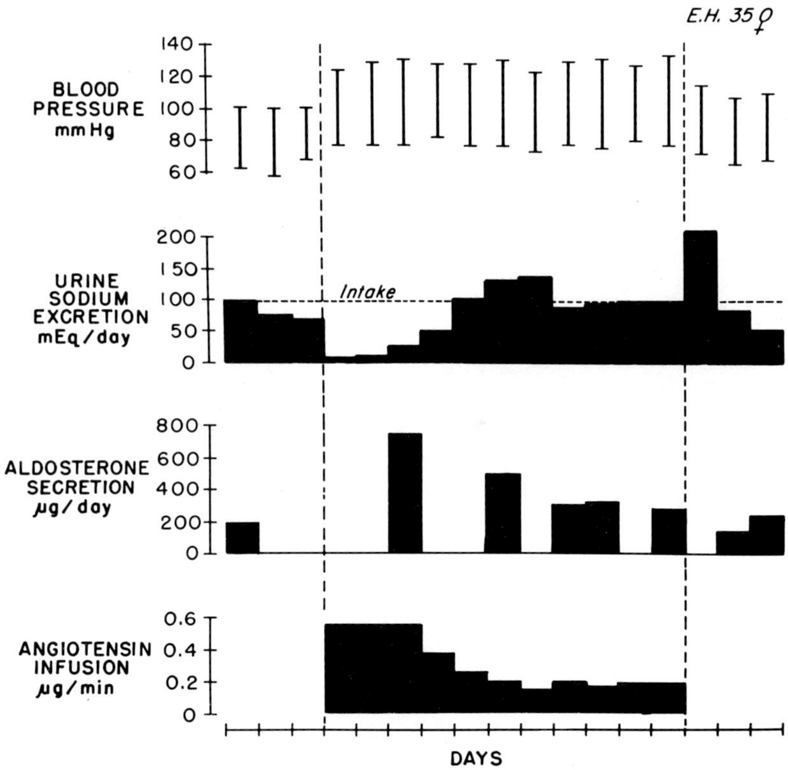

FIG. 2. Prolonged continuous angiotensin infusion in a normal subject for 11 days. The dose of angiotensin was adjusted to keep a mildly pressor response. Angiotensin II induced a marked and selective increase in the adrenal cortical secretion of aldosterone, together with consequent sodium retention. As sodium was retained, angiotensin became more pressor. Because of this increasing pressor sensitivity to angiotensin, the dose was serially reduced to a point where aldosterone secretion returned to control levels. Thus the pressor sensitivity to angiotensin increased as sodium retention progressed. The results indicate that angiotensin, unlike norepinephrine, can produce and then sustain hypertension in progessively smaller amounts as sodium-volume gain turns off the need for angiotensin. (From ref. 47).

iology. Accordingly, the gross renin excesses, generally detected in the more severe hypertensions such as malignant or renovascular hypertension, could suggest a causal or sustaining role. The confusion only arises when one considers essential hypertension as a single process. This "condition" accounts for at least 85% of hypertensive patients.

At the root of this misunderstanding, too, was oversight of the fact that the renin system, like other endocrinologic control systems, does not function in unilateral isolation but is reactive to other forces, internal and external, affecting its servocontrol of blood pressure and electrolyte balance. Just as a normal level of serum insulin is best defined in relationship to the concurrent influence of glucose, so a normal level of renin can be best defined only in relationship to the concurrent influence of dietary sodium intake.

This is illustrated by the development of a protocol called "renin-sodium profiling" in which renin levels are indexed to the current state of sodium balance as determined by a 24-hr sodium excretion analysis (18,19). The nomograms obtained from normal subjects (see Fig. 3) display a wide range of renin values depending on sodium intake. This follows the classic reactive behavior of an endocrinologic control system responding to that which it has been assigned to control. From a practical standpoint this nomogram means that to understand the role of renin

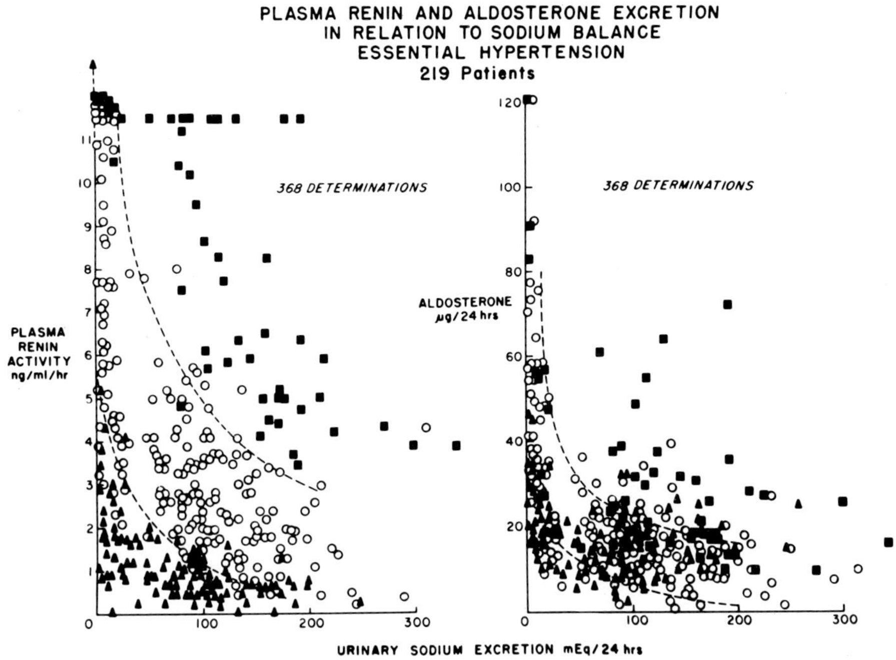

FIG. 3. Relation of renin activity in plasma samples obtained at noon and 24-hr urinary excretion of aldosterone to concurrent daily rate of sodium excretion. For these subjects, the data describe a similar dynamic hyperbolic relationship between the secretion of each hormone and the daily rate of sodium excretion. (From ref. 23.)

in hypertension its activity is best interpreted in terms of the concurrent effects of sodium intake on the behavior of the system.

A sounder basis now existed for assessing high, normal, or low renin levels in hypertensive patients. For one, considering the reactive nature of renin production, it was reasonable to question the meaning of a "normal" renin level in a hypertensive patient. In such a patient, a level like that in a normotensive subject, which suggests business as usual, is not normal at all but may represent the operation of a badly informed renin system. This is because numerous studies show that elevating either pressure or sodium-volume status in normal animals or people routinely suppresses renin values. Accordingly, only a renin level much lower than that of a normal subject at the same state of salt balance can truly be said to represent a normal or appropriate reactive response of the renin system to hypertension.

With this tool the role of the renin system in the various hypertensive disorders could now be reexamined.

THE RENIN SYSTEM IN MALIGNANT HYPERTENSION

The process of malignant hypertension is triggered by the development of a critical degree of renal damage due to causes not always clear, but usually associated with antecedent chronic hypertension. The deficit in renal perfusion downstream from an obliterative arteriolar lesion produces an artifactual local hypotension in the kidneys, which triggers a massive release of renin (11). By its joint vasoconstrictive and sodium-retentive effects this increased activity of the renin system produces a massive increase in blood pressure. Normally this would shut off the renin production, but the compromised damaged kidney cannot perceive the systemic hypertension; it continues to pour out more renin in the blind impression that the local hypotension is systemic.

The huge excesses of circulating renin induce large excesses of aldosterone secretion (13), which would normally work to cause sodium retention, thereby tending to restore renal perfusion and reduce renin secretion. However, the marked angiotensin-induced vasoconstriction and systemic hypertension induce pressure natriuresis and hemoconcentration. The pressure natriuresis and diuresis of malignant hypertension (20) and also of severe two-kidney Goldblatt disease (21) are likely mediated via pressure transmission to those nephrons whose blood supply is still intact or unobstructed, by a direct tubular action of angiotensin (22) and perhaps also by induction of the very recently recognized atrial hormone secretion (23).

Accordingly, malignant hypertension (like severe Goldblatt hypertension) typically presents as a "dry" hypertension. Natriuretic mechanisms responding properly when they can, in the surviving intact nephrons, work to eliminate sodium and fluid and produce hemoconcentration. This becomes a "dry" underperfusion hypertension.

Thus, the sum effects of the volume depletion and renin-mediated vasoconstriction are hemoconcentration, with azotemia, increased blood viscosity, poor flow to the microcirculation, acrocyanosis, and deepened tissue ischemia. The local renal defects underlying the condition are thereby extended and compounded. The misinformed renin system boosts its production of renin. The vicious downward spiral accelerates, culminating in fibrinoid, necrotizing arteriolitis and an early demise from irreversible vascular damage in the heart, brain, and kidneys (11).

The above description of the process of malignant hypertension is supported by several observations. Diffuse vasculitis and death will result in a day or two in rats overloaded by simultaneous injections of renin and aldosterone (15). Also, the experience from dialysis wards shows that the blood pressure of malignant hypertensive patients can be lowered virtually to normal and their arteriolar necrosis reversed by a bilateral nephrectomy (23).

An equally convincing demonstration of the causal role of the renin system can be made by pharmacologic blockade. Renin system blockers, such as propranolol and captopril, can alone normalize and maintain the blood pressure of an impressive proportion of malignant hypertensive patients, some in encephalopathic crisis (24). In others, the addition of diuretics may be required for normalization, illustrating the joint participation of renin and sodium retention.

THE RENIN SYSTEM IN RENOVASCULAR HYPERTENSION

There are two general types of renovascular hypertension, a category perhaps accounting for up to 15% of all clinical hypertension. The first type is unilateral renal disease, which, if the contralateral kidney can be demonstrated to be unaffected, is curable by surgery (i.e., nephrectomy or vascular repair) or by balloon angioplasty. The second type, bilateral renal arterial disease, is often approachable nowadays by balloon angioplasty. Both types may have equal levels of hypertension, but final diagnosis and differentiation between the two is greatly aided by study of the renin system.

Unilateral Renovascular Disease

A pure experimental analog of human unilateral renovascular disease can be found in the two-kidney Goldblatt model, in which one renal artery of the animal is clipped and the other kidney left intact (25). Assays of plasma renin activity will generally be excessively high. The affected kidney, suffering a perfusion deficit due to a stenotic renal artery, interprets the situation as systemic hypotension and responds by releasing renin. The generation of angiotensin results in vasoconstriction, which raises blood pressure. The raised blood pressure shuts off renin release in the unaffected contralateral kidney but not in the affected kidney, because beyond the clip, the perfusion deficit and reduced filtration, albeit improved, still continue. High renin secretion from the affected kidney and low to absent renin in the contralateral kidney, a highly specific diagnostic duet, can be verified by measurements of renal vein blood samples.

Although the affected kidney cannot respond with appropriate natriuresis, the contralateral kidney, exposed to systemic hypertension, is in pressure-induced natriuresis, thereby more than canceling aldosterone's sodium-retaining effect and tending to maintain blood volume at low normal levels, although without successfully reducing blood pressure. Thus, pressure natriuresis plus an appropriate suppression of renin in the contralateral kidney cannot counterbalance the uncontrolled release of renin from the affected kidney.

The renin dependency of this unilateral hypertension of a renovascular lesion can be demonstrated in animals (26) or in patients by the prompt corrective response of the blood pressure to renin system blockade. Such a hypotensive response in a patient with high peripheral renin, particularly to a test dose of the specific angiotensin-converting enzyme inhibitor, captopril (27), is highly suggestive and provides sound reason for pursuing the possibility of curable renovascular hypertension. The 60-min response of the plasma renin to captopril is an even more sensitive and specific indicator (27). Patients with renovascular disease exhibit a sharp rise in plasma renin not seen in essential hypertension, and this can occur even when the acute blood pressure response is not apparent. Finally, a renal vein study before and following the acute administration of captopril (27,28) provides the definitive evidence for lateralization of the hypersecretion, as confirmed with more precision after converting enzyme inhibition, which produces a pronounced increase in renin release from the ischemic kidney.

Thus, the renin system is so clearly involved in unilateral renovascular hypertension that it provides the basis for definitive diagnosis and making management decisions. Normally, each renal vein renin level is approximately 25% higher than the renal arterial level (29), and this increment determines the peripheral level. Accordingly, with renin secretion totally suppressed in the contralateral kidney of unilateral renal disease, the one affected kidney must now produce a 50% increment in renin secretion in order to sustain the peripheral renin level. Thus, if the culpable kidney exhibits a 50% or greater increment from its renal vein, it can be concluded that the contralateral kidney is totally suppressed in its production of renin, and is thus behaving normally and is most probably capable of good function in the event of nephrectomy. The degree of elevation in renin concentrations above the 50% support value then becomes a fairly reliable indicator of the extent of renal ischemia in the suspect kidney (29).

The ability to use such relatively innocuous measurements to define curable renovascular hypertension, together with the development of balloon angioplasty as an alternative to surgery (30,31), appears to be identifying a far greater frequency of curable renovascular disease than was ever supposed. Many such patients, now cured by a nonsurgical angioplastic procedure, would in earlier days have been deemed to have essential hypertension and might have been kept on antihypertensive drugs for the rest of their lives.

Bilateral Renal Arterial Disease

In the patient with bilateral renal arterial disease, peripheral renin levels are most often either normal or low (31). This also prevails in the experimental one-kidney Goldblatt model, in which one kidney is clipped and the other removed (25). In the model or in the human with two compromised kidneys, the perfusion defect likely initially stimulates renin production because of a reduced total glomerular filtration capacity, but at the same time, it also results in an inability to excrete sodium and water freely or to react properly with natriuresis to the increased pressure. There is no functioning contralateral kidney, as in unilateral renal disease, to provide an adequate sodium and water runoff.

The result is a buildup of body sodium and volume to the point where pressure is nearly restored in the compromised kidneys. As a result, renin production is depressed to normal or even subnormal levels. This restoration of equilibrium in the kidney is accomplished at the cost of systemic volume expansion and systemic hypertension. Here, the hypertension is sustained by the influence of sodium (32) rather than renin-angiotensin, even though sodium was not involved in its primary etiology.

The sodium dependency of this hypertension in the presence of a masked renin factor can be demonstrated in experimental animals. Infusion of an angiotensin blocker or antibody produces no fall in blood pressure (26,33). Neither does sodium depletion produce a fall in blood pressure, but it does raise the renin level sharply, converting the sodium-dependent hypertension to a renin-dependent one (33). After such sodium depletion the blood pressure now can be promptly normalized by giving an angiotensin-blocking drug. Thus, in this model, reciprocation of two pressor mechanisms can be demonstrated; one is sodium dependent and the other one is renin mediated. The system appears to be trying to maintain pressure equilibrium in the compromised organ by whatever means are available, either renin- or sodium-dependent hypertension. The behavior of the renin system, participating in and reacting to this process, provides the clue.

THE RENIN SYSTEM IN PRIMARY AND PSEUDOPRIMARY ALDOSTERONISM

Primary aldosteronism, or Conn's syndrome, is due to an autonomous oversecreting solitary adrenal tumor (34). Pseudoprimary aldosteronism describes a subgroup characterized instead by diffuse bilateral adrenocortical hyperplasia (35,36). Together, these conditions probably account for less than 1% to 2% of hypertensive patients. In both disorders there is sustained oversecretion of aldosterone, producing a clinical syndrome in which there is evidence of maintained sodium and volume retention above the normal range with "escape" from further sodium-retaining action of the hormone. The "escape" is evidenced by an unusual capacity to excrete additional sodium chloride (37) and by a state of chronic potassium deficiency. As one might expect, considering the reactive nature of the renin system described above, plasma renin activity is maximally suppressed.

The diagnostic triad for both rare forms of mineralocorticoid hypertension is (a) high aldosterone levels with (b) resultant sodium-volume expansion and resultant *low renin levels* and (c) resultant hypokalemia. The abnormalities tend to be more marked in the primary or adenomatous form. Primary aldosteronism can be cured by removing the offending tumor, but there is no known cure as yet for the pseudoprimary form, since even total adrenalectomy may not be corrective. Discriminating between the two disorders involves specialized radiographic techniques sometimes requiring demonstration of unilateral as opposed to bilateral hypersecretion of aldosterone. Clues can be derived from studies exploiting the fact that such bilateral hyperplasia cases respond to stimuli, such as posture (i.e., renin release), so that in the upright plasma aldosterone increases whereas in patients with adenoma it is unaffected (38). A more recent variation of this strategy shows that patients with hyperplasia respond to captopril with a fall in aldosterone where patients with tumor do not (27).

There are some rare interesting variations on this pathophysiologic theme. Excessive ingestion of licorice, which contains a steroid-like substance that mimics aldosterone action, can produce a syndrome mimicking primary aldosteronism (39). Aldosteronism-like syndromes can also be produced by other mineralocorticoids, notably desoxycorticosterone (40), and possibly by certain adrenal androgens, excesses of which might occur in adrenal enzyme deficiencies (41,42). In all of these, however, aldosterone will be suppressed by the induced renal sodium retention and resultant suppression of renin secretion.

On the other hand, the hypertensions of glucocorticoid excess, such as occur in Cushing's syndrome or prolonged ingestion of synthetic glucocorticoids including the oral contraceptives, may be accompanied by *elevated* production or activity of angiotensin. This can be attributed partly to elevated plasma renin substrate levels (43), possibly induced by glucocorticoid, and to a direct augmentation of vascular responsiveness to angiotensin. This participation of the renin system in these states can usually be verified by a depressor response to specific angiotensin blockade (44).

This brief discussion of the role of the adrenal cortex in clinical and experimental hypertension is intended solely for the purpose of reviewing the unique pathophysiological features of mineralocorticoid hypertensions that lead to the production of a state of long-term vasoconstriction, apparently requiring antecedent sodium retention, and so regularly accompanied by marked suppression of plasma renin activity. Indeed, experimental mineralocorticoid hypertension does not occur if salt is withheld from the diet, nor does the suppression of plasma renin activity (45). More recent experimental evidence indicates too that this form of arteriolar vasoconstriction is exquisitely sensitive to calcium channel or α-adrenergic blockade. These drugs produce dramatic correction of mineralocorticoid hypertension, whereas the antirenin system agents, converting enzyme inhibitors, and β-blockers are totally ineffective.

As discussed below, all of these characteristics also appear to obtain in the vasoconstriction occurring in low-renin forms of essential hypertension.

WET AND DRY: TWO FORMS OF VASOCONSTRICTION

The mechanisms of the more extreme form of hypertension described so far suggest a spectrum of etiology with definable degrees of renin system involvement. At one pole of the spectrum hypertension is sustained (and possibly caused) by the vasoconstrictor forces of the renin system's active agent, angiotensin II. At the other pole the hypertension is sustained by a nonrenin vasoconstrictive force acting on arterioles, which instead appears almost surely to involve the pressor influence of dietary sodium and the possible joint participation of norepinephrine. The predominance of activity of one element at either pole maximally depresses activity of the other; and in the middle regions of the spectrum both of these two vasoconstrictive forces may well assert their influence.

Either polar force by itself is capable of producing the exalted peripheral resistance that is the common characteristic of all hypertension. But the similarity ends there, for the conditions imposed by these two mechanisms are radically different in their implications for risk, survival, and treatment.

The vasoconstriction ordered by angiotensin II, the active component evoked from renin secretion, results in a "dry" hypertension (46,47). It is characterized by a peripheral resistance higher than that imposed by the other form. Since angiotensin stimulates aldosterone production even while it directly constricts arterioles, aldosterone secretion is correspondingly high. Nevertheless, plasma volume is relatively low (given a reasonable renal capacity for "pressure" diuresis), as is cardiac output. A by-product of this reactive diuresis is comparatively elevated blood viscosity, with other evidences of hemoconcentration—higher blood urea, hematocrit, hemoglobin, and total protein values. Understandably, tissue perfusion is lower and the patient is susceptible to postural hypotension.

In the hypertension imposed by the nonrenin vasoconstrictor mechanism, antecedent sodium-volume excess appears to be a key prerequisite, and α-adrenergic influences also may be circumstantially implicated. In this form of vasoconstriction, peripheral resistance is generally less dramatically elevated. Plasma renin activity is low to absent, whereas aldosterone production is variable from low to high (a finding of considerable research interest). This type of hypertension can be called a "wet" hypertension, because it is associated with a higher plasma volume and cardiac output and with lower hematocrit, blood urea, and viscosity values. Postural hypotension is absent, and all of these parameters allow the eponym of "wet" hypertension to be applied. The implication here is that, because of better rheology, tissue perfusion and nutrition are better maintained and ischemic injury tends to be avoided.

Accordingly, the renin-mediated dry forms of hypertension have been shown to have a far higher incidence of vascular sequelae: stroke, heart attack, renal damage, retinopathy, and en-

High Renin (vasoconstricted)		Low Renin (less vasoconstricted)
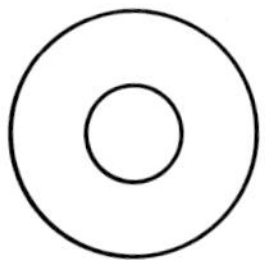	Arterioles	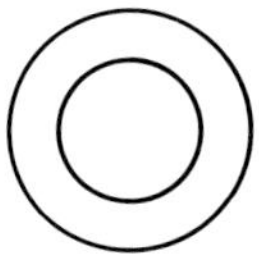
Higher	Peripheral resistance	High
High	Aldosterone	Low to high
Low	Plasma volume	High
Low	Cardiac output	High
High	Hematocrit	Low
High	Blood urea	Low
High	Blood viscosity	Low
Low	Tissue perfusion	High
Yes	Postural hypotension	No
	Clinical Examples	
High renin essential Renovascular and malignant		Low renin essential Primary aldosteronism
	Vascular Sequelae	
(+)	Stroke	(−)
(+)	Heart attack	(−)
(+)	Renal damage	(−)
(+)	Retinopathy-encephalopathy	(−)
	Treatments	
No	Diuretics	Yes
Yes	Antirenin drugs	No
Yes	Direct vasodilators	±
Yes	Adrenergic blockers	±

FIG. 4. Relatively predominant features of high blood pressure mechanisms. (Redrawn from ref. 47.)

cephalopathy (16,19). The reasons for this may probably be laid to the poor perfusion and tissue nourishment associated with the turgid blood supply, resulting in fragile vessels. Rheological study suggests that the friction generated by the viscous blood may share responsibility for the greater blood pressures associated with this type of hypertension. Conversely, the relative cardiac protection afforded by low-renin wet hypertension, with its comparatively luxurious blood volume and cardiac output, may stem from a more congenial rheology and better flow and tissue nourishment.

The differences between these two major mechanisms of hypertension and the culpability of renin in one and not the other are demonstrated dramatically by the more extreme pathologies. Soaring plasma renin values with reduced blood flow and cardiac output can readily be shown in such "dry" hypertensions as malignant hypertension or malignant scleroderma; indeed, in the latter the extremities are black for want of perfusion (48). That renin-induced vasoconstriction is the source of the trouble is shown by the ability to promptly reverse these effects by renin system blockade. A number of other clinical and experimental paradigms support the concept of the characteristics of this renin-mediated form of hypertension. Thus, patients with renin-secreting tumors or acute renal artery occlusion also exhibit severe hypertension with vascular damage (2,16). The animal model of acute renal artery clipping produced by Byron and Wilson (16) is another case in point, in which renal artery clipping illustrates the companion acute development of renin-mediated cerebral vasospasm and encephalopathy.

In primary aldosteronism, on the other hand, "wet" hypertension finds its paradigm; runaway sodium retention builds up massive fluid accumulations, with high blood volumes (37) and abundant flow and cardiac output, and it causes a reactive shutdown of the renin system. Total correction of the situation can be achieved in both experimental and clinical forms by rigid dietary sodium deprivation or by diuretics, and permanent cure by surgically removing the offending adrenocortical tumor. Plasma renin values are very low, and so renin-system-blocking drugs, such as β-blockers and converting enzyme inhibitors, are conspicuously ineffective. Accordingly, the source of this vasoconstriction must be sought in other mechanisms.

As discussed above, the existence of at least two vasoconstrictor mechanisms, one mediated by renin and the other by nonrenin forces, also is interestingly demonstrated by Goldblatt's experimental models. In the animal, when renin secretion is stimulated by clipping a single kidney while leaving the other intact, a "dry" hypertension results because the properly functioning unclipped kidney is unable to fully compensate for the renin-induced runaway vasoconstriction and hypertension by jettisoning sodium and water (26). If the unclipped kidney is removed (or both kidneys are clipped), the resultant reduced filtration rate causes an inability to excrete sodium and water, leading to accumulation of fluid (32) and a reactive shutdown of renin secretion; this is a sodium volume-induced or "wet" hypertension. However, if the latter animal is deprived of salt (33) and thus the ability to retain fluid, renin secretion increases reciprocally; in short, the animal converts itself from a sodium-dependent to a renin-dependent hypertensive, thereby moving from one pole of the hypertensive (i.e., vasoconstriction) spectrum to the other.

In these Goldblatt models it is as if the damaged kidney *requires* hypertension and will maintain it by one of two means available to it. Considered in the light of the knowledge that vasoconstriction is the common characteristic of all hypertension, expressed universally by an increased peripheral resistance, one can conclude that two vasoconstrictive mechanisms are available for the long-term maintenance of hypertension. One is related to excess renin secretion, and the other is a nonrenin pressor mechanism in some way related to sodium retention and, as is discussed below, perhaps involving α-adrenergic activity.

These animal models find their human counterpart in unilateral and bilateral renovascular disease. Here, too, the level of renin activity in the periphery and renal veins help makes the diagnosis (31). As in the animal, the human patient with low-renin bilateral disease is salt retentive but may be converted by salt deprivation to renin-mediated hypertension.

Still another demonstration of this kind of reciprocation of two pressor mechanisms can be revealed in patients with congestive heart failure (49). Just as in hypertensive disorders, here, too, there is a broad splay of renin values, from very low to very high. Diuretics were stopped in a group of such patients to try to learn more about the basis for their wide splay in renin system activity. Surprisingly, we found that a modest high-salt diet converted the high-renin patients to a low-renin state, and a low-salt diet was able to reverse the condition. In fact, modest salt feeding to these patients at times suppressed previously high renin values to levels as low as those seen in full-blown low-renin essential hypertension or primary aldosteronism. In some cases the change in renin values approached 20-fold.

The fascinating finding is that, once again, whatever the renin status, their blood pressure remained the same. Indeed, peripheral resistance, measured with cardiac catheterization before and after salt feeding, remained virtually unchanged. It was only the mechanism of its mediation that changed. Moreover, as one might expect, the patients with high renin heart failure are uniquely sensitive to unloading (i.e., reduced peripheral resistance) with a specific antirenin system agent such as enalaprilat given intravenously. Conversely, too, enalapril may be ineffective in low-renin congestive heart failure, where a calcium-channel-blocking drug will produce prompt reduction in peripheral resistance with improvement in cardiac performance (50). Thus, once again, it is possible to demonstrate and characterize the two different mechanisms of vasoconstriction.

RENIN SYSTEM PATTERNS IN ESSENTIAL HYPERTENSION

It is reasonable to speculate that the two vasoconstrictor mechanisms demonstrated by renin profiling in the more specific forms of hypertension and in their experimental counterparts, and in congestive heart failure too, might also be operative within essential hypertension, an umbrella category covering some 85% of patients with hypertension.

When renin profiling is correctly performed and indexed in patients with essential hypertension, it is found that approximately 20% have high renin and approximately 30% low renin values, with the remaining half distributed in between (19). Does this indicate that renin has nothing to do with essential hypertension, or does it instead suggest a vasoconstrictive spectrum like the one identified in the more defined hypertensive forms described above?

The question has aroused some considerable controversy in the past, perhaps due to an earlier abundance of faulty renin assays, and to lack of agreement on a proven renin blockade. Thus, even though data using propranolol and saralasin to block renin secretion or activity were mutually reinforcing (1,2), many scientists preferred to suspect nonspecificity rather than to implicate renin in pathogenesis. These conflicts have settled, however, with the advent of converting enzyme inhibitors, which demonstrably interfere with the conversion of the angiotensin I to its active vasoconstrictive form. This interference explains the hypotensive action, or lack of it, of these agents, and it has verified earlier findings with the less powerful renin-system-blocking drugs, propranolol (24) and saralasin (51). It turns out that converting enzyme inhibitors are impressively depressor in high-renin patients with essential hypertension and that they also identify a renin factor in the majority of patients with medium renin levels (52–55). Accordingly, in such patients, the renin profile becomes diagnostic with regard to the mechanisms of the hypertension and quickly leads to specific therapy.

In fact, converting enzyme inhibitors are so effective in blocking the renin system that they are even effective in lowering the blood pressure to some degree in some low-renin patients (55). However, this should not be the basis for suspecting nonspecificity of drug action, because the lesser amounts of renin circulating in such patients still can contribute to the blood pressure level. This is especially true because low-renin patients by definition comprise a range of renin values. What is especially relevant is the fact that captopril, like its forerunner converting enzyme inhibitor, teprotide, is totally ineffective in lowering pressure when renin levels are very low or absent, such as in primary aldosteronism and in experimental and DOC-salt hypertension, or in anephric humans or animals. Furthermore, many claims for effectiveness in low-renin states (56) are based on the administration of drugs to low-renin patients already treated with diuretics, which raise renin levels to enable a "false positive" response.

Altogether the experience (57) indicates a remarkably good correlation between the height of pretreatment plasma renin levels and the blood pressure response, or lack of it, to converting enzyme inhibitors, especially when one considers the inherent noise or error in casual blood pressure measurements. Thus, a plasma renin value is a reliable guide for both diagnosis and therapy of increasing value as the measurements deviate more from the normal range. Claims to the contrary based on the recent findings of the possible existence of renin in certain extravascular sites should not yet be used as a basis for doubting the meaning of plasma measurements. This is because active renin and aldosterone are both virtually absent in anephric people, thereby demonstrating the purely renal origin of circulating renin pressor systems (58).

Accordingly, a renin profile that documents a low to absent renin value is equally diagnostic and just as important. It points to nonrenin pressor mechanisms. Confirming the concept, renin system blockade by converting enzyme inhibitors or β-blockers is of little therapeutic value. Nonetheless, the renin profile is of no less importance in guiding specific therapy. In this area some interesting new agents are available and challenging new concepts are being developed.

That sodium retention plays a dominant role in low-renin essential hypertension scarcely needs proof in view of the impressive performance of diuretics in this category compared with their spotty results in high-renin patients (56). The diuretic correction of this hypertension is associated with a rise of renin levels to normal. Moreover, whenever it has been studied, hypertensive patients with low renin values have been found to exhibit larger blood and extracellular fluid volumes than do the normal or high-renin patients (2). However, the mechanisms through which sodium retention exerts its pressor effects are devious and not completely understood (59). Indeed, in just the last few years it has become apparent that there may be more than one pathway to the source of low-renin hypertension. The first of these indications has come from the worldwide experience (60,61) showing that calcium influx-blocking agents can be depressor and are most predictably so in low-renin patients with essential hypertension. In this regard, Dr. Lawrence Resnick has made some exciting findings in his work tracking the relationship of calcium and magnesium metabolism in untreated essential hypertension. He has shown (62) that serum ionized calcium is directly related to plasma renin whereas serum magnesium is inversely related. He has also demonstrated (63) that in hypertensive subjects, a high salt diet reduces plasma ionized calcium (most probably because of influx to the cell) to levels similar to those seen in low-renin essential hypertension, whereas salt restriction does the reverse. We can begin to suggest the possibility that the influence of dietary sodium on blood pressure (i.e., on vasoconstriction) may be mediated by companion or induced changes in these divalent cations.

The sodium-calcium relationship takes on additional dimensions with the realization that cytosolic calcium is a critical actor in the neural theater (64) and that neural blockade is yet another avenue through which vasopressor phenomena may be influenced. What makes this avenue especially attractive now is the availability of the newer α_1-adrenergic blockers like prazosin and indoramin, going directly for the α-receptors with a specificity unconnected with the widespread side effects associated with the earlier ganglionic blockers. Indoramin, the newest of this class, is particularly interesting because of an antihistamine-like sedative effect and an antiarrhythmic action that appears to limit the reflex tachycardia that sometimes appears with prazosin.

It is highly significant that the depressor effects of these agents, too, are particularly selective among the low-renin patients, those also preferred by calcium channel blockers and diuretics. Our group, led by Dr. John P. Nicholson, demonstrated marked orthostatic decreases in blood pressure as a first-dose response to prazosin, the degree of which was inversely correlated with the baseline plasma renin activity (65). Furthermore, the α-antagonism stimulated renin secretion, again demonstrating the reciprocation between renin and nonrenin pressor phenomena.

Exploiting these relationships, Nicholson and colleagues (66) have recently shown that the antihypertensive effectiveness of a calcium-channel-blocking drug is not helped by sodium depletion and may actually be enhanced by concurrent liberalization of salt intake. This approach could lead to new, more palatable modes of therapy.

A PHARMACOLOGIC ROADMAP FOR PHYSIOLOGICALLY BASED THERAPY OF HUMAN HYPERTENSION

Since renin profiling can be used to sort out different pathophysiologic mechanisms in different patients, one can further exploit this information not only to diagnose curable renal or cerebral forms but also to design simpler and more specific therapies using a minimum number of drugs. Although it is beyond the scope of this chapter to discuss drug therapy in detail, the basis for the application of this new knowl-

Table 1. *Relationship of baseline renin profile to effectiveness of antihypertensive drugs*

The baseline renin profile predicts the effectiveness or lack of it of the five major types of antihypertensive agents:	
1. β-receptor blockers	Increasingly effective in medium- and high renin but ineffective in low-renin states
2. Converting enzyme inhibitors	
3. Diuretics	Effective in low-renin and ineffective in high-renin states
4. α-receptor blockers	
5. Calcium channel blockers	
This research defines *two* fundamentally different mechanisms of long-term vasoconstriction revealed by renin profiling. One is renin dependent, the other sodium and volume mediated. Each is accompanied by characteristic changes in calcium and magnesium metabolism.	
During therapy, reactive changes in the renin profile explain the development of resistance to antihypertensive drugs.	

edge in long-term therapy is summarized in Table 1.

CONCLUSION

Despite isolated pockets of skepticism, it is fairly well established by now that a relative or an absolute overactivity of the renin system can indeed cause or sustain diastolic hypertension. Surely it is the culprit in the virulent hypertension associated with the autonomous production of renin in renal and extrarenal neoplasms. Equally compelling is the evidence of its culpability in malignant hypertension and renovascular disease, where uncontrolled excesses of renin production result from compromised renal perfusion. Although its primary culpability in other forms of hypertension may be moot, its active participation or lack of it, as evidenced by heterogeneity in renin profiles, is not. The modern understanding of hypertension is, at long last, characterized by the selective and specific attention to possible etiologies and by less abrasive and more effective treatments. It is thus no longer appropriate to endorse a single recipe for all hypertension.

The awareness of the central role of the renin system in hypertensive phenomena has allowed application of this knowledge for construction of an analytical model for biochemical definition of the heterogeneity common in pathophysiology for all human hypertension, including essential hypertension. This analytical approach is now rationalizing the management of hypertension. The ability to reverse high- and medium-renin forms with antirenin system therapy alone is a case in point. And a low renin profile is no less informative, for it identifies those patients whose vasoconstriction will respond instead to a diuretic alone or to a monotherapy with a calcium-channel- or α-adrenergic blocking agent.

Moreover, because it identifies and quantifies which, and to what extent, one of two mechanisms for long-term vasoconstriction is at work, renin-sodium profiling of untreated new patients permits, at the outset, the diagnosis or exclusion of curable renovascular disease among patients presenting with medium or high values. A follow-up captopril test and then a renal vein study with angiography can lead to cure of many patients who might otherwise be treated blindly with drugs for a lifetime.

At the same time, this new level of understanding and therapy becomes a first approximation, allowing us to frame new questions that will surely take us closer to full understanding of causation. Thus, we need to learn why the renin system becomes overactive in high- and medium-renin states and why with systemic hypertension it fails to turn itself off. And in low-renin states we need to learn why sodium retention occurs and why another form of vasoconstriction related to sodium and calcium transport takes over. The answers to these questions may involve the revelation of still other endocrine and neural pathways.

REFERENCES

1. Laragh, J. H. (1981): The renin-angiotensin-aldosterone system for blood pressure regulation and for subdividing patients to reveal and analyze different forms of hypertension. In: *Frontiers in Hypertension Research,* edited by J. H. Laragh, F. R. Bühler, and D. W. Seldin, pp. 183–194. Springer-Verlag, New York.
2. Laragh, J. H., Letcher, R. L., and Pickering, T. G. (1979): Renin profiling for modern diagnosis and treatment of hypertension. *JAMA,* 241:151–156.
3. Tigerstedt, R., and Bergman, P. G. (1898): Niere and Kreislafu. *Scand. Arch. Physiol.,* 8:223–271.
4. Goldblatt, H. J., Lynch, R. F., Hanzal, R. F., et al. (1934): Studies on experimental hypertension. Production of persistent elevation of systolic blood pressure by means of renal ischemia. *J. Exp. Med.,* 49:347–379.
5. Page, I. H. (1939): On the nature of the pressor action of renin. *J. Exp. Med.,* 70:521–542.
6. Braun-Menendez, E., Fasciolol, J. C., Leloir, L. F., et al. (1969): La substancia hipertensora de la sangre del rinon isquemiado. *Rev. Soc. Argent. Biol.,* 15:420–430.
7. Skeggs, L. T., Jr., March, W. H., Kahn, H. R., et al. (1954): The existence of two forms of hypertension. *J. Exp. Med.,* 99:275–282.
8. Skeggs, L. T., Jr., Dorer, E. R., Kahn, J. R., et al. (1976): The biochemistry of the renin-angiotensin system and its role in hypertension. *Am. J. Med.,* 60:737–748.
9. Ng, K. K. F., and Vane, J. R. (1968): Fate of angiotensin I in the circulation. *Nature,* 218:144–140.
10. Laragh, J. H., Angers, M., Kelly, W. G., and Lieberman, S. (1960): Hypotensive agents and pressor substances. The effect of epinephrine, norepinephrine, angiotensin II and others on the secretory rate of aldosterone in man. *JAMA,* 174:234–240.
11. Laragh, J. H. (1960): The role of aldosterone in man: Evidence for regulation of electrolyte balance and arterial pressure by renal-adrenal system which may be involved in malignant hypertension. *JAMA,* 174:293–295.
12. Biron, P., Koiw, E., Nowaczynski, W., et al. (1961): The effects of intravenous infusions of valine-5-angiotensin II and other pressor agents on urinary electrolyte and corticosteroids, including aldosterone. *J. Clin. Invest.,* 40:338–347.
13. Laragh, J. H., Ulick, S., Januszewicz, V., Kelly, W. G., and Lieberman, S. (1960): Electrolyte metabolism and aldosterone secretion in benign and malignant hypertension. *Ann. Intern. Med.,* 53:259–272.
14. Laragh, J. H., Cannon, P. J., and Ames, R. P. (1963): Aldosterone secretion and various forms of hypertensive vascular disease. *Ann. Intern. Med.,* 59:117–120.
15. Conn, J. W. (1955): Primary aldosteronism. *J. Lab. Clin. Med.,* 45:661–667.
16. Laragh, J. H. (1981): Hypertension, vasoconstriction, and the causation of cardiovascular injury: The renin-sodium profile as an indicator of risk. In: *Frontiers in Hypertension Research,* edited by J. H. Laragh, F. R. Bühler, and D. W. Seldin, pp. 383–385. Springer-Verlag, New York.

16a. Laragh, J. H. (1985): Atrial natriuretic hormone the renin-aldosterone axis, and blood pressure-electrolyte homeostasis. *N. Engl. J. Med.,* 313: 1330–1340.

17. Ames, R. P., Borkowski, A. J., Sicinski, A. M., and Laragh, J. H., (1965): Prolonged infusions of angiotensin II and norepinephrine and blood pressure, electrolyte balance, aldosterone and cortisol secretion in normal man and in cirrhosis with ascites. *J. Clin. Invest.,* 44:1171–1186.
18. Laragh, J. H., Sealey, J. E., and Sommers, S. C. (1966): Patterns of adrenal secretion and urinary excretion of aldosterone and plasma renin activity in normal and hypertensive subjects. *Circ. Res.,* 18,19(*Suppl.* I):I158–I174.
19. Brunner, H. R., Laragh, J. H., Baer, L., Newton, M. A., Goodwin, F. T., Krakoff, L. R., Bard, R. H., and Bühler, F. R. (1972): Essential hypertensions: Renin and aldosterone, heart attack and stroke. *N. Engl. J. Med.,* 286:441–449.
20. Berlyne, G. M., Nilwarangkur, S., Janabi, K., and Cooper, H. (1965):Nocturnal nephrogenic diabetes insipidus. *Q. J. Med.,* 34:463–479.
21. Möhring, J., Petri, M., Szokol, M., Haack, D., and Möhring, B. (1976): Effects of saline drinking on malignant course of renal hypertension in rats. *Am. J. Physiol.,* 230:849–857.
22. Laragh, J. H., Cannon, P. J., Bentzel, C. J., Sicinski, A. M., and Meltzer, J. I. (1963): Angiotensin II, norepinephrine and the renal transport of electrolytes and water in normal man and in cirrhosis with ascites. *J. Clin. Invest.,* 42:1179–1192.
23. Laragh, J. H., Baer, L., Brunner, H. R., Bühler, F. R., Sealey, J. E. and Vaughan, E. D., Jr. (1972): Renin, angiotensin and aldosterone system in pathogenesis and management of hypertensive vascular disease. *Am. J. Med.,* 52:633–652.
24. Bühler, F. R., Laragh, J. H., Baer, L., Vaughan, E. D., Jr., and Brunner, H. R. (1972): Propranolol inhibition of renin secretion. A specific approach to diagnosis and treatment of renin-dependent hypertensive diseases. *N. Engl. J. Med.,* 287:1209–1214.
25. Laragh, J. H., Sealey, J. E., Bühler, F. R., Vaughan, E. D., Jr., Brunner, H. R., Gavras, H., and Baer, L. (1975): The renin axis and vasoconstriction volume analysis for understanding and treating renovascular and renal hypertension. *Am. J. Med.,* 58:4–13.
26. Brunner, H. R., Kirshman, H. D., Sealey, J. E., and Laragh, J. H. (1971): Hypertension of renal origin: Evidence for two different mechanisms. *Science,* 174:1344–1346.
27. Müller, F. B., Sealey, J. E., Case, D. B., Atlas, S. A., Pickering, T. G., Pecker, M. S., Preibisz, J. J., and Laragh, J. H. (1986): The captopril test for identifying renovascular disease in hypertensive patients. *Am. J. Med.,* 80:633–644.
28. Vaughan, E. D., Jr., Bühler, F. R., Laragh, J. H., Sealey, J. E., Baer, L., and Bard, R. H. (1973): Renovascular hypertension: Renin measurements to indicate hypersecretion and contralateral suppression, estimate renal plasma flow and score for surgical curability. *Am. J. Med.,* 55:402–414.
29. Sealey, J. E., Bühler, F. R., Laragh, J. H., and Vaughan, E. D., Jr. (1973): The physiology of renin secretion in essential hypertension: Estimation

of renin secretion rate and renal plasma flow from peripheral and renal vein renin levels. *Am. J. Med.*, 55:391–401.
30. Sos, T. A., Pickering, T. G., Sniderman, K., Saddenki, S., Case, D. B., Silane, M. F., Vaughan, E. D., Jr., and Laragh, J. H. (1983): Percutaneous transluminal renal angioplasty in renovascular hypertension due to atheroma or fibromuscular dysplasia. *N. Engl. J. Med.*, 309:274–279.
31. Pickering, T. G., Sos, T. A., Vaughan, E. D., Jr., Case, D. B., Sealey, J. E., Harshfield, G. A., and Laragh, J. H. (1984): Predictive value and changes of renin secretion in hypertensive patients with unilateral renovascular disease undergoing successful renal angioplasty. *Am. J. Med.*, 76:398–404.
32. Tobian, L., Coffee, K., and McCrea, P. (1969): Contrasting exchangeable sodium in rats with different types of Goldblatt hypertension. *Am. J. Physiol.*, 217:458–460.
33. Gavras, H., Brunner, H. R., Vaughan, E. D., Jr., and Laragh, J. H. (1973): Angiotensin-sodium interaction in blood pressure maintenance of renal hypertensive and normotensive rats. *Science*, 180:1369–1371.
34. Conn, J. W. (1964): Plasma renin activity in primary aldosteronism. Importance in differential diagnosis and in research of essential hypertension. *JAMA*, 190:222–225.
35. Laragh, J. H., Ledingham, H. G. G., and Sommers, S. C. (1967): Secondary aldosteronism and reduced plasma renin in hypertensive disease. *Trans. Assoc. Am. Physicians*, 80:168–182.
36. Baer, L., Sommers, S. C., Krakoff, L. R., Newton, M. A., and Laragh, J. H. (1970): Pseudo-primary aldosteronism: An entity distinct from true primary aldosteronism. *Circ. Res.*, 26,27(*Suppl.* I):203–220.
37. Biglieri, E. G., and Forsham, P. H. (1961): Studies on the expanded extracellular fluid and the responses to various stimuli in primary aldosteronism. *Am. J. Med.*, 34:564–576.
38. Biglieri, E. G., and Lopez, J. M. (1976): Clinical and laboratory diagnosis of adrenocortical hypertension. *Cardiovasc. Med.*, 1:335–341.
39. Conn, J. W., Rovner, D. R., and Cohen, E. L. (1968): Licorice-induced pseudo-aldosteronism. *JAMA*, 205:492–496.
40. Biglieri, E. G., Stockigt, J. R., and Schambelan, M. (1972): Adrenal mineralocorticoids causing hypertension. *Am. J. Med.*, 52:523–532.
41. Liddle, G. W., and Sennett, J. A. (1974): New mineralocorticoids in the syndrome of low-renin essential hypertension. *J. Steroid Biochem.*, 6:751–753.
42. Ulick, S., and Ramirez, L. C. (1976): Adrenocortical factors in hypertension—The significance of 16-oxygenated C-19 steroids. *J. Steroid Biochem.*, 7:953–961.
43. Krakoff, L. R. (1973): Plasma renin substrate: Measurement by radioimmunoassay of angiotensin I concentration in syndromes associated with steroid excess. *J. Clin. Endocrinol. Metab.*, 37:110–118.
44. Dalakos, T. G., Anderson, G. H., and Streeten, D. H. P. (1976): Mechanisms of the hypertension in Cushing's syndrome (Abstr.) *Clin. Res.*, 24:271A.
45. Goodwin, R. J., Knowlton, A. I., and Laragh, J. H. (1969): Absence of renin suppression by deoxycorticosterone acetate in rats. *Am. J. Physiol.*, 216:1476–1480.
46. Laragh, J. H. (1973): Vasoconstriction-volume analysis for understanding and treating hypertension: The use of renin and aldosterone profiles. *Am. J. Med.*, 55:261–274.
47. Laragh, J. H., Sealey, J. E., Niarchos, A. P., and Pickering, T. G. (1982): The vasoconstriction-volume spectrum in normotension and in the pathogenesis of hypertension. *Fed. Proc.*, 41:2415–2423.
48. Lopez-Ovejero, J. A., Saal, S. D., D'Angelo, W. A., Cheigh, J. S., Stenzel, H., and Laragh, J. H. (1979): Reversal of scleroderma vascular and renal crisis by oral angiotensin converting enzyme blockade. *N. Engl. J. Med.*, 300:1417–1418.
49. Cody, R. J., Covit, A. B., Schaer, G. L., Laragh, J. H., Sealey, J. E., and Feldschuh, J. (1986): Sodium and water balance in chronic congestive heart failure. *J. Clin. Invest.*, 77:1441–1452.
50. Cody, J. R., Laragh, J. H., Atlas, S. A., and Case, D. B. (1983): Converting enzyme inhibition to identify and treat renin-mediated or sodium-volume related forms of increased peripheral resistance in hypertension and in congesive heart failure. *J. Hypertension*, 1(*Suppl.* 1):77–84.
51. Brunner, H. R., Gavras, H., Laragh, J. H., and Keenan, R. (1974): Hypertension in man. Exposure of the renin and sodium components using angiotensin II blockade. *Circ. Res.*, 34(*Suppl.* I):35–43.
52. Gavras, H., Brunner, H. R., Laragh, J. H., Sealey, J. E., Gavras, I., and Vukovitch, R. A. (1974): An angiotensin converting enzyme inhibitor to identify and treat vasoconstrictor and volume factors in hypertensive patients. *N. Engl. J. Med.*, 291:817–821.
53. Case, D. B., Wallace, J. M., Keim, H. J., Weber, M. A., Sealey, J. E., and Laragh, J. H. (1977): Possible role of renin in hypertension as suggested by renin-sodium profiling and inhibition of converting enzyme. *N. Engl. J. Med.*, 296:641–646.
54. Case, D. B., Atlas, S. A., Laragh, J. H., Sealey, J. E., Sullivan, P. A., and McKinstry, D. N. (1978): Clinical experience with blockade of the renin-angiotensin-aldosterone system by an oral converting enzyme inhibitor (SQ 14,225, Captopril) in hypertensive patients. *Prog. Cardiovasc. Dis.*, 21:195–206.
55. Laragh, J. H. (1978): The renin system in high blood pressure, from disbelief to reality: Converting enzyme blockade for analysis and treatment. *Prog. Cardiovasc. Dis.*, 21:159–166.
56. Case, D. B., Wallace, J. M., Kein, J. H., Weber, M. A., Drayer, J. I. M., White, R. P., Sealey, J. E., and Laragh, J. H. (1976): Estimating renin participation in hypertension. Superiority of converting enzyme inhibitor over saralasin. *Am. J. Med.*, 61:790–796.
57. Laragh, J. H., Case, D. B., Atlas, S. A., and Sealey, J. E. (1980): Captopril compared with other anti-renin system agents in hypertensive patients. Its triphasic effects on blood pressure and its use to identify and treat the renin factor. *Hypertension*, 2:586–593.
58. Laragh, J. H. (1984): The meaning of plasma renin measurements: Renin and sodium volume-mediated (low renin) forms of vasoconstriction in experimental and human hypertension and in the oedematous states

of nephrosis and heart failure. *J. Hypertension, 2(Suppl. 1)*:141–150.

59. Laragh, J. H., and Pecker, M. S. (1983): Dietary sodium and essential hypertension: Some myths, hopes and truths. *Ann. Intern. Med.*, 98:735–743.
60. Erne, P., Bolli, P., Bertel, O., Hulthen, U. L., Kiowski, W., Müller, F. B., and Bühler, F. R. (1983): Factors influencing the hypotensive effects of calcium antagonists. *Hypertension,* 5(*Suppl.* II):II97–II102.
61. Resnick, L. M., Nicholson, J. P., Sealey, J. E., and Laragh, J. H. (1983): Acute and long term effects of calcium channel blockade on divalent ions, blood pressure and plasma renin activity. *Clin. Res.*, 31:253A.
62. Resnick, L. M., Laragh, J. H., Sealey, J. E., and Alderman, M. H. (1983): Divalent cations in essential hypertension. Relations between serum ionized calcium, magnesium, and plasma renin activity. *N. Engl. J. Med.*, 309:888–891.
63. Resnick, L. M., Nicholson, J. P., and Laragh, J. H. (1985): Alterations in calcium metabolism mediate dietary salt sensitivity in essential hypertension. *Trans. Assoc. Am. Physicians,* 98:313–332.

dietary salt sensitivity in essential hypertension. *Trans. Assoc. Am. Physicians,* 98:313–332.

64. van Zwieten, P. A., van Meel, J. C. A., and Timmermans, P. B. M. W. M. (1983): Functional interaction between calcium antagonists and the vasoconstriction induced by the stimulation of post-synaptic α-adrenoceptors. *Circ. Res.* (*Suppl.* I), 52:I77–I80.
65. Nicholson, J. P., Resnick, L. M., Pickering, T. G., Marion, R., Sullivan, P., and Laragh, J. H. (1985): Relationship of blood pressure response and the renin-angiotensin system to first-dose prazosin. *Am. J. Med.*, 78:241–244.
66. Nicholson, J. P., Resnick, L. M., and Laragh, J. H. (1986): Dietary sodium and the antihypertensive action of verapamil in essential hypertension (*submitted for publication*).

The Kidney in Hypertension, edited by
Norman M. Kaplan, Barry M. Brenner,
and John H. Laragh. Raven Press,
New York © 1987.

The Kidney in the Pathogenesis of Hypertension: Role of the Renal Nerves

John P. Koepke, Ulla C. Kopp, and Gerald F. DiBona

Department of Internal Medicine, University of Iowa College of Medicine, and Veterans Administration Medical Center, Iowa City, Iowa 52242

The sympathetic nervous system has long been thought to be critical in the pathophysiology of hypertension. In a recent comprehensive analysis of the physiological aspects of primary hypertension, Folkow (19) described three major interdependent causative elements: hereditary predisposition, environmental influences, and structural cardiovascular adaptations. Of the environmental element, two major factors are distinguished: excitatory environmental (psychoemotional) stress and dietary salt (NaCl) intake. Environmental stress may be translated into increased sympathetic nervous system activity via the limbic-hypothalamic-bulbar autonomic centers. Elevated dietary salt intake can augment sympathetic nervous system activity responses to environmental stress. The critical importance of the sympathetic nervous system in the pathophysiology of hypertension has been reviewed by Abboud (1). Increased sympathetic nervous system activity may lead to hypertension through four major mechanisms: (a) increased vascular resistance resulting from sustained arteriolar constriction; (b) increased cardiac rate, stroke volume, and output; (c) sodium retention and renin release, and (d) vascular muscle defects. Any of these factors, alone or in combination, may lead to structural cardiovascular adaptations and established hypertension.

A major hypothesis is that abnormal renal function is critical for the initiation, development, or maintenance of primary hypertension (9). The maintenance of sodium and water balance by the kidneys is believed to be primary in long-term control of arterial pressure. In the normal system, an increase in arterial pressure leads to an increased urinary excretion of sodium and water, consequently reducing blood volume until arterial pressure returns to normal. In hypertension, it is hypothesized that factors disrupt the maintenance of sodium and water balance by the kidneys such that an elevated arterial pressure is required to reestablish and maintain normal sodium and water balance. Several types of renal dysfunction could contribute to the hypertensive state, including increased renal vascular resistance, increased renal retention of sodium and water, and increased release of renin, catecholamines, prostaglandins, or other vasoactive substances. The kidney possesses extensive efferent and afferent innervation, which is known to be important in the physiological regulation of these renal functions.

How the sympathetic nervous system interacts with renal function in the pathophysiology of hypertension is the major focus of this chapter. Increased efferent renal sympathetic nerve activity can increase renal sodium retention, which may be important in the initiation, maintenance, or exacerbation of hypertension. In addition, alterations in afferent renal sympathetic nerve activity, subserving renal mechanoreceptors and chemoreceptors, can modulate sympathetic nervous system activity via central neural connections. Evidence concerning the role of efferent and afferent renal sympathetic innervation in the initiation, maintenance, or exacerbation of hypertension will be reviewed in this chapter.

RENAL NEUROANATOMY AND NEUROPHYSIOLOGY

Efferent Renal Nerves

Relative to its size, the kidney has a richer innervation than almost any other organ (10,54). The renal nerves emanate from the celiac plexus, the thoracic and lumbar branches of the splanchnic nerves, the superior and inferior mesenteric plexus, the intermesenteric nerves, and the superior hypogastric plexus (54). These nerve fibers and their interconnections make up the renal plexus, which lies in a relatively uniform association with the aorticorenal ganglion. The aorticorenal ganglion is the largest ganglion associated with the renal plexus and lies near the junction of the aorta and the renal artery (57). From the renal plexus, the renal nerves course along the renal artery and vein to enter the hilus of the kidney.

Within the kidney, prominent adrenergic nerve bundles are associated with the afferent and efferent glomerular arterioles, surrounding tubules, and the renin-secretory juxtaglomerular granular cells (3). The tubules receive a distinct innervation with nerve fibers closely following the contour of both proximal and distal tubules and the thick ascending limb of Henle's loop. A recent quantitative study of rat cortical nephrons by Barajas and colleagues (4) shows that the greatest number of innervated profiles is in the proximal tubules, followed by the thick ascending limb of Henle's loop, the distal convoluted tubule, and the collecting duct.

The efferent renal nerves can regulate urinary sodium and water excretion by (a) changing intrarenal hemodynamics (e.g., renal blood flow, glomerular filtration rate) through changes in renal vascular resistance; (b) changing renin release from the juxtaglomerular granular cells through increased formation of angiotensin II; or (c) through a direct effect on the innervated renal tubules (11). Increases in renal sympathetic nerve activity resulting from direct electrical stimulation cause frequency-dependent decreases in renal blood flow, which are mediated by renal vascular α_1-adrenoceptors. Increased renal sympathetic nerve activity, however, produced by carotid baroreflex activation, does not produce renal vasoconstriction. In contrast, environmental stress in conscious rats, dogs, and humans can cause marked renal vasoconstriction with decreased renal blood flow and glomerular filtration rate. In general, decreased renal sympathetic nerve activity results in renal vasodilation only when basal renal sympathetic nerve activity is elevated.

Increases or decreases in renal sympathetic nerve activity, which do not affect renal perfusion pressure, glomerular filtration rate, total renal blood flow, or its distribution, cause parallel changes in net renal tubular sodium and water reabsorption, with reciprocal changes in urinary sodium and water excretion (11). Renal micropuncture studies point to the proximal convoluted tubule and thick ascending loop of Henle as specific nephron segments responsible for these responses; other evidence implicates the distal convoluted tubule and collecting duct as well (11). Pharmacological studies show that the direct effect of the renal sympathetic nerves on renal tubular sodium and water excretion is mediated via α_1-adrenoceptors.

Increased renal sympathetic nerve activity increases renin release, with subsequent increased formation of angiotensin II, a powerful vasoconstrictor and antinatriuretic hormone (11). There are several levels of interaction among renal sympathetic nerve activity, renin release, renal hemodynamics, and urinary sodium excretion (11,43,62). At high frequencies of renal nerve stimulation (2.0–2.5 Hz), renin release is mediated by activation of both β- and α-adrenoceptors; the former is due to a direct effect on the juxtaglomerular granular cells, and the latter is due to renal vasoconstriction in series with prostaglandin release. At frequencies of renal nerve stimulation (ca 1.0 Hz) that do not change renal hemodynamics, but decrease urinary sodium excretion, renin release is mediated predominantly by β_1-adrenoceptors. Similarly, β_1-adrenoceptors mediate renin release at levels of renal nerve stimulation (ca 0.5 Hz) that have no effect on renal hemodynamics or urinary sodium excretion. Even lower levels of renal nerve stimulation (<0.25 Hz), which have no effect on renal hemodynamics, urinary sodium excretion, or renin release, enhance the renin release response to nonneural stimuli, such as decreased renal arterial pressure.

Afferent Renal Nerves

Both myelinated and unmyelinated nerve fibers are present in the kidney at the outer stripe of the outer zone of the medulla, in the periarterial loose connective tissue, and in the subepithelial connective tissue of the calyces (24). Afferent renal nerve fibers project into ipsilateral dorsal root ganglia and dorsal horn in the spinal cord (between T_7 and L_2) as well as to medullary sites (7). Although renal sensory receptors (mechanoreceptors and chemoreceptors) have been identified with neurophysiological techniques, a detailed ultrastructural description is not yet available.

The afferent renal sympathetic nerves participate in a wide variety of renorenal and renosystemic reflexes (24,42,55). Renal mechanoreceptors are stimulated by altering intrarenal pressure, such as by increased ureteral or renal venous pressure or by compression of the kidney. Renal chemoreceptors are stimulated by renal ischemia (R1), such as marked renal vasoconstriction, hypotension, or systemic asphyxia, or by altering the ionic composition of the medullopapillary interstitium (R2), such as isobaric retrograde ureteropelvic perfusion with hypertonic saline. The term renorenal reflexes refers to the response of one kidney to an alteration in the same or the contralateral kidney. The functional changes in the contralateral kidney are mediated by the contralateral efferent renal sympathetic nerves. Electrophysiological studies show that afferent renal nerves project to nuclei in the medulla and hypothalamus known to regulate body fluid and cardiovascular homeostasis. Direct electrical stimulation of the afferent renal nerves results in an integrated cardiovascular response, which is abolished by lesioning periventricular tissue in the anteroventral third ventricle. Thus, the afferent renal nerves, through connections with medullary and hypothalamic autonomic centers, modulate sympathetic neural discharge to the kidney and to other vascular beds, thereby regulating body fluid homeostasis and cardiovascular function.

RENAL NERVES IN PATHOPHYSIOLOGY OF HYPERTENSION

Efferent Renal Nerves

Increased sympathetic nervous system activity to the kidney is critical in the development, maintenance, and exacerbation of hypertension. As early as 1945, Kottke and associates (46) and Kubicek and colleagues (47,48) showed that long-term electrical stimulation of the renal artery nerves or splanchnic nerves in conscious dogs increased renal vascular resistance and mean arterial pressure. The hypertension was sustained throughout renal artery nerve stimulation and was reversible on termination of stimulation. The mechanism of this hypertension was not clarified, since no measurements of sodium balance, renin-angiotensin system activity, or sympathetic nervous system activity were made. More recent studies confirm the importance of increased sympathetic nervous system activity to the kidney in the production of sustained hypertension. Long-term infusion of norepinephrine into the renal artery of uninephrectomized conscious dogs produces hypertension for the duration of the infusion (8,25). The hypertension resulting from chronic infusion of norepinephrine into the renal artery is associated with decreased renal plasma flow, positive sodium balance, and increased total peripheral resistance; glomerular filtration rate remains normal and the renin-angiotensin system is not involved, since pharmacological blockade of angiotensin II receptors has no effect on the arterial pressure response to renal arterial infusion of norepinephrine (25).

If sympathetic neural input to the kidneys is important in the pathophysiology of hypertension, then interruption of efferent renal sympathetic nerve activity should influence the development of hypertension. Support for this hypothesis comes from studies of genetic models of hypertension: surgical denervation of the kidneys delays the onset and attenuates the severity of hypertension in spontaneously hypertensive rats (Okamoto strain) and New Zealand hypertensive rats (16,34,63). The development of hypertension in genetic hypertension models is associated with increased renal retention of sodium; both the hypertension and increased renal sodium retention are inhibited by surgical denervation of the kidneys. The eventual development of hypertension in renal-denervated spontaneously hypertensive rats or New Zealand hypertensive rats is associated with parallel increase in renal sodium retention and increased renal norepinephrine content, indicating the reinnervation of the kidneys (16,34,63). In these studies, plasma and renal renin activity or urinary prostaglandin E_2 or kallikrein excretion are similar between renal-denervated and sham-operated animals, indicating that the attenuation in the hypertensive process is likely not due to differences in the activity of the renin-angiotensin, renal prostaglandin, or renal kallikrein systems.

With repeated surgical denervation of the kidneys at 3-week intervals to prevent renal reinnervation in prehypertensive spontaneously hypertensive rats, hypertension is significantly attenuated compared with sham-treated spontaneously hypertensive rats (56). In contrast, if hypertension is allowed to become well established before denervation of kidneys in the spontaneously hypertensive rats, no changes in arterial pressure or renal sodium retention are observed (63). These studies indicate that the renal sympathetic nerves are important in initiating but not maintaining established hypertension in the spontaneously hypertensive rat.

The importance of the renal nerves in the pathophysiology of hypertension is also demonstrated in the deoxycorticosterone acetate (DOCA)-NaCl hypertensive rat, a sodium-dependent model of hypertension. Renal denervation prior to the start of DOCA-NaCl treatment delays the onset of hypertension (29). Associated with the inhibition of hypertension is a decreased renal sodium retention, compared with sham-denervated DOCA-NaCl hypertensive rats; as renal reinnervation occurs (as judged by increased renal norepinephrine content), hypertension and increased renal sodium retention progress to sham-denervated DOCA-NaCl hypertensive levels. Surgical denervation of the kidneys after 3 weeks of DOCA-NaCl treatment reduces both renal sodium retention and arterial pressure (28). In this study (28), renal precapillary arteriolar wall-to-lumen ratios in sham DOCA-NaCl hypertensive rats are higher compared with vessels of similar size in hindlimb and cremaster muscle. In renal-denervated rats, however, renal precapillary arteriolar wall-to-lumen ratios are the same as in vessels of similar size in hindlimb and cremaster muscle. The observation that renal denervation in 3-week DOCA-NaCl hypertensive rats decreases renal precapillary arteriolar wall-to-lumen ratio but has no effect on renal arteriole wall-to-lumen ratio suggests that the renal sympathetic nerves selectively influence the renal precapillary arteriole at this stage of DOCA-NaCl hypertension (28). Such an increase in renal precapillary wall-to-lumen ratio in DOCA-NaCl hypertensive rats could lead to increased renal vascular resistance, thereby contributing to the increased renal sodium retention. Similar to spontaneously hypertensive rats, denervation of the kidneys in DOCA-NaCl hypertensive rats with established hypertension (10 weeks of DOCA-NaCl treatment) has no effect on the hypertension or renal sodium retention (28). Hence, increased efferent renal sympathetic nerve activity with renal sodium retention appears to be critical for the initiation and the development of hypertension in spontaneously hypertensive rats and DOCA-NaCl hypertensive rats, but does not contribute significantly to the established phases of hypertension in these models.

Direct recordings of multifiber renal or splanchnic sympathetic nerve activity and of single fiber renal sympathetic nerve activity in conscious or anesthetized rats support the hypothesis that efferent renal sympathetic nerve activity is greater in spontaneously hypertensive rats than in normotensive Wistar-Kyoto rats (22,52,53). Direct measurements of postganglionic multifiber nerve activity in anesthetized prehypertensive spontaneously hypertensive rats suggest that sympathetic activity to the kidney may be much more elevated than activity to other vascular beds (58).

The control of renal function by the renal sympathetic nerves is influenced by an interaction among environmental stress, dietary sodium intake, and genetic predisposition to hypertension (35). Environmental stress (air jet to head) in conscious spontaneously hypertensive rats increases heart rate, mean arterial pressure, and renal sympathetic nerve activity (Fig. 1). In addition, air stress decreases urine flow rate and urinary sodium excretion in spontaneously hypertensive rats (37,53). In sharp contrast, air stress has little or no effect on these measures in conscious normotensive Wistar-Kyoto rats (37,53). A genetic predisposition to develop hypertension, therefore, is associated with a propensity to respond to environmental stress with increased renal sympathetic nerve activity and renal sodium retention. High dietary sodium intake, another environmental factor, enhances the increased renal sympathetic nerve activity and antinatriuretic responses to air stress in conscious spontaneously hypertensive rats, but has no additional effects in Wistar-Kyoto rats (37) (Figs. 2 and 3). The importance of the renal sympathetic nerves in the antinatriuretic response to air stress in conscious spontaneously hypertensive rats is indicated by studies showing that surgical renal denervation abolishes the antinatriuretic response to air stress in spontaneously hypertensive rats on either normal or high-sodium intakes (37) (Fig. 2).

Similar to spontaneously hypertensive rats, in conscious DOCA-NaCl hypertensive rats, a sodium-dependent model of hypertension, air stress increases renal sympathetic nerve activity and decreases urinary sodium excretion, indicating that a genetic predisposition is not a necessary condition for environmental stress to influence the neural control of renal function (40). However, the interaction between environmental stress and DOCA-NaCl treatment is critical, since air stress has no effect on renal sympathetic nerve activity or urinary sodium excretion in sham DOCA-NaCl normotensive rats (40). Moreover, renal denervation prevents the antinatriuretic response to air stress in conscious DOCA-NaCl hypertensive rats, emphasizing the importance of the renal sympathetic nerves in the antinatriuretic response (40).

The renal mechanisms of the antinatriuretic response to air stress in conscious spontaneously hypertensive rats and DOCA-NaCl hypertensive rats include an increased renal tubular reabsorption of sodium (36,37,40). Glomerular filtration rate and plasma sodium concentration are unaffected by air stress, indicating an unchanged filtered sodium load. Hence, the decrease in both absolute and fractional excretion of sodium points to an increased renal tubular reabsorption of sodium during air stress in conscious spontaneously hypertensive rats and DOCA-NaCl hypertensive rats (36,37,40). Moreover, since effective renal plasma flow and mean arterial pressure are unchanged by air stress in DOCA-NaCl hypertensive rats, renal vascular resistance is not changed, eliminating it as a mechanism of the renal responses to air stress. However, in spontaneously hypertensive rats on a high sodium intake, the greater increase in renal sympathetic nerve activity resulting from air stress compared with spontaneously hypertensive rats on normal sodium intake is associated with reduced glomerular filtration rate and effective renal plasma flow (37). Hence, the interactions among environmental stress, high sodium intake, and genetic predisposition to hypertension have a greater influence on the neural control of renal function than any factor alone.

The central nervous system controls renal sympathetic nerve activity and renal function in conscious spontaneously hypertensive rats and DOCA-NaCl hypertensive rats. In conscious spontaneously hypertensive rats, the intracerebroventricular administration of $\beta_{1,2}$- (propranolol, timolol) or β_2- (ICI 118,551) adrenoceptor antagonists or α_2-adrenoceptor agonists (cloni-

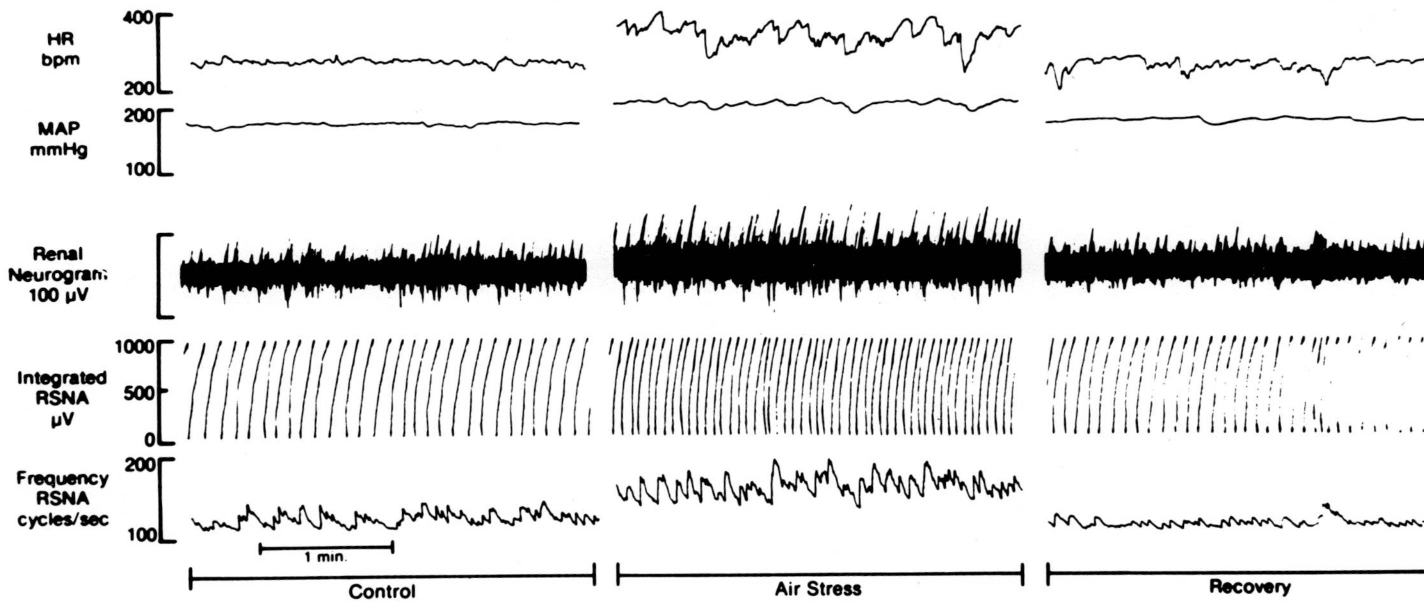

FIG. 1. Original tracing from a conscious spontaneously hypertensive rat. Air stress increases heart rate (HR), mean arterial pressure (MAP), renal neurogram activity, integrated renal sympathetic nerve activity (RSNA), and frequency discharge RSNA. During the recovery period each measure returns to control levels. Each tracing represents minutes 5, 6, and 7 of each 10-min control, air stress, and recovery period.

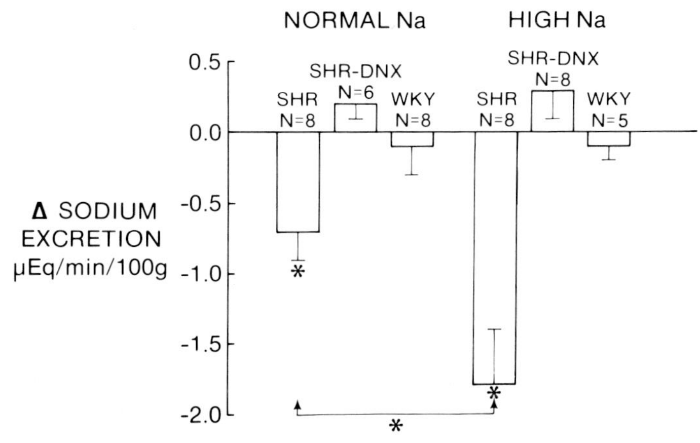

FIG. 2. The antinatriuretic response to air stress is enhanced in conscious spontaneously hypertensive rats (SHR) on a high sodium intake compared with SHR on a normal sodium intake. Renal denervation (DNX) abolishes the antinatriuretic response to air stress in SHR on normal or high sodium intake. Air stress has no effect on urinary sodium excretion in conscious normotensive Wistar-Kyoto rats (WKY) on normal or high sodium intake. (From ref. 37).

dine, guanabenz) inhibits the increased renal sympathetic nerve activity and antinatriuretic responses to air stress (36,38). The administration of ICI 118,551 (but not guanabenz) into the posterior hypothalamus inhibits, and the administration of isoproterenol into the posterior hypothalamus enhances, the renal sympathetic nerve activity and antinatriuretic responses to air stress

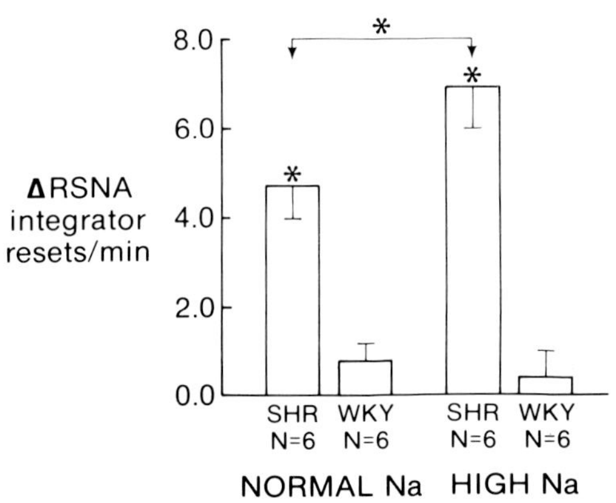

FIG. 3. The renal sympathetic nerve activity (RSNA) response to air stress was enhanced in conscious spontaneously hypertensive rats (SHR) on a high sodium intake. Air stress has no effect on RSNA in conscious normotensive Wistar-Kyoto rats (WKY) on normal or high sodium intake. (From ref. 37).

in conscious spontaneously hypertensive rats (39), suggesting a site-specificity for central β_2-adrenoceptors. Conversely, the administration of guanabenz (but not ICI 118,551) into the central amygdaloid nucleus prevents the renal sympathetic nerve activity and antinatriuretic responses to air stress in conscious spontaneously hypertensive rats (41). The potential importance of hypothalamic β-adrenoceptors in the increased renal sympathetic nerve activity and antinatriuresis to air stress in DOCA-NaCl hypertensive rats is suggested by previous studies. The density of β-adrenoceptors in the hypothalamus is greater in DOCL-NaCl hypertensive rats than in sham DOCA-NaCl normotensive rats (65). In addition, electrical stimulation of the posterior hypothalamus elicits a greater increase in abdominal sympathetic nerve activity and arterial pressure in DOCA-NaCl hypertensive rats than in sham DOCA-NaCl normotensive rats (61). Together, these studies point to a greater sensitivity of the central nervous system to neurogenic stimuli in conscious spontaneously hypertensive rats and DOCA-NaCl hypertensive rats than in control normotensive rats.

An increase in the sensitivity of the kidney to renal sympathetic nerve activity may also contribute to the antidiuretic and antinatriuretic response to neurogenic stimuli in conscious spontaneously hypertensive rats and DOCA-NaCl hypertensive rats. For example, high sodium intake in stroke-prone spontaneously hypertensive rats increases the vascular smooth muscle response to norepinephrine (14,15). Similarly, high sodium intake in stroke-prone spontaneously hypertensive rats increases the peripheral release of norepinephrine and impairs peripheral neuronal norepinephrine reuptake, resulting in higher baseline plasma norepinephrine concentrations and exaggerated increases in plasma norepinephrine concentrations during cold exposure (15). With respect to DOCA-NaCl hypertensive rats, the pressor response to intravenous injection of norepinephrine is greater than in sham DOCA-NaCl normotensive rats, suggesting an increased sensitivity of the peripheral vasculature in DOCA-NaCl hypertensive rats (61).

There may be a selective activation of sympathetic nervous system activity to the kidneys during exposure to environmental stress in conscious spontaneously hypertensive rats and DOCA-NaCl hypertensive rats. In conscious DOCA-NaCl hypertensive rats, air stress increases renal sympathetic nerve activity, but has no effect on mean arterial pressure or heart rate (40). In conscious spontaneously hypertensive rats, the increased renal sympathetic nerve activity and antinatriuretic response to air stress are abolished by central β-adrenoceptor blockade, but the mean arterial pressure and heart rate responses are unchanged (36,38,39). Similarly, high dietary sodium intake enhances the renal sympathetic nerve activity and antinatriuretic responses to air stress in conscious spontaneously hypertensive rats, but has no additional effect on the mean arterial pressure or heart rate responses (37). Certainly, any rigorous test of whether sympathetic outflow to the kidneys can be changed selectively over that to other vascular beds requires simultaneous measurement of sympathetic outflow to the other vascular beds.

Environmental (stress, sodium intake) and genetic factors may interact to promote increased renal sympathetic nerve activity and renal sodium retention, resulting in the production or exacerbation of hypertension. Long-term stimulation of the central nervous system with chronic environmental stress produced hypertension in borderline hypertensive rats (i.e., F_1 generation of crossbred spontaneously hypertensive rat × Wistar-Kyoto rat) and increases the severity of hypertension in spontaneously hypertensive rats (17,49). High dietary sodium intake further exacerbates the hypertension in spontaneously hypertensive rats resulting from environmental stress (17). Surgical renal denervation delays the onset of chronic stress hypertension in borderline hypertensive rats, implicating the renal sympathetic nerves in chronic stress hypertension (50).

Spontaneously hypertensive rats have an exaggerated natriuretic response to intravenous saline volume expansion, which is associated with an exaggerated inhibition of renal sympathetic nerve activity compared with normotensive Wistar-Kyoto rats (12,20,60). Bilateral renal denervation reduces the magnitude of the natriuretic response to volume expansion in spontaneously hypertensive rats to that of normotensive Wistar-Kyoto rats (13). These observations suggest that the greater inhibition of efferent renal sympathetic nerve activity in spontaneously hypertensive rats contributes to the exaggerated natriuretic response by directly reducing renal tubular sodium reabsorption.

These studies in experimental animal models are complemented by studies in normotensive and hypertensive humans. In the study by Light and associates (51), the effects of a stressful competitive task on urinary sodium excretion are compared in a group of normotensives with a parental history of hypertension (or borderline hypertension) and a group of normotensives with no parental history of hypertension (51). Additionally, the subjects are divided on the basis of responding to the psychological stress with little or no increase in heart rate, or a large increase in heart rate, which is mediated by increased sympathetic nervous system activity. Of greatest interest is the finding that the psychological stress causes an antinatriuresis only in subjects with a parental history of hypertension who are also high heart rate responders (51). In a study by Hollenberg and colleagues (21), the renal blood flow response to a stressful nonverbal IQ test is measured in hypertensive and normotensive subjects, some of whom have a parent with hypertension. This stressful psychological stimulus decreases renal blood flow in the hypertensive subjects; normotensive subjects with a parental history of hypertension respond similarly, although to a smaller degree; and normotensive subjects without a parental history of hypertension are least responsive to the stressful task (21). An increased renal vascular resistance is one of the most consistent findings in primary hypertension (5,21,23). The increased renal vascular resistance in such patients is decreased by either phentolamine (α-adrenoceptor antagonist) or splanchnic blockade (L_1 spinal anesthesia); the presence of normal renal vascular reactivity to norepinephrine suggests that the increased renal vascular resistance is due to increased efferent renal sympathetic nerve activity. Further evidence of increased efferent renal sympathetic nerve activity in hypertensive patients comes from measurements of renal venous norepinephrine outflow, which can be used as an index of renal sympathetic nerve activity (59). Renal venous norepinephrine outflow is increased in hypertensive patients, some of whom have normal peripheral venous plasma norepinephrine concentrations (6). In addition, norepinephrine outflow from the kidney in patients with hypertension is greater than that from heart or liver (6), suggesting a disproportionately greater sympathetic activation of the kidneys than other organ systems.

Afferent Renal Nerves in Hypertension

The afferent renal nerves are important in several models of experimental hypertension. In renovascular hypertension, such as that produced by one-kidney, one-clip in rats (Goldblatt hypertension), renal denervation attenuates the hypertension (31). The antihypertensive effect of renal denervation in one-kidney, one-clip hypertension in rats is not mediated by changes in sodium or water balance, glomerular filtration rate, or renin-angiotensin system activity, suggesting that interruption of efferent renal sympathetic nerve activity does not contribute to the attenuated hypertension (31). Other studies indicate that increased afferent renal nerve activity contributes to one-kidney, one-clip renovascular hypertension by increasing peripheral sympathetic outflow. Plasma norepinephrine concentration is elevated in one-kidney, one-clip hypertensive rats compared with normotensive controls; renal denervation 2 weeks after clipping decreases plasma norepinephrine concentration to normal levels (33). In addition, the norepinephrine content of the hypothalamus is elevated in one-kidney, one-clip hypertensive rats compared with control rats or renal-denervated hypertensive rats (64). One-clip, one-kidney hypertensive rats have an enhanced sympathoadrenal response to environmental stress, which returns to control levels after renal denervation (32). The importance of the afferent renal nerves in one-kidney, one-clip hypertension is clearly shown in a study employing selective denervation of afferent renal nerves. In one-kidney, one-clip hypertensive rats, lesion of the eighth thoracic through the second lumbar dorsal root nerves (T_8–L_2 dorsal rhizotomy) on the side of the remaining kidney lowers arterial pressure by approximately 50% (2), similar to renal afferent/efferent denervation. The specific and critical importance of afferent renal nerves, as opposed to nonrenal afferent nerves, in this study is shown by the finding that T_8–L_2 dorsal rhizotomy on the side contralateral to the remaining kidney has no effect on arterial pressure in one-kidney, one-clip hypertensive rats (2). Together, these studies indicate that increased afferent renal nerve activity in one-kidney, one-clip hypertensive rats signal the central nervous system to increase sympathetic nervous system activity leading to hypertension.

Several recent studies have examined the hypothesis that adenosine, which is readily released by ischemic kidney cells, serves as a stimulus to activate renal chemoreceptors, thereby increasing afferent renal nerve activity. In conscious dogs, renal artery infusion of adenosine increases mean arterial pressure and plasma norepinephrine, suggesting an increased sympathetic nervous system activity (30). After surgical renal denervation, intrarenal infusion of adenosine has no effect on mean arterial pressure or plasma norepinephrine concentration (30). In anesthetized dogs, intrarenal adenosine infusion increases multifiber afferent renal nerve activity (26). The latency in onset of afferent renal nerve activity is much shorter when adenosine is infused into the renal pelvis compared with intrarenal adenosine infusion (26). Consistent with these observations, urinary adenosine concentration is elevated in one-kidney, one-clip hypertensive rats, and lowering urinary adenosine concentration with intrarenal infusion of adenosine deaminase attenuates the hypertension (27). These studies support the hypothesis that stimulation of renal chemoreceptors located within or near the renal pelvis by adenosine increases afferent renal nerve activity, and consequently sympathetic outflow, leading to hypertension.

The elevated mean arterial pressure resulting from acute unilateral renal artery stenosis in rats with sinoaortic denervation and inhibition of the renin-angiotensin system depends on the afferent renal nerves (18). In these rats, acute unilateral renal artery stenosis increases mean arterial pressure and vascular resistance in hindquarter, mesenteric, and contralateral renal circulations. These responses are prevented by surgical denervation of the stenotic kidney, suggesting mediation via the afferent renal nerves (18); however, dorsal rhizotomy was not performed to confirm this conclusion. This study suggests that increased afferent renal nerve activity produces hypertension in conscious rats via increased resistance in several vascular beds.

Consistent with impaired carotid and cardiopulmonary baroreflexes in spontaneously hypertensive rats (1), renorenal reflexes are also impaired. In normotensive rats, stimulation of renal mechanoreceptors (increased ureteral pressure) in one kidney (ipsilateral kidney), increases ipsilateral afferent renal nerve activity (Fig. 4) (42). The responses of the contralateral kidney to ipsilateral stimulation of renal mechanoreceptors include decreased efferent renal nerve activity, diuresis, and natriuresis (Fig. 4) (42). Denervation of either kidney prevents the contralateral diuresis and natriuresis resulting from stimulation of ipsilateral renal mechanoreceptors (42). In contrast, in spontaneously hypertensive rats, stimulation of ipsilateral renal mechanoreceptors has no effect on contralateral efferent renal nerve activity, urine flow rate, or urinary sodium excretion (44). The specific defect in the impaired renorenal reflex in spontaneously hypertensive rats may be at the renal mechanoreceptor level, since increased ureteral pressure in spontaneously hypertensive rats fails to alter ipsilateral afferent renal nerve activity (44). The intact renorenal reflex in normotensive rats, therefore, may promote normotension, since an increased afferent renal nerve activity in one kidney promotes decreased sodium retention in the other kidney. Conversely, the impaired renorenal reflex in spontaneously hypertensive rats could promote hypertension, since the stimulation of renal mechanoreceptors is not able to decrease renal sodium retention as effectively.

CONCLUSION

The renal efferent and afferent nerves are important in the pathophysiology of hypertension. Increased efferent renal sympathetic nerve activity in Okamoto spontaneously hypertensive rats, New Zealand hypertensive rats, and DOCA-NaCl hypertensive rats contributes to the development of hypertension by increasing renal sodium and water retention. In addition, efferent renal sympathetic nerve activity is influenced by an interaction among genetic predisposition to hypertension and environmental factors (stress, dietary salt intake). Environmental stress increases renal sympathetic nerve activity and decreases urinary sodium retention to a greater degree in spontaneously hypertensive rats (genetic model) or in DOCA-NaCl hypertensive rats (sodium-dependent model) than in normotensive control rats. Moreover, in spontaneously hypertensive rats on a high dietary sodium intake, the increased renal sympathetic nerve activity and antinatriuretic responses to environmental stress are enhanced. Central nervous

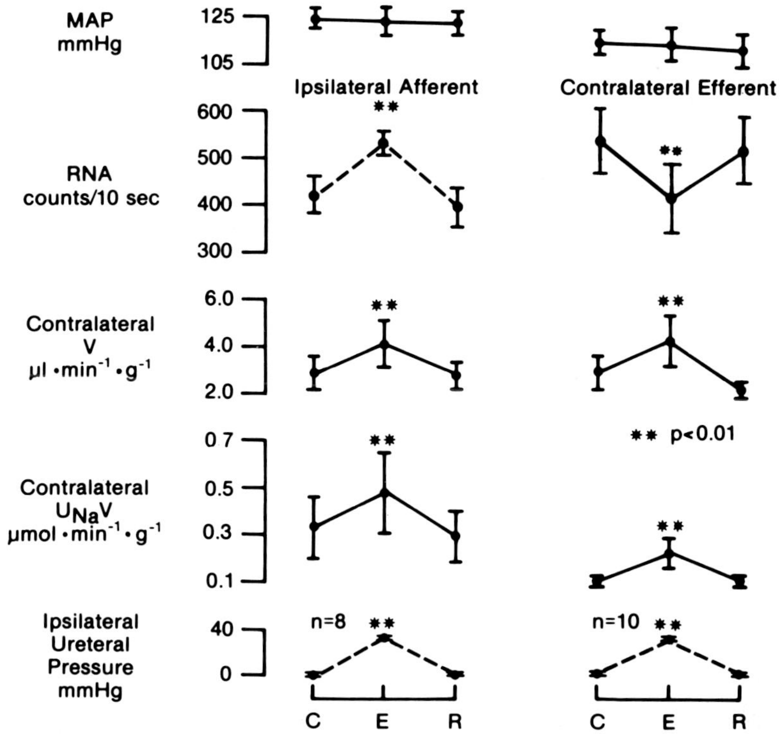

FIG. 4. Mechanoreceptor stimulation with increased ureteral pressure increases ipsilateral afferent renal nerve activity (RNA), decreases contralateral efferent RNA, and increases contralateral urine flow rate (V) and urinary sodium excretion ($U_{Na}V$). (MAP) mean arterial pressure (From ref. 45).

system α_2- and β_2-adrenoceptors are important in the neural control of renal function in conscious hypertensive rats. Efferent renal sympathetic nerves are also important in human primary hypertension.

In experimental renovascular hypertension, the afferent renal nerves contribute to the development of hypertension. The afferent renal nerves contribute to renovascular hypertension primarily by reflex modulation of the activity of the sympathetic nervous system. The intrarenal accumulation of adenosine may stimulate renal chemoreceptors and alter afferent renal nerve activity in renovascular hypertension. Moreover, spontaneously hypertensive rats do not respond to renal mechanoreceptor stimulation with increased afferent renal nerve activity and contralateral natriuresis as efficiently as normotensive Wistar-Kyoto rats; thus, an impaired renorenal reflex may contribute to hypertension in spontaneously hypertensive rats by favoring renal sodium retention.

REFERENCES

1. Abboud, F. M. (1982): The sympathetic system in hypertension. *Hypertension*, 4 (*Suppl.* II):II208–II225.
2. Aboukarsh, N., Sripairojthikoon, W., and Wyss, J. M. (1985): Further analysis of the effect of dorsal rhizotomy on Goldblatt hypertension. *Neurosci. Abstr*, 11:1000.
3. Barajas, L. (1978): Innervation of the renal cortex. *Fed. Proc.*, 37:1192–1201.
4. Barajas, L., Powers, K., and Wang, P. (1984): Innervation of the renal cortical tubules: A quantitative study. *Am. J. Physiol.*, 247:F50–F60.
5. Brod, J., Fencl, V., Hejl, Z., Jirka, J., and Ulrych, M. (1962): General and regional hemodynamic patterns underlying essential hypertension. *Clin. Sci.*, 23:339–349.
6. Brown, M. J., Jenner, D. A., Allison, D. J., and Dollery, C. T. (1981): Variations in individual organ release of noradrenaline measured by an improved radioenzymatic technique: Limitations of peripheral

nervous measurements in the assessment of sympathetic nervous activity. *Clin. Sci.*, 61:585–590.
7. Ciriello, J., and Calaresu, F. R. (1983): Central projections of afferent renal fibers in the rat: An antegrade transport study of horseradish peroxidase. *J. Auton. Nerv. Syst.*, 8:273–285.
8. Cowley, A. W., Jr., and Lohmeier, T. E. (1979): Changes in renal vascular sensitivity and arterial pressure associated with sodium intake during long-term intrarenal norepinephrine infusion in dogs. *Hypertension*, 1:549–558.
9. Cowley, A. W., Jr., and Roman, R. J. (1983): Renal dysfunction in essential hypertension—Implications of experimental studies. *Am. J. Nephrol.*, 3:59–72.
10. DeMuylder, G. G. (1952): *The "Neurility" of the Kidney*. Blackwell, Oxford.
11. DiBona, G. F. (1982): The functions of the renal nerves. *Rev. Physiol. Biochem. Pharmacol.*, 94:76–181.
12. DiBona, G. F., and Rios, L. L. (1978): Mechanism of exaggerated diuresis in spontaneously hypertensive rats. *Am. J. Physiol.*, 235:F409–F416.
13. DiBona, G. F., and Sawin, L. L. (1986): Exaggerated natriuresis in experimental hypertension. *Proc. Soc. Exp. Biol. Med.*, 182:43–51.
14. Dietz, R., Schomig, A., Haebra, H., Mann, J. F. E., Rascher, W., Luther, J. B., Grunherz, N., and Gross, F. (1978): Studies on the pathogenesis of spontaneous hypertension of rats. *Circ. Res.*, 43(*Suppl.* I):98–106.
15. Dietz, R., Schomig, A., Rascher, W., Strasser, R., Luth J. B., Ganten, U., and Kubler, W. (1982): Contribution of the sympathetic nervous system to the hypertensive effects of high sodium diet in stroke-prone spontaneously hypertensive rats. *Hypertension*, 4:773–781.
16. Diz, D. I., Nasjletti, A., and Baer, P. G. (1982): Renal denervation at weaning retards development of hypertension in New Zealand genetically hypertensive rats. *Hypertension*, 4:361–368.
17. Ely, D. L., and Weigand, J. (1983): Stress and high sodium effects on blood pressure and brain catecholamines in spontaneously hypertensive rats. *Clin Exp. Hypertens.*, A5:1559–1587.
18. Faber, J. E., and Brody, M. J. (1985): Afferent renal nerve-dependent hypertension following acute renal artery stenosis in the conscious rat. *Circ. Res.*, 57:676–688.
19. Folkow, B. (1982): Physiological aspects of primary hypertension. *Physiol. Rev.*, 62:347–504.
20. Francisco, L. L., Sawin, L. L., and DiBona, G. F. (1981): Renal sympathetic nerve activity and the exaggerated natriuresis of the spontaneous hypertensive rat. *Hypertension*, 3:134–138.
21. Hollenberg, N. K., Williams, G. H., and Adams, D. F. (1981): Essential hypertension: Abnormal renal vascular and endocrine responses to a mild psychological stimulus. *Hypertension*, 3:11–17.
22. Iriuchijima, J. (1980): Sympathetic discharge rate in spontaneously hypertensive rats. *Jpn. Heart J.*, 14:330–356.
23. Kaplan, N. M. (1979): The role of kidney in hypertension. *Hypertension*, 1:456–461.
24. Katholi, R. E. (1983): Renal nerves in the pathogenesis of hypertension in experimental animals and humans. *Am. J. Physiol.*, 245:F1–F14.
25. Katholi, R. E., Carey, R. M., Ayers, C. R., Vaughan, E. D., Yancey, M. R., and Morton, C.L. (1977): Production of sustained hypertension by chronic intrarenal norepinephrine infusion in conscious dogs. *Circ. Res.*, 40(*Suppl.* I):118–126.
26. Katholi, R. E., Hageman, G. R., Whitlow, P. L., and Woods, W. T. (1983): Hemodynamic and afferent renal nerve response to intrarenal adenosine in the dog. *Hypertension*, 5(*Suppl.* I):149–154.
27. Katholi, R. E., McCann, W. P., and Woods, W. T. (1985): Intrarenal adenosine produces hypertension via renal nerves in the one-kidney, one-clip rat. *Hypertension*, 7(*Suppl.* I):88–93.
28. Katholi, R. E., Naftilan, A. J., Bishop, S. P., and Oparil, S. (1983): Role of renal nerves in maintenance of DOCA-salt hypertension in the rat: Influence on renal vasculature and sodium excretion. *Hypertension*, 5:427–435.
29. Katholi, R. E., Naftilan, A. J., and Oparil, S. (1980): Importance of renal sympathetic tone in the development of DOCA-salt hypertension in the rat. *Hypertension*, 2:266–273.
30. Katholi, R. E., Whitlow, P. L., Hageman, G. R., and Woods, W. T. (1984): Intrarenal adenosine produces hypertension by activating the sympathetic nervous system via the renal nerves in the dog. *J. Hypertension*, 2:349–359.
31. Katholi, R. E., Winternitz, S. R., and Oparil, S. (1981): Role of renal nerves in the pathogenesis of one-kidney renal hypertension in the rat. *Hypertension*, 3:404–409.
32. Katholi, R. E., Winternitz, S. R., and Oparil, S. (1982): Decrease in sympathetic nervous system activity and attenuation in response to stress following renal denervation in the one-kidney one-clip Goldblatt hypertensive rat. *Clin. Exp. Hypertens.*, A4:707–716.
33. Katholi, R. E., Winternitz, S. R., and Oparil, S. (1982): Decrease in peripheral sympathetic nervous system activity following renal denervation or unclipping in the one-kidney one-clip Goldblatt hypertensive rat. *J. Clin. Invest.*, 69:55–61.
34. Kline, R. L., Stuart, P. J., and Mercer, P. F. (1980): Effect of renal denervation on arterial pressure and renal norepinephrine concentration in Wistar-Kyoto and spontaneously hypertensive rats. *Can. J. Physiol. Pharmacol.*, 58:1384–1388.
35. Koepke, J. P. (1985): Renal responses to stressful environmental stimuli. *Fed. Proc.*, 44:2823–2827.
36. Koepke, J. P., and DiBona, G. F. (1985): Central β-adrenergic receptors mediate renal nerve activity during stress in conscious spontaneously hypertensive rats. *Hypertension*, 7:350–356.
37. Koepke, J. P., and DiBona, G. F. (1985): High sodium intake enhances renal nerve and antinatriuretic responses to air stress in spontaneously hypertensive rats. *Hypertension*, 7:357–363.
38. Koepke, J. P., and DiBona, G. F. (1986): Central adrenergic receptor control of renal function in conscious hypertensive rats. *Hypertension*, 8:133–141.
39. Koepke, J. P., Jones, S., and DiBona, G. F. (1986): Hypothalamic beta-2 adrenoceptor control of renal sympathetic nerve activity and urinary sodium excretion in conscious spontaneously hypertensive rats. *Circ. Res.*, 58:241–248.

40. Koepke, J. P., Jones, S., and DiBona, G. F. (1986): Renal nerve activity and renal function during environmental stress in DOCA-NaCl rats. *Am. J. Physiol.*, 251:R289–R294.
41. Koepke, J. P., Jones, S., and DiBona, G. F. (1987): Alpha-2 adrenoceptors in amygdala control renal sympathetic nerve activity and renal function in conscious spontaneously hypertensive rats. *Brain Res.* (*in press*).
42. Kopp, U. C. (1985): Renorenal reflexes: Neural and functional responses. *Fed. Proc.*, 44:2834–2839.
43. Kopp, U. C., and DiBona, G.F. (1984): Interaction between neural and nonneural mechanisms controlling renin secretion rate. *Am. J. Physiol.*, 246:F620–F626.
44. Kopp, U. C., Smith, L. A., and DiBona, G. F. (1987): Impaired renorenal reflexes in spontaneously hypertensive rats. *Hypertens.*, 9:69–75.
45. Kopp, U. C., Olson, L. A., and DiBona G. F. (1984): Renorenal reflex responses to mechano- and chemoreceptor stimulation in the dog and rat. *Am. J. Physiol.*, 246:F67–F77.
46. Kottke, F. J., Kubicek, W. G., and Visscher, M. B. (1945): The production of arterial hypertension by chronic renal artery-nerve stimulation. *Am. J. Physiol.*, 145:38–47.
47. Kubicek, W. G., and Kottke, F. J. (1946): Glomerular filtration rate and renal plasma flow during renal and splanchnic nerve stimulation in dogs in relation to arterial hypertension. *Fed. Proc.*, 5:58.
48. Kubicek, W. G., Kottke, F. J., Laker, D. J., and Visscher, M.B. (1953): Renal function during arterial hypertension produced by chronic splanchnic nerve stimulation in the dog. *Am. J. Physiol.*, 174:397–400.
49. Lawler, J. E., Barker, G. F., Hubbard, J. W., and Schaub, R.F. (1981): Effects of stress on blood pressure and cardiac pathology in rats with borderline hypertension. *Hypertension*, 3:496–505.
50. Lawler, J. E., Cox, R. H., Sanders, B. J., Mitchell, V. P., and Baer, P. G. (1985): Renal denervation can prevent stress-induced hypertension in the borderline hypertensive rat. *Neurosci. Abstr.* 11:999.
51. Light, K. C., Koepke, J. P., Obrist, P. A., and Willis, P. W., IV (1983): Psychological stress induces sodium and fluid retention in men at high risk for hypertension. *Science*, 220:429–431.
52. Lundin, S., Ricksten, S.-E., and Thoren, P. (1984): Interaction between "mental stress" and baroreceptor reflexes concerning effects on heart rates, mean arterial pressure and renal sympathetic activity in spontaneously hypertensive rats. *Acta Physiol. Scand.*, 120:273–281.
53. Lundin, S., and Thoren, P. (1982): Renal function and sympathetic activity during "mental stress" in normotensive and spontaneously hypertensive rats. *Acta Physiol. Scand.*, 115:115–124.
54. Mitchell, G. A. G. (1950): The nerve supply of the kidneys. *Acta Anat.*, 10:1–37.
55. Moss, N. G. (1982): Renal function and renal afferent and efferent nerve activity. *Am. J. Physiol.*, 243:F425–F433.
56. Norman, R. A., Jr., and Dzielak, D. J. (1982): Role of renal nerves in the onset and maintenance of spontaneous hypertension. *Am. J. Physiol.*, 41:111–114.
57. Norvell, J. E. (1968): The aorticorenal ganglion and its role in renal innervation. *J. Comp. Neurol.*, 133:101–112.
58. Okamoto, K., Nosako, S., Yamori, Y., and Matsumoto, M. (1967): Participation of renal factors in the pathogenesis of hypertension in the spontaneously hypertensive rat. *Jpn. Heart J.*, 8:168–180.
59. Oliver, J. A., Pinto, J., Sciacca, R. R., and Cannon, P. J. (1980): Basal norepinephrine overflow into the renal vein: Effect of renal nerve stimulation. *Am. J. Physiol.*, 239:F371–F377.
60. Ricksten, S. E., Yao, T., DiBona, G. F., and Thoren, P. (1981). Renal nerve activity and exaggerated natriuresis in conscious spontaneously hypertensive rats. *Acta Physiol. Scand.*, 112:161–167.
61. Takeda, K., and Bunag, R. D. (1980): Augmented sympathetic nerve activity and pressor responses in DOCA hypertensive rats. *Hypertension*, 2:97–101.
62. Thames, M. D., and DiBona, G. F. (1979): Renal nerves modulate the secretion of renin mediated by non-neural mechanisms. *Circ. Res.*, 44:645–652.
63. Winternitz, S. R., Katholi, R. E., and Oparil, S. (1980): Role of the renal sympathetic nerves in the development and maintenance of hypertension in the spontaneously hypertensive rat. *J. Clin. Invest.*, 66:971–978.
64. Winternitz, S. R., Katholi, R. E., and Oparil, S. (1982): Decrease in hypothalamic norepinephrine content following renal denervation in the one-kidney, one-clip Goldblatt hypertensive rat. *Hypertension*, 4:369–373.
65. Yamada, S., Yamamura, H., and Roeske, W. R. (1980): Alterations in central and peripheral adrenergic receptors in deoxycorticosterone/salt hypertensive rats. *Life Sci.*, 27:2405–2416.

The Kidney in Hypertension, edited by Norman M. Kaplan, Barry M. Brenner, and John H. Laragh. Raven Press, New York © 1987.

Role of Intraglomerular Hypertension in the Initiation and Progression of Renal Disease

Sharon Anderson and Barry M. Brenner

Department of Medicine, Brigham and Women's Hospital, and Harvard Medical School, Boston, Massachusetts 02115

Systemic hypertension has long been recognized as a significant component of progressive renal disease, in that elevated systemic arterial pressure is both cause and consequence of chronic renal disease. The incidence of systemic hypertension in patients with serious renal disease approaches 90% (38). The incidence of renal failure attributable to "benign" essential hypertension, without an accelerated phase, is harder to define, but may be as high as 10% (43,50). However, although uncontrolled systemic hypertension is a known risk factor for the progressive deterioration of renal function in patients with renal disease (43,45), clinical studies have not uniformly demonstrated slowing of progressive renal disease with antihypertensive therapy. Recent studies in animal models of hypertensive renal disease have provided insight into this question by elucidating the complex and variable relationship between systemic and glomerular hypertension. The findings that systemic and glomerular hypertension are not necessarily co-occurrences, and that therapeutic interventions may affect systemic and glomerular capillary pressures independently, help to explain the renal response to systemic hypertension and to antihypertensive therapy, in a number of different circumstances.

EXPERIMENTAL MODELS OF HYPERTENSIVE RENAL DISEASE

Classically, systemic hypertension was believed to cause glomerular obsolescence as a consequence of ischemia, with decreased glomerular perfusion resulting from vascular disease in the preglomerular vasculature (39). However, recent studies have suggested the contrary, namely that glomerular capillary hyperperfusion and hypertension, rather than ischemia, initiate glomerular structural injury. Evidence in support of this pathogenetic mechanism comes from experimental studies of hypertensive renal disease, which may be usefully subdivided into categories based on the presence or absence of systemic and/or glomerular hypertension (Table 1).

Systemic Hypertension with Glomerular Hypertension

Afferent arteriolar resistance (R_A) determines the fraction of systemic pressure that is transmitted to the glomerular capillary network. In 1968 Hill and Heptinstall (29) proposed that it was a failure of afferent arteriolar vasoconstriction, rather than atherosclerotic narrowing, that allowed the development of sclerosis in the glomeruli of uninephrectomized rats with steroid-induced hypertension. More recently, Azar and co-workers extended this concept in micropuncture studies of salt-sensitive Holtzman hypertensive rats (4) (Table 1). In these rats, failure of R_A to increase in the face of systemic hypertension resulted in glomerular capillary hyperperfusion and hypertension, and the subsequent development of glomerular sclerosis. More recent studies have revealed a similar

Table 1. *Systemic and glomerular hypertension in experimental renal disease*

Authors	Model/strain	*SBP*	R_A	$\overline{P}_{GC}$
Adrendshorst & Beierwaltes (3) Azar et al. (6)	SHR	↑	↑	↔
Schweitzer & Gertz (55)	Goldblatt (unclipped kidney) (severe)	↑	↑	↑
Steiner et al. (59)	Goldblatt (unclipped kidney) (moderate)	↑	↔	↑
Azar et al. (4,5)	Holtzman "post-salt"	↑	↓	↑
Azar et al. (7)	Dahl salt-sensitive	↑	↓	↑
Baer & Bianchi (8)	Milan hypertensive	↑		↑
Dworkin et al. (20)	Mineralocorticoid-salt	↑	↓	↑
Dworkin & Feiner (18)	SHR/uninephrectomy	↑	↓	↑
Hostetter et al. (31) Anderson et al. (1,2) Meyer et al. (40)	Extensive renal ablation	↑	↓	↑
Hostetter et al. (32) Zatz et al. (69,70)	Diabetes mellitus	↔	↓	↑
Deen et al. (17)	Uninephrectomy	↔	↓	↑
Gushwa et al. (27)	Anti-GBM disease	↔	↓	↑

(SBP) Systemic blood pressure; (R_A) afferent arteriolar resistance; ($\overline{P}_{GC}$) glomerular capillary hydraulic pressure; (↑) increased; (↔) normal; (↓) decreased.

hemodynamic pattern, with transmission of high systemic pressures into the glomerular capillary network, in mineralocorticoid-salt hypertension (20), a salt-sensitive hypertensive model of nephrotoxic serum nephritis (47), and in the unclipped kidneys of rats with Goldblatt hypertension (55,59).

Perhaps the most extensively studied model of hypertensive renal disease is that produced by surgical excision of renal mass. Reduction of functioning nephron number leads to an increase in the single nephron glomerular filtration rate (SNGFR) in the remaining nephrons (17,31). Vascular resistance is reduced in both afferent and efferent arterioles, allowing an increase in the glomerular capillary plasma flow rate, Q_A. Because the decrease in afferent arteriolar resistance (R_A) is proportionately greater than that in efferent arteriolar resistance (R_E), the hydraulic pressure in the glomerular capillary ($\overline{P}_{GC}$) increases. Together, these increases in Q_A and $\overline{P}_{GC}$ account for compensatory single nephron hyperfiltration. Uninephrectomy in the rat does not produce systemic hypertension (13,17), but more extensive (>70%) reduction of renal mass leads to severe systemic hypertension, and a syndrome of progressive azotemia, proteinuria, and eventual glomerular sclerosis (1,48,57).

Brenner and colleagues have suggested that these compensatory elevations of glomerular capillary pressures and flows, though serving to maintain total kidney function for a period of time, are in fact maladaptive, and are responsible for the eventual development of proteinuria and glomerular structural injury in the remaining nephrons (16). Support for this concept comes from the demonstration that dietary protein restriction, which limits the adaptive increases in SNGFR, Q_A, and $\overline{P}_{GC}$, results in striking amelioration of the development of proteinuria and glomerular sclerosis in rats with extensive renal ablation (30,40,48) and mineralocorticoid-salt hypertension (20). Of note, dietary protein restriction is associated with reduction of systemic hypertension in the latter model, but has no effect on the high systemic pressures in rats with remnant kidneys. Thus, reduction of glomerular capillary pressures and flows exerts a beneficial effect even in the face of continued systemic hypertension.

Systemic Hypertension Without Glomerular Hypertension

Another example of systemic hypertension without glomerular capillary hypertension occurs in the spontaneously hypertensive rat (SHR), a commonly studied animal model of human essential hypertension. As Arendshorst and Beierwaltes (3) demonstrated, the glomerulus is protected from high systemic pressure in this model by relative afferent arteriolar vasoconstriction (Table 1). Despite the severe systemic hypertension, the superficial nephrons of the young SHR exhibit relatively low values for Q_A, and normal values for $\overline{P}_{GC}$ and SNGFR, together with relative resistance against the development of proteinuria and glomerular structural injury. In these rats, the juxtamedullary glomeruli, which have higher plasma flow rates and presumably higher capillary pressures, are the major source of the observed proteinuria and are also susceptible to glomerular sclerosis (22). Therefore, the relative afferent arteriolar vasoconstriction and consequent absence of glomerular capillary hypertension in the majority of the cortical glomeruli may explain the absence of severe progressive renal disease. Of note, the relative intrarenal vasoconstriction frequently noted in patients with benign essential hypertension (25) may be a reflection of an analogous renal hemodynamic pattern in these patients, thus providing an attractive explanation for the relatively infrequent occurrence of renal failure in these patients as well.

The importance of afferent arteriolar vasoconstriction in protection against glomerular structural damage in this model is clearly demonstrated when this protective vasoconstriction is abolished by uninephrectomy. As Dworkin and Feiner have recently demonstrated (18), removal of one kidney in young SHRs results in lowering of R_A in the remaining kidney, thereby allowing transmission of systemic hypertension to the glomeruli and elevation of $\overline{P}_{GC}$. This hemodynamic alteration is associated with a sharp increase in proteinuria, and acceleration of glomerular sclerosis. When the uninephrectomized SHR is fed a low (6%) protein diet, afferent arteriolar vasoconstriction is preserved, $\overline{P}_{GC}$ is maintained at normal levels, and glomerular structural injury is prevented. Thus, prevention of glomerular capillary hypertension appears to be an essential element in protection against glomerular injury in this model.

Glomerular Hypertension Without Systemic Hypertension

In contrast to extensive ablation of renal mass, uninephrectomy in the rat does not result in systemic hypertension (13,17). Nevertheless, the modest increases in glomerular capillary hyperperfusion and hypertension are associated with modest acceleration of the glomerular sclerosis seen in this condition (13,30,60). Similarly, glomerular capillary hypertension and eventual glomerular sclerosis have been noted in the normotensive kidneys of rats with anti-GBM antibody mediated glomerulonephritis (27).

A more prominent clinical example of glomerular hypertension without systemic hypertension is that seen in diabetes mellitus. In the insulin-treated rat with streptozotocin-induced diabetes mellitus, systemic arterial pressure is normal, but moderate hyperglycemia is accompanied by single nephron hyperfiltration, due to elevated values for Q_A and $\overline{P}_{GC}$ (32,69,70), the same hemodynamic pattern as in the remnant kidney rats. In these diabetic rats, intraglomerular hyperperfusion and hypertension also lead to glomerular sclerosis in the absence of systemic hypertension (69,70). As in the remnant kidney, therapeutic interventions that limit the adaptive increases in glomerular capillary pressures and flows retard the development of albuminuria and glomerular structural injury. As reported by Zatz and co-workers (70), dietary protein restriction limited glomerular capillary pressures and flows, and eventual glomerular sclerosis, in diabetic rats in the absence of any improvement in metabolic control. The critical role of glomerular capillary hypertension was further highlighted using another therapeutic intervention, the angiotensin I converting enzyme inhibitor (CEI) enalapril. A modest, 20-mm Hg reduction of systemic arterial pressure within the normal range was associated with normalization of $\overline{P}_{GC}$, without affecting the supranormal values for SNGFR and Q_A (69). Thus, control of glomerular hypertension results in protection against glomerular injury in this normotensive model as well. The clinical importance of these glomerular hemodynamic processes has been suggested by the observations that those patients with Type I diabetes with overt hyperfiltration at the time of diagnosis are more likely to progress to diabetic nephropathy (44), and that administration of the CEI captopril to patients with established diabetic nephropathy, in doses that do not affect systemic blood pressure, results in reduced urinary protein excretion over the short term (62).

Finally, uninephrectomy hastens glomerular injury, even in the absence of systemic hypertension, in such diverse forms of experimental renal disease as nephrotoxic serum nephritis, diabetes mellitus, puromycin aminonucleoside nephrosis, and lupus-like nephropathy (14,56,64,67). Presumably, unilateral nephrectomy adds to the hemodynamic burden of glomerular capillaries previously subjected to various injurious stresses, thereby accelerating glomerular destruction.

EFFECTS OF SUPERIMPOSED HYPERTENSION ON EXPERIMENTAL RENAL DISEASE

Although a number of studies have suggested that superimposition of systemic hypertension aggravates the course of experimental glomerulonephritis, many of these studies lacked the appropriate nonnephritic hypertensive controls (reviewed in 10). Recently, carefully performed studies have helped to clarify this issue. Neugarten and co-workers (46) compared otherwise normal rats with two-kidney, one-clip hypertension to nephritic rats with the same level of hypertension, and found that the combination of nephritis and hypertension resulted in glomerular injury far worse than that seen with either hypertension or nephritis alone. In the remnant kidney, further elevation of $\overline{P}_{GC}$ with superimposition of clip hypertension has been reported to accelerate glomerular sclerosis (63). Similarly, glomerular injury was accelerated in hypertensive, salt-sensitive Dahl rats with ferritin-antiferritin immune-complex glomerular injury (53). Since both clip hypertension and Dahl salt-sensitive hypertension are known to result in reduction of afferent arteriolar vasoconstriction and elevation of $\overline{P}_{GC}$ (7,59), it would appear that intraglomerular hypertension contributes to the accelerated injury associated with systemic hypertension in these models.

This point is further emphasized by recent studies involving the SHR. Systemic hypertension in the SHR does not appear to aggravate the course of experimental glomerulonephritis (49,53,58). Although glomerular hemodynamics were not assessed in these studies, it is reasonable to speculate that the relatively high values for R_A in the SHR prevented glomerular capillary hypertension, and thus protected the glomeruli from any synergistic deleterious effect of hypertension and glomerulonephritis. Thus, it appears that in renal parenchymal disease, as in the previous studies of renal ablation and diabetes mellitus, systemic hypertension exerts its detrimental effect by producing or accentuating glomerular capillary hypertension, rather than by a syndrome of acceleration of extraglomerular vascular injury and/or glomerular ischemia.

EFFECTS OF ANTIHYPERTENSIVE THERAPY IN EXPERIMENTAL RENAL DISEASE

Early studies of the effects of antihypertensive therapy in modulating the progression of experimental hypertensive renal disease gave conflicting and sometimes disappointing results (Table 2). In the SHR, triple drug therapy with reserpine, hydralazine, and hydrochlorothiazide was reported to protect against glomerular sclerosis when administered for 6 months (24), but a subsequent study found that this regimen only delayed, rather than prevented, the appearance of proteinuria and glomerular sclerosis (21). In the partially nephrectomized rat, Purkerson and co-workers (51) found only a modest reduction in glomerular sclerosis despite excellent control of systemic hypertension using this same triple drug regimen.

A hemodynamic explanation for the failure of triple therapy to prevent progressive renal disease has been provided by recent micropuncture studies of this regimen in several models of experimental renal disease. In the case of

Table 2. *Effects of antihypertensive therapy in experimental renal disease*

Authors	Therapy	*SBP*	$\overline{P}_{GC}$	*FGS*
	Extensive renal ablation			
Hostetter et al. (30,31) Meyer et al. (40)	Low protein diet	↔	↓	↓
Anderson et al. (1,2) Meyer et al. (40)	CEI	↓	↓	↓
Anderson et al. (2)	Triple therapy	↓	↔	↔
	Diabetes mellitus			
Zatz et al. (70)	Low protein diet	↔	↓	↓
Zatz et al. (69)	CEI	↓	↓	↓
	Mineralocorticoid-salt			
Dworkin et al. (20)	Low protein diet	↓	↓	↓
Dworkin et al. (19)	Triple therapy	↓	↔	↔
	Nephrotoxic serum nephritis/saline			
Neugarten et al. (47)	Triple therapy	↓	↓	↓

(*SBP*) Systemic blood pressure; ($\overline{P}_{GC}$) glomerular capillary hydraulic pressure; (*FGS*) focal glomerular sclerosis; (CEI) enalapril; (↔) no change; (↓) decreased.

saline-dependent hypertension in a model of nephrotoxic serum nephritis, Neugarten and co-workers (47) found that this regimen normalized systemic and glomerular capillary pressures, and exerted modest but by no means complete protection against renal injury. In contrast, Anderson and co-workers (2) documented extensive glomerular sclerosis despite excellent control of systemic hypertension with this regimen in rats subjected to one and two-thirds nephrectomy.

In this study, reduction of systemic pressure resulted in even further reduction in afferent arteriolar resistance, with no change in efferent arteriolar resistance, as compared with untreated rats with remnant kidneys. Accordingly, $\overline{P}_{GC}$ was maintained at very high levels in the rats made normotensive with triple therapy, and maintenance of glomerular capillary hypertension was associated with the development of proteinuria and eventual glomerular sclerosis. A similar failure of this regimen to limit $\overline{P}_{GC}$ and glomerular injury has been reported in mineralocorticoid-salt hypertension (19). Though glomerular hemodynamics were not studied, failure to control $\overline{P}_{GC}$ may also explain the failure of this regimen to limit proteinuria and glomerular structural injury in the SHR with renal ablation (54) and in Wistar rats with clip hypertension (41).

The hemodynamic consequences of this drug regimen are consistent with the known effects of these drugs on the renin-angiotensin system. Both the vasodilator hydralazine and the diuretic hydrochlorothiazide stimulate the renin-angiotensin system, and angiotensin II serves to enhance efferent arteriolar tone (15). Though hemodynamics were not studied, it is conceivable that the inclusion of the β-blocker metoprolol, which should suppress renin activity, explains the reported efficacy of a slightly different triple therapy regimen in preventing glomerular injury in spontaneously hypertensive rats with diabetes (52).

Alternatively, antihypertensive therapy that normalizes glomerular capillary pressure affords virtually complete protection against progressive glomerular injury. This has been convincingly demonstrated in studies using CEI therapy in experimental models of hypertensive renal disease. In rats with one and two-thirds nephrectomy, administration of enalapril resulted in control of systemic and glomerular hypertension, and marked limitation of the development of proteinuria and glomerular sclerosis (1,2). Reduction of systemic arterial pressure with CEI results in further lowering of R_A, as does triple therapy. In contrast to triple therapy, however, CEI also produces relaxation of R_E, and therefore results in normalization of $\overline{P}_{GC}$ (2). This reduction of R_E with CEI is consistent with inhibition of endogenous angiotensin II formation and action (15). Of note, however, the efficacy of CEI in reducing systemic or glomerular pressure is not dependent on prior stimulation of the circulating renin-angiotensin system, since plasma renin levels are normal or even low in rats with renal ablation (1,2) and diabetes mellitus (11). Though glomerular hemodynamics were not studied, therapy with CEI has also been reported to lessen glomerular injury in Heyman nephritis (33), the partially nephrectomized SHR (54), and clip hypertension (41).

Little is known of the intrarenal hemodynamic consequences of antihypertensive therapy with other available agents. Preliminary reports have suggested a protective effect in partially nephrectomized rats treated with verapamil (28), clonidine (68), or guanethidine plus hydralazine (66), but not with the calcium channel blocker fenoldipine (34). Clearly, further studies of the effect of these agents on glomerular capillary pressure are needed to clarify the potential role of these antihypertensive agents.

The foregoing studies with dietary protein restriction and with CEI therapy suggest that control of glomerular capillary hypertension, with or without control of systemic hypertension, is protective against the development of glomerular structural injury. In the majority of these studies, therapy has been initiated prior to or shortly after the process of renal injury is initiated. Recently Meyer and co-workers (40) investigated whether dietary protein restriction or CEI therapy would effectively control glomerular hypertension, and limit glomerular injury, even when therapy was delayed until hypertension and glomerular injury were established. Rats were subjected to one and two-thirds ablation and received no therapy, early CEI therapy, or late therapy with protein restriction or CEI, which was withheld until 8 weeks after ablation. Untreated rats demonstrated glomerular capillary hyperfiltration, hyperperfusion, and hypertension with progressive proteinuria and eventually extensive glomerular sclerosis. Early CEI therapy again controlled systemic and glomerular hypertension, and markedly limited the development of proteinuria and glomerular sclerosis. Rats receiving late therapy demonstrated systemic hypertension and progressive proteinuria up to the 8-week time point, when therapy was initiated. Thereafter, CEI controlled systemic blood pressure to normal levels, and both CEI and low-protein therapy controlled $\overline{P}_{GC}$ to near-normal levels. Reduction of $\overline{P}_{GC}$ was associated with stabilization of proteinuria, and limitation of glomerular sclerosis at levels previously seen just prior to this intervention. Thus, control of glomerular capillary hypertension may provide protection even when, as is the usual clinical case, therapy is not initiated until systemic hypertension and some degree of glomerular injury have been established.

THE PROGRESSION OF HUMAN RENAL DISEASE

Taken together, the experimental studies described above suggest that glomerular capillary hemodynamic derangements, and particularly glomerular capillary hypertension, initiate glomerular injury when nephron number is reduced and accelerate glomerular injury following other insults to the kidney. Studies in humans, though necessarily less direct, support the view that hyperperfused nephrons ultimately fail. Morphologic studies in human renal disease have demonstrated hypertrophy (presumably reflecting hyperperfusion and hyperfiltration) of those nephrons least damaged by disease (26). Clinical studies have demonstrated progressive loss of the renal function associated with increasing glomerular sclerosis in patients whose initiating disease process has remitted spontaneously or been controlled therapeutically. For example, patients with bilateral cortical necrosis may temporarily recover stable, albeit reduced, renal function before proceeding to end-stage renal failure (37). Recovery of renal function is frequently incomplete in acute renal failure of other etiologies, and in some of these cases progressive loss of renal function also follows initial recovery (23). Patients with vesicoureteric reflux who have developed significant impairment of renal function and glomerular disease manifested by proteinuria may progress to renal failure despite control of systemic hypertension, and surgical correction of the reflux (65). Likewise, patients with analgesic nephropathy, sometimes said to exhibit stable renal insufficiency, in fact often progress to renal failure despite discontinuation of analgesic medications (36). Progressive glomerular sclerosis in the absence of continuing immunologic injury has been demonstrated in certain patients after initial recovery from acute poststreptococcal glomerulonephritis (9). Hemodynamic factors might also explain the observation that pregnancy, which raises glomerular filtration and renal blood flow rates in normal women, frequently accelerates loss of renal function in those with preexisting renal disease (35).

SUMMARY

Recent experimental evidence has helped to clarify the role of systemic hypertension in the initiation and progression of renal disease. When afferent arteriolar resistance is lowered in the course of adaptation to reduction in functioning renal mass, enhanced transmission of systemic pressure results in glomerular capillary hypertension. Intraglomerular hypertension and hyperperfusion may be responsible for the accelerated glomerular injury in human as well as experimental renal disease.

Since elevated glomerular capillary pressures and flows cause progressive glomerular sclerosis in patients with renal insufficiency, therapies aimed at correcting these glomerular hemodynamic derangements may be useful in preserving renal function over the long term. One such therapy is dietary protein restriction, which may limit glomerular capillary hypertension and hyperperfusion despite its lack of effect on systemic hypertension. Promising results suggesting that protein restriction indeed slows the progression of a variety of renal disorders have recently been published (reviewed in 42).

Other therapies directed toward limiting glomerular capillary hypertension and hyperperfusion may ultimately prove more effective or more palatable than dietary protein restriction. Although long-term, prospective studies of the effects of antihypertensive therapy on progressive renal disease remain to be performed, recent preliminary reports suggest that therapy with CEI (12) or calcium channel blockers (61) may be effective in controlling systemic hypertension and stabilizing renal function in patients with renal insufficiency. Clearly, long-term controlled studies are needed to establish whether these beneficial effects of specific antihypertensive agents on renal blood flow and function, as compared with the more general beneficial effects of control of systemic hypertension, confer protection in the patient with progressive renal disease. In view of new evidence regarding systemic and glomerular hypertension, attention must be paid to the intrarenal hemodynamic consequences of antihypertensive therapy. Pharmacologic reduction of glomerular capillary hypertension may confer special benefit to the hypertensive patient at risk for progressive renal disease.

REFERENCES

1. Anderson, S., Meyer, T. W., Rennke, H. G., and Brenner, B. M. (1985): Control of glomerular hypertension limits glomerular injury in rats with reduced renal mass. *J. Clin. Invest.*, 76:612–619.
2. Anderson, S., Rennke, H. G., and Brenner, B. M. (1986): Therapeutic advantage of converting enzyme inhibitors in arresting progressive renal disease associated with systemic hypertension in the rat. *J. Clin. Invest.*, 77:1993–2000.
3. Arendshorst, W. J., and Beierwaltes, W. H. (1979): Renal and nephron hemodynamics in spontaneously hypertensive rats. *Am. J. Physiol.*, 236:F246–F251.
4. Azar, S., Johnson, M. A., Hertel, B., and Tobian, L. (1977): Single-nephron pressures, flows and resistances in hypertensive kidneys with nephrosclerosis. *Kidney Int.*, 12:28–40.
5. Azar, S., Johnson, M. A., Iwai, J., Bruno, L., and Tobian, L. (1978): Single nephron dynamics in "postsalt" rats with chronic hypertension. *J. Lab. Clin. Med.*, 91:156–166.
6. Azar, S., Johnson, M. A., Scheinman, J., Bruno, L., and Tobian, L. (1979): Regulation of glomerular capillary pressure and filtration rate in young Kyoto hypertensive rats. *Clin. Sci.*, 56:203–209.

7. Azar, S., Weller, D., Bruno, L., Livingston, S., and Iwai, J. (1977): Single nephron dynamics in the normotensive Dahl rat on high salt intake (Abstr.). *Clin. Res.*, 25:504A.
8. Baer, P. G., and Bianchi, G. (1978): Renal micropuncture study of normotensive and Milan hypertensive rats before and after development of hypertension. *Kidney Int.*, 13:452–466.
9. Baldwin, D. S. (1977): Poststreptococcal glomerulonephritis: A progressive disease? *Am. J. Med.*, 62:1–11.
10. Baldwin, D. S., and Neugarten, J. (1986): Blood pressure control and progression of renal insufficiency. In: *The Progressive Nature of Renal Disease, Vol. 14*, edited by W. E. Mitch, B. M. Brenner, and J. H. Stein, pp. 81–110. Churchill Livingstone, New York.
11. Ballermann, B. J., Skorecki, K. L., and Brenner, B. M. (1984): Reduced glomerular angiotensin II receptor density in early untreated diabetes mellitus in the rat. *Am. J. Physiol.*, 247:F110–F116.
12. Bauer, J. H., and Gaddy, P. (1985): Effect of enalapril alone, and in combination with hydrochlorothiazide, on renin-angiotensin-aldosterone, renal function, salt and water excretion, and body fluid composition. *Am. J. Kidney Dis.*, 4:222–232.
13. Beukers, J. J. B., Hoedemaeker, P. J., and Weening, J. J. (1986): Converting enzyme inhibition prevents the development of proteinuria and focal glomerular sclerosis in uninephrectomized Wistar rats (Abstr.). *Kidney Int.*, 29:265A.
14. Beyer, M. M., Steinberg, A. D., Nicastri, A. D., and Friedman, E. A. (1977): Unilateral nephrectomy: Effect on survival in NZB/NZW mice. *Science*, 198:511–513.
15. Blantz, R. C., Konnen, K. S., and Tucker, B. J. (1976): Angiotensin II effects upon the glomerular microcirculation and ultrafiltration coefficient of the rat. *J. Clin. Invest.*, 57:419–434.
16. Brenner, B. M., Meyer, T. W., and Hostetter, T. W. (1978): Dietary protein intake and the progressive nature of kidney disease. *N. Engl. J. Med.*, 307:652–660.
17. Deen, W. M., Maddox, D. A., Robertson, C. R., and Brenner, B. M. (1974): Dynamics of glomerular ultrafiltration in the rat. VII. Response to reduced renal mass. *Am. J. Physiol.*, 227:556–562.
18. Dworkin, L. D., and Feiner, H. D. (1986): Glomerular injury in uninephrectomized spontaneously hypertensive rats. A consequence of glomerular capillary hypertension. *J. Clin. Invest.*, 77:797–809.
19. Dworkin, L. D., Feiner, H. D., and Randazzo, J. (1985): Evidence for hemodynamically mediated glomerular injury despite antihypertensive therapy in rats with desoxycorticosterone-salt hypertension (Abstr.). *Kidney Int.*, 27:189A.
20. Dworkin, L. D., Hostetter, T. H., Rennke, H. G., and Brenner, B. M. (1984): Hemodynamic basis for glomerular injury in rats with desoxycorticosterone-salt hypertension. *J. Clin. Invest.*, 73:1448–1461.
21. Feld, L.G., Van Liew, J. B., Brentjens, J. R., and Boylan, J. W. (1981): Renal lesions and proteinuria in the spontaneously hypertensive rat made normotensive by treatment. *Kidney Int.*, 20:606–614.
22. Feld, L.G ., Van Liew, J. B., Galaske, R. G., and Boylan, J. W. (1977): Selectivity of renal injury and proteinuria in the spontaneously hypertensive rat. *Kidney Int.*, 12:332–343.
23. Finn, W. F. (1983): Recovery from acute renal failure. In: *Acute Renal Failure*, edited by B. M. Brenner and J. M. Lazarus, pp. 753–774. Saunders, Philadelphia.
24. Freis, E. D., Ragan, D., Pillsbury, H., and Mathews, M. (1972): Alteration of the course of hypertension in the spontaneously hypertensive rat. *Circ. Res.*, 31:1–7.
25. Goldring, W., Chasis, H., Ranges, H. A., and Smith, H. W. (1941): Effective renal blood flow in subjects with essential hypertension. *J. Clin. Invest.*, 20:637–653.
26. Gottschalk, C. W. (1971): Function of the chronically diseased kidney: The adaptive nephron. *Circ. Res.*, 28(*Suppl.* 1):1–13.
27. Gushwa, L. C., Wilson, C. B., and Blantz, R. C. (1984): Chronic effects of concomitant hypertension on glomerular hemodynamics in a model of anti-glomerular basement membrane nephritis (Abstr.). *Clin. Res.*, 32:533A.
28. Harris, D. C. H., Hammond, W. S., Burke, T. J., and Schrier, R. W. (1986): Protective effect of verapamil on progression of experimental chronic renal failure (Abstr.). *Kidney Int.*, 29:319A.
29. Hill, G. S., and Heptinstall, R. H. (1968): Steroid-induced hypertension in the rat. *Am. J. Pathol.*, 52:1–20.
30. Hostetter, T. H., Meyer, T. W., Rennke, H. G., and Brenner, B. M. (1986): Chronic effects of dietary protein on renal structure and function in the rat with intact and reduced renal mass. *Kidney Int.*, 30:509–517.
31. Hostetter, T. H., Olson, J. L., Rennke, H. G., Venkatachalam, M. A., and Brenner, B. M. (1981): Hyperfiltration in remnant nephrons: A potentially adverse response to renal ablation. *Am. J. Physiol.*, 241:F85–F93.
32. Hostetter, T. H., Troy, J. L., and Brenner, B. M. (1981): Glomerular hemodynamics in experimental diabetes mellitus. *Kidney Int.*, 19:410–415.
33. Hutchison, F. N., Schambelan, M., and Kaysen, G. A. (1986): Enalapril blocks increased albuminuria resulting from high protein intake in nephrotic rats (Abstr.). *Kidney Int.*, 29:320A.
34. Jackson, B., Cubela, R., and Debrevi, L. (1986): Preservation of renal function in the rat remnant kidney model of chronic renal failure by blood pressure reduction (Abstr.). *Kidney Int.*, 29:867A.
35. Kincaid-Smith, P. (1975): *The Kidney: A Clinico-Pathological Study*, pp. 222–239. Blackwell Scientific, Oxford.
36. Kincaid-Smith, P. (1980): Analgesic abuse and the kidney. *Kidney Int.*, 17:250–260.
37. Kleinknecht, C., Grünfeld, J. P., Gomez, P. C., Moreau, J. F., and Garcia-Torres, R. (1973): Diagnostic procedures and long-term prognosis in bilateral renal cortical necrosis. *Kidney Int.*, 4:390–400.
38. Lazarus, J. M., Hampers, C. L., and Merrill, J. P. (1974): Hypertension in chronic renal failure. *Arch. Intern. Med.*, 133:1059–1066.

39. McManus, J. F. A., and Lupton, C. H., Jr. (1960): Ischemic obsolescence of renal glomeruli. The natural history of the lesions and their relation to hypertension. *Lab. Invest.*, 9:413–434.
40. Meyer, T. W., Anderson, S., Rennke, H. G., and Brenner, B.M. (1986): Reversing glomerular hypertension stabilizes established glomerular injury. *Kidney Int.* (*in press*).
41. Michel, J. B., Dussaule, J. C., Choudat, L., Auzan, C., Nochy, D., Corvol, P., and Menard, J. (1986): Effects of antihypertensive treatment in one-clip, two kidney hypertension in rats. *Kidney Int.*, 29: 1011–1020.
42. Mitch, W. E. (1984): The influence of diet on the progression of renal insufficiency. *Annu. Rev. Med.*, 35:249–264.
43. Mitchell, H. C., Graham, R. M., and Pettinger, W. A. (1980): Renal function during long-term treatment of hypertension with minoxidil. Comparison of benign and malignant hypertension. *Ann. Intern. Med.*, 93:676–681.
44. Mogensen, C. E., and Christensen, C. K. (1984): Predicting diabetic nephropathy in insulin-dependent patients. *N. Engl. J. Med.*, 311:89–93.
45. Moyer, J. H., Heider, C., Pevey, K. and Ford, R. V. (1958): The effect of treatment on the vascular deterioration associated with hypertension, with particular emphasis on renal function. *Am. J. Med.*, 24:177–192.
46. Neugarten, J., Feiner, H. D., Schacht, R. G., Gallo, G. R., and Baldwin, D. S. (1982): Aggravation of experimental glomerulonephritis by superimposed clip hypertension. *Kidney Int.*, 22:257–263.
47. Neugarten, J., Kaminetsky, B., Feiner, H. D., Schacht, R. G., Liu, D. T., and Baldwin, D. S. (1985): Nephrotoxic serum nephritis with hypertension: Amelioration by antihypertensive therapy. *Kidney Int.*, 28:135–139.
48. Olson, J. L., Hostetter, T. H., Rennke, H. G., Brenner, B. M., and Venkatachalam, M. A. (1982): Altered glomerular permselectivity and progressive sclerosis following extreme ablation of renal mass. *Kidney Int.*, 22:112–126.
49. Olson, J. L., Wilson, S. K., and Heptinstall, R. H. (1986): Relation of glomerular injury to preglomerular resistance in experimental hypertension. *Kidney Int.*, 29:849–857.
50. Papper, S., and Vaamonde, C. A. (1971): Nephrosclerosis. In: *Diseases of the Kidney, Vol. 2*, edited by M. B. Strauss and L. G. Welt, pp. 735–768. Little, Brown, Boston.
51. Purkerson, M. L., Hoffsten, P. E., and Klahr, S. (1976): Pathogenesis of the glomerulopathy associated with renal infarction in rats. *Kidney Int.*, 9:407–417.
52. Rabkin, R., Petersen, J., Kitaji, J., Marck, B., Murphy, W., and Muirhead, E. E. (1984): Effect of antihypertensive therapy on the kidney in spontaneously hypertensive rats with diabetes (Abstr.). *Kidney Int.*, 25:205A.
53. Raij, L., Azar, S., and Keane, W. F. (1985): Role of hypertension in progressive glomerular immune injury. *Hypertension*, 7:398–404.
54. Raij, L., Chiou, X., Owens, R., and Wrigley, B. (1985): Therapeutic implications of hypertension-induced glomerular injury. Comparison of enalapril and a combination of hydralazine, reserpine, and hydrochlorothiazide in an experimental model. *Am. J. Med.*, 79(*Suppl.* 3C):37–41.
55. Schweitzer, G., and Gertz, K. H. (1979): Changes of hemodynamics and glomerular ultrafiltration in renal hypertension of rats. *Kidney Int.*, 15:134–143.
56. Seyer-Hansen, K. (1978): Renal hypertrophy in experimental diabetes: A comparison to compensatory hypertrophy. *Diabetologia*, 14:325–328.
57. Shimamura, T., and Morrison, A. B. (1975): A progressive glomerulosclerosis occurring in partial five-sixths nephrectomized rats. *Am. J. Pathol.*, 79:95–106.
58. Stein, H. D., Sterzel, R. B., Hunt, J. D., Pabst, R., and Kashgarian, M. (1986): No aggravation of the course of experimental glomerulonephritis in spontaneously hypertensive rats. *Am. J. Pathol.*, 122:520–530.
59. Steiner, R. W., Tucker, B. J., Gushwa, L. C., Gifford, J., Wilson, C. B., and Blantz, R. C. (1982): Glomerular hemodynamics in moderate Goldblatt hypertension in the rat. *Hypertension*, 4:51–57.
60. Striker, G. E., Nagle, R. B., Kohnen, P. W., and Smuckler, E. A. (1969): Response to unilateral nephrectomy in old rats. *Arch. Pathol.*, 87:439–442.
61. Sunderrajan, S., Reams, G. P., and Bauer, J. H. (1986): Reversible renal vascular changes in essential hypertension with diltiazem (Abstr.). *Proc. Am. Soc. Hypertension*, 36A.
62. Taguma, Y., Kitamoto, Y., Futaki, G., Ueda, H., Monma, H., Ishikazi, M., Takahashi, H., Sekino, H., and Sasaki, Y. (1985): Effect of captopril on heavy proteinuria in azotemic diabetics. *N. Engl. J. Med.*, 313:1617–1620.
63. Tapia, E., Franco, M., Calleja, C., Cermeno, J. L., Bobadilla, N.A., Perez, J.M., Gabbai, F., and Herrera-Acosta, J. (1986): Role of glomerular pressure and flow in renal damage of Goldblatt hypertension with partial renal ablation (Abstr.). *Kidney Int.*, 29:260A.
64. Teodoru, C. V., Saifer, A., and Frankel, H. (1959): Conditioning factors influencing evolution of experimental glomerulonephritis in rabbits. *Am. J. Physiol.*, 196:457–460.
65. Torres, V. E., Velosa, J. A., Holley, K. E., Kelalis, P. P., Stickler, G. B., and Kurtz, S. B. (1980): The progression of vesicoureteral reflux nephropathy. *Ann. Int. Med.*, 92:776–784.
66. Tsuruda, H., Okuda, S., Onoyama, K., Oh, Y., and Fujishima, M. (1986): Effect of blood pressure on the progress of renal deterioration in rats with renal mass reduction. *J. Lab. Clin. Med.*, 107:43–50.
67. Velosa, J. A., Glasser, R. J., Nevins, T. E., and Michael, A. F. (1977): Experimental model of focal sclerosis. II. Correlation with immunopathologic changes, macromolecular kinetics, and polyanion loss. *Lab. Invest.*, 36:527–534.
68. Wilke, W. L., Fettman, M. J., and Tan, A. A. (1986): Abatement of the progression of chronic renal disease in the rat by clonidine (Abstr.). *Kidney Int.*, 29:327A.

69. Zatz, R., Dunn, B. R., Meyer, T. W., Anderson, S., Rennke, H.G., and Brenner, B.M. (1986): Prevention of diabetic glomerulopathy by pharmacological amelioration of glomerular capillary hypertension. *J. Clin. Invest.*, 77:1925–1930.

70. Zatz, R., Meyer, T. W., Rennke, H. G., and Brenner, B. M. (1985): Predominance of hemodynamic rather than metabolic factors in the pathogenesis of diabetic glomerulopathy. *Proc. Natl. Acad. Sci. USA*, 82:5963–5967.

The Kidney in Hypertension, edited by
Norman M. Kaplan, Barry M. Brenner,
and John H. Laragh. Raven Press,
New York © 1987.

Pathology of the Kidney in Hypertension

Michael Kashgarian

Department of Pathology, Yale University School of Medicine, New Haven, Connecticut 06510

The role that the renal vessels play in the pathogenesis of essential hypertension has been debated for many years. The interplay between the kidney and the cardiovascular systems was recognized as far back as 1868 in Johnson's report on Bright's disease (19). He associated the thickening of the walls of the arterioles of the granular kidney of Bright's disease with cardiac hypertrophy. Shortly thereafter Gull and Sutton (15) described generalized small vessel disease, which they called "arteriocapillary fibrosis," and suggested that the vascular disease was a primary pathologic change responsible for hypertension. The description of two types of contracted kidneys—inflammatory and arteriosclerotic—by Jores in 1904 (21) provided an anatomical basis for differentiating secondary hypertension associated with renal disease from primary essential hypertension.

By the early twentieth century, three apparently divergent theories began to emerge. One postulated that renal disease was primary and that associated vascular disease and hypertension were its results. The second suggested that renal disease was part of a primary diffuse vascular disease and that progressive vascular sclerosis increased peripheral resistance resulting in systemic hypertension. The third maintained that essential hypertension itself was a primary disease and that the vascular diseases seen in all organs were a result rather than a cause. Even from the simplistic analysis of the formula that relates mean arterial pressure to a product of the cardiac output and the total peripheral resistance, it can be seen that the structure of the small vessels is an important determinant in the pathogenesis of systemic hypertension.

The unique importance of the small vessels of the kidney was emphasized by Fishberg (8). He described a pattern of vascular damage in patients with chronic hypertension not associated with inflammatory or obstructive renal disease where the small vessels of the kidney showed sclerosis in the absence of vascular disease of similar intensity in other organs. Fahr (7) further distinguished the vascular lesions of hypertension into compensated benign, decompensated benign, and malignant nephrosclerosis. These early morphological studies have been confirmed in numerous studies over the years. The uniqueness of the relationship between the kidney and hypertension was emphasized by Moritz and Oldt (29) in a now classic paper in which they state, "Arteriolar sclerosis occurs as a primary pathological change. When the renal arterioles become sclerotic, hypertension is invariably present. This was in the kidneys and no comparable correlation could be found in any other organs or tissue." Furthermore, combining their morphological observations with the then recently published studies of experimental hypertension by Goldblatt (13), they concluded, "The effect of renal arteriolar sclerosis in human hypertension appears to be the functional analog of the renal arterial clamp in experimental hypertension. Arteriolar sclerosis is the most common cause of chronic hypertension." These observations are now generally interpreted as being part of both cause and effect in chronic hypertension. In the two-kidney, one-clip model of experimental hypertension, the hypertension that develops will disappear with the removal of the clip in the early phase. Late removal of the clip has no effect and hypertension persists, but if the contralateral unclipped kidney is then removed, blood pressure is normalized. Examination of the small vessels of both kidneys reveals that the arteriolar sclerosis is present in the unprotected unclipped kidney, whereas the vessels of the clipped kidney appear normal and have been protected from the vascular disease of hypertension (12). Indeed, early studies by Hueck (18) suggested that the existence of hypertension of only a few weeks could result in structural changes in the arteriolar walls. More recently, morphometric studies by Tracy and coworkers (40) have confirmed that the renal arteriolar lesions are related to the severity and length of hypertension, whereas Bohle and coworkers (2,28) have begun to separate out the effects of hypertension on preglomerular and postglomerular vasculature in an attempt to separate direct effects of increased pressure from changes due to ischemia. The interrelationship of the vascular disease with the endocrine role of the kidney in relation to the renin-angiotensin system, the effects of antidiuretic hormone, the prostaglandin system, and other vasoactive or ion-transport-related systems further complicates and enhances the role of the kidney in hypertension.

Aside from the virtues of any of these theories relative to the primary or secondary nature of the renal vascular lesions, it is clear that the microangiopathy of hypertension is a distinct and perhaps unique lesion that involves the kidney preferentially. It is, therefore, of importance to understand the anatomical and biochemical nature of the arteriolar changes seen in hypertension.

MICROVASCULAR DISEASE OF THE KIDNEY IN HYPERTENSION

The vessels most susceptible to pathologic change in hypertension are the small arteries and arterioles. The preglomerular vessels tend to be more prominently affected than the postglomerular arterioles. Small arteries of a diameter of 50 to 150 μm are characterized by one to three layers of vascular smooth muscle in the media. The endothelium is separated from the media by a fenestrated internal elastic lamina. The endothelium or intima consists of a single layer of endothelial cells on an opposed basement membrane. The arterioles are vessels that have outer diameters measuring 50 μm or less with only a single layer of smooth muscle and no elastic lamina. The endothelial cells of both small arteries and arterioles are joined by incomplete tight junctions. The cytoplasm contains the usual complement of cytoplasmic organelles including coated pits and pinocytotic vesicles. The incomplete tight junctions and pinocytotic vesicles may represent an anatomic correlate of a double system of pores for transendothelial transport of low- and high-molecular-weight substances.

The vascular pathology of the small vessels of the kidney falls into three general categories—hyaline arteriolar sclerosis, myointimal hypertrophy and hyperplasia, and fibrinoid necrosis. Hyaline arteriolar sclerosis is seen in all forms of hypertension, whereas hyperplastic arteriolosclerosis and necrotizing arteriolitis have been considered hallmarks of malignant hypertension.

HYALINE ARTERIOLOSCLEROSIS

Perhaps the most interesting microvascular pathology is the lesion of hyaline arteriolosclerosis (6). Indeed, the lesion has been described by Zollinger (46) as playing the role of the great sphinx of renal pathology. Hyaline is derived from the Greek *hyalos,* meaning glass. It has been given this description because the walls of the vessels are thickened by the deposition of homogeneous glassy material, which is eosinophilic (Fig. 1). Ultrastructurally (Fig. 2) the deposition of hyaline is associated with atrophy of the smooth muscle cells and by irregular thickening of the basement membrane and collagen as well as a homogeneous dense material which by immunofluorescent studies contains plasma proteins, including immunoglobulins and

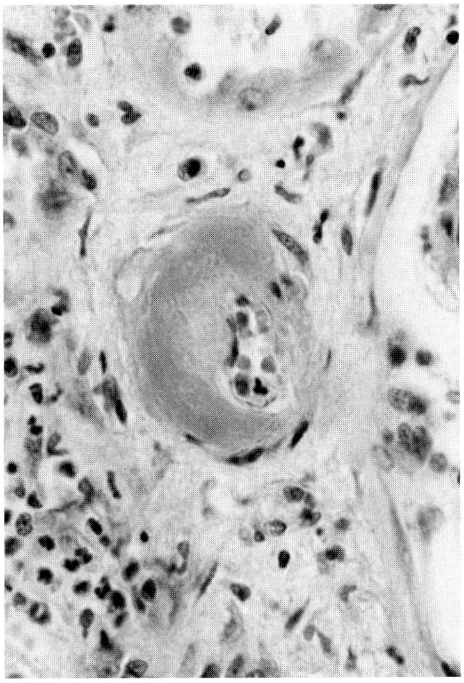

FIG. 1. Photomicrograph of a glomerular arteriole with striking hyaline arteriolar sclerosis. The vessel wall is thickened by the deposition of a homogeneous amorphous "glassy" material. There is evidence of atrophy of the cells of the arteriolar wall and narrowing of the lumen. ×600.

complement. Although mild hyaline arteriolosclerosis is often encountered in aged patients having moderate systolic hypertension, it is most prominently seen in patients with hypertension or diabetes. The changes associated with aging are usually minimal and focal and are generally not associated with elevations of diastolic pressure. The lesion in patients with hypertension is usually more dramatic. Its presence is unrelated to age and appears to have a relationship to both severity and duration of the hypertension. Although occasional patients with essential hypertension show minimal changes, this is related either to duration, lability, or lack of severity of the hypertension.

The exact biochemical nature and origin of hyaline is still not completely understood. It appears to be composed largely of glycoproteins mixed with collagenous matrix. Histochemically, it avidly takes the periodate acid Schiff (PAS) stain and has positive Millon and sulfhydryl reactions. Lipid is also present diffusely mixed with the glycoprotein and collagenous matrix. Rokitansky (35) was the first to propose that this material might be derived from substances filtered from the bloodstream. Hueck (18) later described an insudative lesion derived from plasma constituents that had leaked across injured endothelium into the arteriolar wall (9,36). Others have felt that hyaline originates from the degeneration or necrosis of smooth muscle cells and medial collagen with release of degenerative components into the media of the vessel (27). And finally, it has been suggested that hyaline deposits may be formed by the coalescence of increased amounts of basement membrane material synthesized by endothelial and smooth

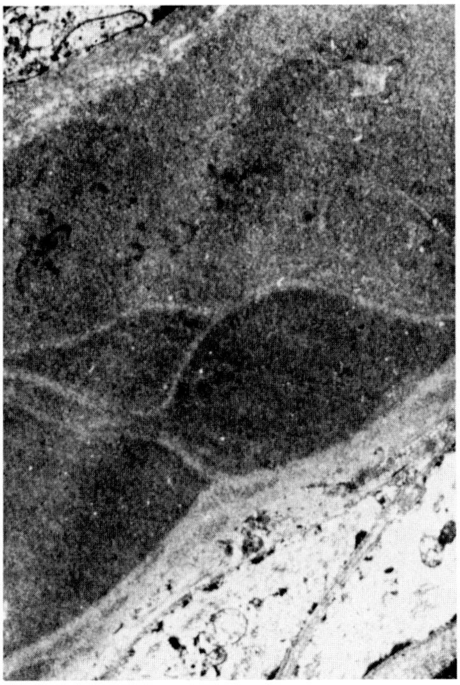

FIG. 2. Electron micrograph of the wall of an arteriole involved with hyaline arteriolar sclerosis. There is splitting and lamination of the basement membrane by deposition of a electron-dense material that comprises the hyaline. Smooth muscle cells cannot be easily identified, and the pericytes are flattened and elongated. ×13,000.

muscle cells (27,44). Since there is some evidence to support each of these concepts, it is likely to be a combination of all. The end result is a thicker and less compliant small vessel, which results in a more or less fixed vascular lumen leading to an elevation of peripheral vascular resistance and relative ischemia of the regions supplied by the vessel.

The interplay between the extracellular matrix and the cellular components of the vessel wall undoubtedly are important in the pathogenesis of hyaline arteriolosclerosis. At the present time at least ten separate types of collagenous proteins have been identified. Of these, at least seven types have been found in the extracellular matrix of vessels or are known to be synthesized by endothelial cells or vascular smooth muscle cells. Type I, III, and VI collagens are found as organized fibrillar collagens in the interstitial connective tissue regions of the vessel wall and adjacent tissues. The basement membrane collagens IV and V are found in the basal lamina that underlies the endothelium and surrounds the vascular smooth muscle cells and pericytes. Type VIII collagen and a heparan-inducible 60-kilodalton collagenous protein are synthesized by bovine endothelial cells and vascular smooth muscle cells in culture. In addition, there are a number of matrix-associated proteins, including the attachment proteins laminin and fibronectin, as well as a variety of glycoproteins, including glycosoaminoglycans. One of these, heparan sulfate proteoglycan, has been demonstrated to be important in regulating the permeability of basement membranes by limiting the penetration of charged macromolecules. The matrix components are synthesized by the various cellular elements of the vessel wall. Unfortunately, except for a few isolated studies, little is known about the alterations in collagen synthesis and structure seen in hypertensive states. The histochemical and morphological studies of hyaline arteriolosclerosis suggest that matrix components comprise at least a part of the material that is deposited (43). Whether this occurs as a result of increased synthesis, increased incorporation of plasma constituents, decreased degradation, or a combination is presently unclear.

Biochemical analysis of the composition of the vascular wall in hypertension has demonstrated a number of interesting changes that relate to the structural abnormalities that have been observed. Sodium, calcium, and water content of the vessel walls is increased, and studies on sodium exchange have suggested that the increased sodium is located in the extracellular matrix (39). Glycosoaminoglycans, the matrix-associated proteins that are potent binders of cations, have also been shown to be increased in experimental hypertension (32) and may provide the binding sites for these cations. Similarly, increased absolute amounts of collagen and elastin have been found (45). Increased incorporation of [^{14}C]lysine into collagenous proteins of the vessel walls of animals with experimental hypertension has indicated that stimulated collagen synthesis is of importance (31). Of particular interest in these experiments of Udenfreund and co-workers (41) is one in which the potent inhibitor of collagen crosslinking, β-aminopropriononitryl, was given to a strain of spontaneously hypertensive rats. It blocked the increase in lysine incorporation into collagen and was associated with amelioration of the systemic hypertension. These experiments tend to suggest that even if vascular collagenosis and sclerosis is not a primary initiating factor in the pathogenesis of hypertension, its presence influences the persistence and perhaps the severity of hypertension.

The connective tissue components of the vessel wall are synthesized by the various cellular elements, and there is an increasing body of evidence that alterations of cytoskeletal structure can stimulate or modulate synthetic activities. Experiments on the effect of vasoactive amines or vascular smooth muscle demonstrate stimulation of metabolism with increases in oxygen consumption, cytochrome oxidase activity, and utilization of glucose (1). Although increased workload imposed by contraction of the smooth muscle cells may partially account for these effects, increased protein synthesis can also account for this observation. Similar effects have also been identified in endothelial and pericytic type cells. On the basis of these experiments, one can postulate that when vasoactive amines induce persistent or intense contraction of medial smooth muscle cells, alterations in the cytoskeleton have a stimulatory effect on protein synthesis and lead to hyaline sclerosis. The amines may also be direct mediators of protein synthesis. Thus, whereas in the early phases of hypertension, removal of the stimulus to contraction and protein synthesis would allow return of the vessel to its normal tone and structure, persistence of the chemical mediation of hypertension may result in increased deposition of hyaline within the vessel wall, with the structural changes yielding a vessel with fixed compliance, resulting in persistence of hypertension.

Conversely, there is additional evidence that growth and differentiation of cells is influenced directly by the composition of the extracellular matrix. Endothelial cells that have been cultured on an extracellular matrix secreted and deposited by other endothelial cells have a different response to growth factors and vasoactive amines than cells grown on artificial substrates (23). Similarly, epithelial cell differentiation has been shown to be influenced by the matrix on which cultured cells are grown (14). Proper orientation, cellular differentiation, and the rate of cell growth have been shown to differ relative to the composition and configuration of the extracellular matrix (16). If one accepts the possibility that at least a portion of the hyaline deposits are derived from plasma macromolecules, alterations induced in the matrix by accumulation of these macromolecules may stimulate medial smooth muscle cells to produce additional matrix and contribute to the progression of the arteriolosclerosis.

This system would be analogous to those arguments which have been advanced to explain the development of glomerulosclerosis. Changes in glomerular hemodynamics or increased transglomerular traffic of plasma proteins with accumulation in the mesangium have been implicated as possibly serving as the stimulus to the proliferation of mesangial cells and matrix, eventuating in glomerulosclerosis (30).

Evidence that there is transudation of plasma proteins into the vessel wall in hyaline arteriolosclerosis associated with hypertension is the finding that IgM and early and late classical complement pathway components can also be identified within the vessel wall (33). A recent study (11) demonstrates that iC3b is bound via an ester linkage to hydroxyl groups on the repeating disaccharide units of hyaluronic acid, one of the major components of the glycosoaminoglycans present in hyaline arteriolosclerosis. Slow, spontaneous activation of either the classical or alternative complement pathway may occur and so provide a stimulus to matrix synthesis and deposition.

Hyaline arteriolosclerosis is also accelerated in patients with diabetes. Recent studies have demonstrated a reduced synthesis of basement membrane heparan sulfate proteoglycans at the same time that proline incorporation into laminin and collagenous protein was increased (34). These findings suggest a possible model to account for the glomerular sclerosis of diabetes. Decreased proteoglycan levels would be expected to make the basement membrane more permeable to anionic proteins, and this change could induce the compensatory synthesis of basement membrane components in an attempt to rectify the increased porosity. The resulting unbalanced synthesis would lead to increased deposition of basement membrane and sclerosis. In other studies, altered microcirculatory dynamics have been demonstrated to influence the rate of development of diabetic glomerular lesions (25). In unclipped normotensive rats, characteristic glomerular lesions develop fully in both kidneys. However, when hypertension is experimentally induced using the two-kidney, one-clip hypertensive model, a distinct asymmetry in the development of lesions is found. In the unclipped kidney exposed to elevated systemic pressure, more severe diabetic glomerular changes are present when compared with normotensive diabetic rats, whereas in the clipped or protected kidney of the hypertensive diabetic rat, there is a lesser degree of glomerulosclerosis when compared to the normotensive diabetic control. These studies suggest that local hemodynamic changes can influence the metabolic alterations and further emphasize the interrelationship between cell, matrix, and hemodynamic and biochemical changes.

MYOINTIMAL HYPERPLASIA

The second morphological abnormality of small arteries and arterioles that can be attributed to elevated systemic pressures is a hyperplastic lesion involving the smooth muscle and intima of these vessels. Hyperplastic arteriolosclerosis is generally associated with acute or persistent severe elevations of blood pressure and therefore is seen more frequently in malignant hypertension than in benign hypertension. Hyperplastic lesions are not unique to the arterioles and occur in small and large arteries as well. In the small vessels, the uniform concentric thickening of the vessel has led to its description as "onion-skinning" (Figs. 3 and 4). The hyperplasia causes marked narrowing of the lumen. Although originally described as intimal thickening, suggesting endothelial proliferation, recent studies have identified the cells involved in the hyperplastic thickening to be modified smooth muscle cells or myointimal cells that originate in the media of the vessel (Fig. 5) and migrate into the intima through the fenestrations of the incomplete internal elastic lamina (4). The vascular smooth muscle in hypertension has been extensively studied. The changes are hypertrophic as well

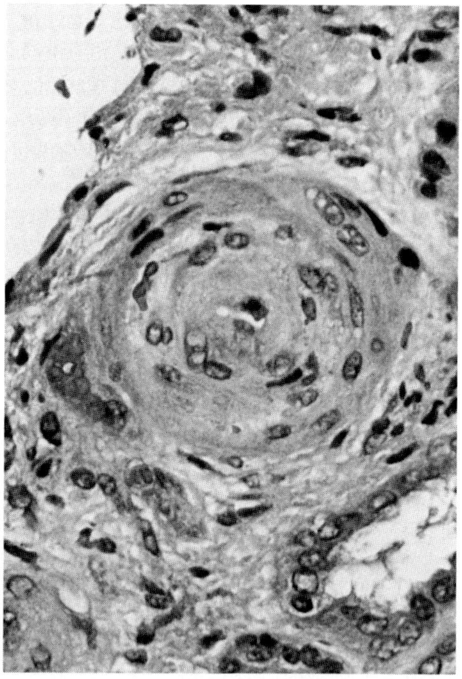

FIG. 3. Photomicrograph of an arteriole with striking myointimal hyperplasia. There is marked narrowing of the lumen by a hyperplasia of the medial cells, as can be seen by the increased numbers of nuclei. In addition, there appears to be an increase of homogeneous matrix material between the cells. ×600.

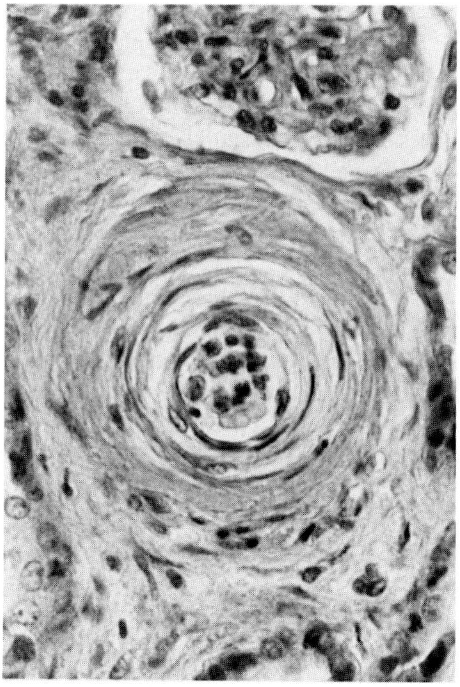

FIG. 4. Photomicrograph of an intralobular artery demonstrating "onion-skinning." The onion-skinning is similar to the myointimal proliferation seen in the arterioles, but the nuclei are more elongated and the proliferating myointimal cells are more spindled in their configuration. ×600.

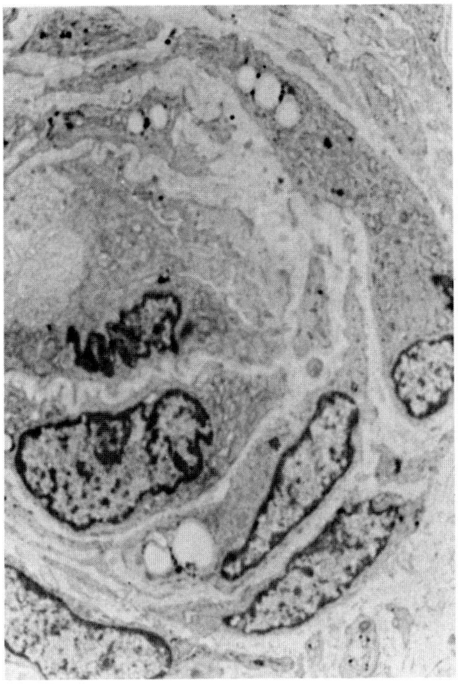

FIG. 5. Electron micrograph of an arteriole with myointimal hyperplasia. The lumen is markedly compromised by the proliferation of cells and reduplication of the basement membranes and matrix. The cells are elongated, contain lipid and sparse organelles, and have features of both smooth muscle cells and endothelial cells. ×4,500.

as hyperplastic. In one study, Freedman and colleagues (10) have reported that in deoxycorticosterone-induced hypertension in the rat surface area and volume of individual smooth muscle cells were increased, demonstrating cellular hypertrophy. Thymidine incorporation is increased, indicating that cell multiplication and hyperplasia are also present. In addition, there is evidence that there is myofiber necrosis with release of debris into the intercellular space associated with an increase in deposition of collagen and glycoproteins. This change is seen as the deposition of a mucoid substance identified by Alcian blue staining. The hyperplastic lesion also demonstrates reduplication of the elastic lamina and an increase in the thickness of the basal lamina.

One interesting mechanism has been postulated to explain this lesion (22). At critical levels the action of vasoactive amines such as angiotensin II, epinephrine, and vasopressin results in an intermittent vascular contraction, producing a "sausage-string" appearance. The turbulence produced in such vessels results in endothelial damage and platelet activation. Platelet factors including thromboxane and platelet growth factor are released and both enhance the intermittent contraction of the vessel and stimulate proliferation and migration of the myointimal cells.

FIBRINOID ARTERIOLAR NECROSIS

The third and perhaps the most dramatic lesion is necrotizing arteriolitis. Fibrinoid necrosis of the arterioles is considered by some to be the hallmark of malignant or accelerated hypertension. The lesion is generally superimposed on existing hyperplastic or hyaline lesions, but it is also occasionally seen as a first event in children and adolescents presenting with severe acute malignant hypertension. Indeed, Linton (24) has hypothesized that a primary arteriolitis resulting in insudation of fibrin into the vascular walls may account for hypertension in such cases. The presence of immunoglobulins within the vessel wall has also led Paronetto (33) to postulate an immunologic mechanism. The lesion consists of obliteration of the normal medial architecture by necrosis with the deposition of a deep eosinophilic granular fibrin-like material (Fig. 6). Ultrastructural examination reveals the fibrillar material embedded in hyaline to have a periodicity considered to be characteristic of fibrin or fibrinogen. Immunofluorescent studies have also confirmed the presence of fibrin in the walls (42). It seems likely that the intramural fibrin comes from the transudation of plasma proteins into the vessel wall secondary to endothelial damage associated with an increased transmural pressor gradient (20,43). The fibrin is sometimes accompanied by extravasation of red blood cells and intraluminal thrombosis. Occasionally, leukocytes may also

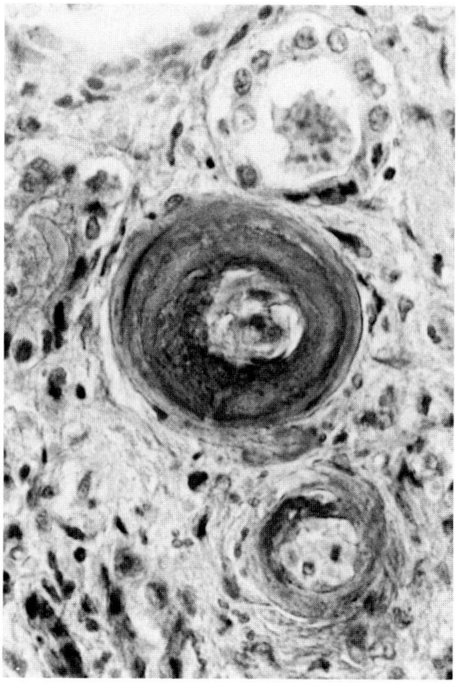

FIG. 6. Photomicrograph of an arteriole with fibrinoid necrosis of the vessel wall. The architecture of the wall is obliterated and destroyed by necrosis, which is accompanied by the deposition of material that stains positively for fibrin. The arteriole in the center shows a concentric deposition of fibrin, whereas the adjacent arteriole contains fibrin in only one portion of the wall. ×600.

be present within the walls, suggesting an inflammatory arteriolitis.

RENAL CONSEQUENCES OF MICROVASCULAR DISEASE

The sequelae of arterial narrowing can be related to the degree and rate at which the narrowing occurs. Acute complete obstruction is associated with infarction, whereas gradual or incomplete obstruction is associated with a decrease in function and subsequent atrophy. Truly mild forms of ischemia may have few or no sequelae. Since the vascular lesions of hypertension primarily affect the small arteries in the preglomerular arterioles, the glomeruli and postglomerular structures are subject to the ischemic changes.

In mild or early hypertension, many glomeruli are normal and there is little evidence of tubular atrophy or interstitial fibrosis. As the hypertension progresses in severity or duration, the same structures begin to demonstrate ischemic changes. The glomerular capillary tufts begin to collapse and show wrinkling and the capillary walls appear thickened by light microscopy (Fig. 7). The tuft gradually undergoes a degree of collapse to the point where the glomeruli appear solid and the nuclei are concentrated, giving a hypercellular appearance. The condensation is followed by glomerular scle-

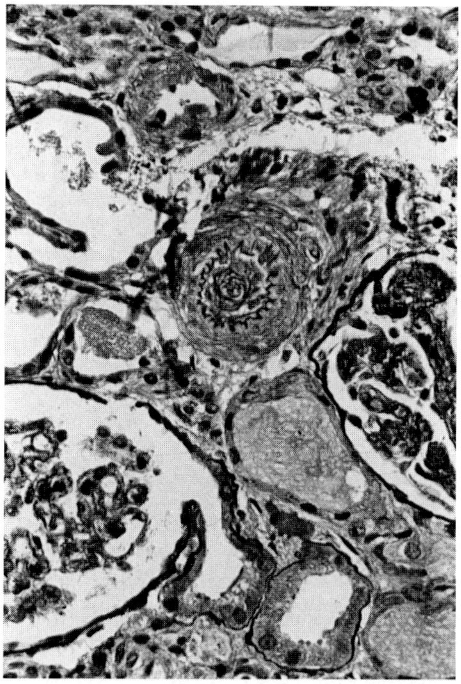

FIG. 7. Photomicrograph of a needle biopsy of a patient with hypertensive nephropathy. The inner lobular artery in the center shows myointimal hyperplasia and reduplication of the elastic lamina. Portions of two glomeruli are present, one of which shows ischemic glomerular capillary collapse with wrinkling of the capillary loops, while the other shows condensation and hyalinization of the glomerular tufts. ×150.

rosis, which initially is segmental but gradually becomes global. Ultrastructurally, the changes initially show collapse of the capillary loop with wrinkling of the basement membrane in the paramesangial region and coalescence of the collapsed basement membrane with the mesangial matrix. There is a gradual increase of mesangial matrix with obliteration of the glomerular capillary lumina, loss of endothelial cells, and increase in basement membrane-like material. Dramatic changes also occur in Bowman's capsule, where there is thickening of Bowman's capsule by the deposition of collagenous material that appears to extend into the urinary space, particularly in the hilar region. Eventually, both the glomerular capillary shrinkage and hyaline sclerosis of Bowman's capsule coalesce, resulting in the global sclerosis of the glomerulus.

The tubules are also affected by ischemia and gradually become atrophic. There is thickening of the tubular basement membrane with either collapse of the tubules and loss of tubular epithelium or dilatation of the tubules with accumulation of hyaline casts in the lumen. The atrophy of the tubules is accompanied by an increase in interstitial collagen, which occasionally is accompanied by a lymphoplasmacytic infiltrate. The reason for the presence of chronic inflammatory cells in ischemic atrophy is not clear.

In 1925 in his treatise on nephrosclerosis, Fahr (7) described changes that differed from both the ischemic alterations of benign nephrosclerosis and the more active necrotic and proliferative lesions associated with malignant nephrosclerosis. He described these changes as being characteristic of what he termed "decompensated benign nephrosclerosis." The glomerular alterations that are present include glomerular cell proliferation, focal capillary loop necrosis, and hyaline change of the glomerular epithelial cell. This lesion had largely been ignored until recently, when Meyer et al. (28) and Bohle and Ratschek (2) rekindled interest with their descriptions of primary hypertensive glomerulopathy and morphometric studies of the sclerotic kidney. In the early stage of what they term hypertensive glomerulopathy, they describe a thickening of the basement membrane of the glomerular capillaries with an irregular increase in mesangial matrix as well as hyaline droplet change in the visceral podocytes. As the lesion progresses, there is an increase in cellularity with adhesion of the glomerular capillaries to each other and to Bowman's capsule, associated with swelling of the endothelial cells and epithelial cells, which appears as apparent epithelial cell proliferation or even crescent formation. The lesion progresses into PAS positive scarring and what has been described as "pseudotubule" formation in Bowman's capsule, and then finally to glomerular hyalinosis. Since this lesion appears more prominently in glomeruli supplied by larger arteries, the authors postulate that the lesion is the result of a direct effect of greatly elevated blood pressure on the glomeruli. They further emphasize that the lesion is seen most commonly in patients who develop secondary malignant hypertension superimposed on longstanding benign essential hypertension.

Thus, in benign hypertension, glomerular damage occurs either as a result of ischemia secondary to narrowing of the preglomerular vessels by arteriolosclerosis, or as a result of direct damage to the glomerular capillaries by increased pressure resulting from an inability of the preglomerular vessels to respond and regulate in a normal fashion. Both forms of glomerular injury could easily correlate with the degree of proteinuria seen in various stages of the course of hypertension, but the direct hypertensive glomerular capillary lesion is more likely to account for the higher levels of proteinuria. Furthermore, it is of interest that recent studies of the Dahl salt-sensitive hypertensive rat (38) have demonstrated that a glomerular lesion can precede the development of hypertension in this model. These results suggest that the glomeruli may play a more important role in both the genesis and progression of hypertension than has been previously suggested. In most patients renal insufficiency is usually mild, but end-stage renal disease can occur and there is increasing evidence that the scarred kidney may continue to play a central role in the perpetuation of hypertension (5).

The glomeruli in malignant nephrosclerosis showed changes in addition to those described for benign and decompensated nephrosclerosis. The fibrinoid necrosis of the afferent arterioles sometimes extends into the glomerulus, and focal necrosis of the glomerular tuft can also be seen. Thrombosis of the capillaries and proliferation of the capillary tuft cells can accompany these changes. Occasionally, well-formed crescents can be found associated with adhesions of the necrotic tuft to Bowman's capsule. These changes can be attributed either to intense ischemia of the glomeruli with subsequent endothelial damage or to a direct action of increased transmural pressure on the glomerular capillary wall. The juxtaglomerular apparatus is frequently enlarged, and there appears to be hyperplasia of the juxtaglomerular cells associated with an increase in granulation.

RENAL ARTERIAL DISEASE

Although small blood vessel disease in the kidney is probably the most important vascular complication from a functional viewpoint, the larger renal arteries also are subject to pathologic change. Atheromatous disease of the major renal arteries is accelerated in patients with hypertension and can perpetuate the disease by creating renal artery stenosis. In addition, it may also be the source of atheromatous emboli, contributing to distal renal parenchymal infarction with its consequent loss of functional renal parenchyma. Arteries down to the arcuate size can show arteriosclerotic changes, but the smaller vessels are more commonly involved in an intimal thickening of the fibroelastic type similar to that seen in the small arteries.

Disease of the major renal arteries becomes of particular importance when it is unilateral and it causes significant stenosis of the renal artery resulting in secondary hypertension (3,37). The lesions can be generally broken down into three major categories: atherosclerosis, dysplastic diseases of the fibromuscular vessels, and a miscellaneous group that includes congenital anomalies, Takayasu's aortitis, and radiation injury. The most common cause of renal artery stenosis is obstruction by an atheromatous plaque involving the orifice of the main renal artery. It is usually associated with severe atheromatous disease of the aorta and as such is seen more frequently in males and patients with diabetes mellitus. The incidence increases with increasing age. The lesion is frequently associated with aneurysmal dilatation of the aorta distal to the renal arteries and with mural thrombosis.

The second group of lesions leading to stenosis are the so-called dysplastic lesions of the renal artery (17) (Table 1). The dysplastic lesions can involve other systemic vessels, suggesting that they may be a genetic disease, but they become clinically important when they cause obstruction of the major renal artery, initiating severe hypertension by creating a Goldblatt kidney. The lesions can be subdivided into six separate groups: intimal fibroplasia, medial fibroplasia, medial hyperplasia, perimedial fibroplasia, medial dissection, and periarterial fibroplasia. The term "fibromuscular dysplasia" has been used to encompass several of these separate cat-

Table 1. *Dysplastic lesions of the renal artery*

	Age and sex incidence	Relative frequency	Lesion
Intimal fibroplasia	1–50 M = F	1–2%	Narrowing by intimal proliferation without lipid
Medial fibroplasia with aneurysms	30–60 F > M	60–70%	"String of beads" alternating stenosis and mural thinning
Medial hyperplasia	30–60 F > M	5–15%	Smooth muscle hyperplasia and thickening
Perimedial fibroplasia	30–60 F > M	15–24%	Fibrosis of outer media occasionally aneurysms
Medial dissection	30–60 F > M	5–15%	Fibrosis of media with dissecting aneurysms
Periarterial fibroplasia	15–50 F > M	1%	Perivascular fibrosis and inflammation

egories, but it appears useful to subclassify them as they may affect different patient populations.

In intimal fibroplasia, the lesion involves only the intima of the vessel, with the elastica and media maintaining a normal architecture. There is hyperplasia of the intima that is essentially indistinguishable from the proliferative stage of atherosclerosis but that is not associated with an increased deposition of lipids. The proliferation can be of such severity as to cause significant narrowing of the lumen. The lesion has been reported in individuals as young as 1 year of age but is most commonly seen in the third and fourth decades. The most common of the medial lesions is medial fibroplasia. This usually results in a multifocal stenotic lesion alternating with microaneurysms, producing a characteristic "string of beads" appearance by renal arteriography (26). Histopathologically, there is atrophy of the muscle and fibrosis of the wall in the region of the small aneurysms alternating with the stenotic lesions, where there is medial muscular hypertrophy with an increase of interstitial collagen. The second most frequently encountered variation of fibromuscular hyperplasia is perimedial fibroplasia. In contrast to medial fibroplasia, segmental aneurysmal dilatation is not present but focal aneurysms occasionally occur. The lesion consists of thickening of the outer half of the media by an increase in fibrous tissue. The muscle is disoriented and there is a generalized thickening of the wall, although the inner portion of the media, elastica, and intima retain a relatively normal architecture. Less commonly seen is medial hyperplasia. Here, there is hyperplasia of the muscle that results in a uniform thickening of the vessel wall and resultant generalized narrowing of the lumen. Periarterial fibroplasia is a rare lesion in which fibrosis of the adventitia occurs, extending into the surrounding adipose and connective tissue and resulting in constriction of the vessel from without rather than from within the vessel wall. The fibrosis is frequently accompanied by an infiltrate of chronic inflammatory cells.

Of the miscellaneous causes of renal artery stenosis, radiation injury probably deserves some discussion. Chronic radiation injury results in loss of the muscle cells and an intense fibrosis of all layers of the vessel wall. It occurs as a distinct event after radiation exposure, usually in the form of radiation therapy for a malignant lesion. Takayasu's aortitis or pulseless disease is a chronic sclerosing aortitis of unknown etiology that can cause renal artery stenosis due to osteal narrowing. An inflammatory infiltrate is seen in addition to the fibrotic lesion, suggesting a possible immunologic mechanism for the aortitis.

In unilateral renal arterial disease, the ischemic kidney generally is smaller than the contralateral kidney and shows diffuse ischemic atrophy. The glomeruli appear small and the tubules are collapsed. Interstitial fibrosis is associated with more marked tubular atrophy if the stenosis is longstanding. The juxtaglomerular apparatus is hyperplastic and there is increased granulation seen with special stains. The small vessels are protected from the hypertension, in contrast to the contralateral kidney where hypertensive microvascular disease is prominent.

In summary, the microangiopathic changes of hypertension have long been recognized to be associated with systemic hypertension. It now seems clear that these changes, and in particular hyaline arteriolosclerosis, probably play an important pathologic role in the progression of the disease. This occurs as a result of fixing peripheral resistance through loss of compliance of the small vessels and through its ischemic effects on the renal parenchyma served by those vessels. Macrovascular disease of the kidney, on the other hand, is of importance in the initiation and perpetuation of renal vascular hypertension by producing a Goldblatt kidney. Both arterial sclerotic and dysplastic lesions of renal artery can result in stenosis, which may be amenable to surgical or intraluminal intravention.

REFERENCES

1. Amer, M. S., Comoll, A. W., and Perhach, J. L. (1974): Aberrations of cyclic-nucleotide metabolism in the hearts and vessels of hypertensive rats. *Proc. Natl. Acad. Sci. USA*, 71:4930–4934.

2. Bohle, A., and Ratschek, M. (1982): The compensated and decompensated form of benign nephrosclerosis. *Pathol. Res. Pract.*, 174:357–367.
3. Breslin, D. J., Swinton, N. W., Libertino, J. A., and Zinman, L. (1982): *Renovascular Hypertension*. Williams and Wilkins, Baltimore.
4. Buck, R. C. (1961): Intimal thickening after ligature of arteries. *Circ. Res.*, 9:418–426.
5. Curtis, J. J., Luke, R. G., Duston, H. P., et al. (1983): Remission of essential hypertension after renal transplantation. *N. Engl. J. Med.*, 309:1009–1015.
6. Dustin, P., Jr. (1962): Arteriolar hyalinosis. *Int. Rev. Exp. Pathol.*, 1:73–138.
7. Fahr, T. (1925): Pathologische Anatomie des Morbus Brightii. In: *Handbuch der Speziellen Pathologischen Anatomie und Histologie,* edited by Henke, F., and Lubarsch, O., pp. 368 ff. Springer Verlag, Berlin.
8. Fishberg, A. M. (1925): Anatomic findings in essential hypertension. *Arch. Intern. Med.*, 35:650–668.
9. Fisher, E. R., Perez, S. E., and Pardo, V. (1966): Ultrastructural studies in hypertension. *Lab. Invest.*, 15:1409–1433.
10. Friedman, S. M., Nakashima, M., and Mar, M. A. (1971): Morphologic assessment of vasoconstriction and vascular hypertrophy in sustained hypertension of the rat. *Microvasc. Res.*, 3:416.
11. Gamble, C. N. (1986): The pathogenesis of hyaline arteriosclerosis. *Am. J. Pathol.*, 122:410–420.
12. Goldblatt, H. (1947): The renal origin of hypertension. *Physiol. Rev.*, 27:120–165.
13. Goldblatt, H., Lynch, J., Hanzal, R. F., et al. (1934): Studies on experimental hypertension I. The production of persistent elevation of systolic blood pressure by means of renal ischemia. *J. Exp. Med.*, 59:347–379.
14. Grospadorowicz, D., Cheng, J., and Livette, M. (1983): Bovine brain and pituitary growth factors: Comparison of their abilities to support the proliferation of human bovine vascular endothelial cells. *J. Cell Biol.*, 97:1677–1685.
15. Gull, W. W., and Sutton, H. G. (1872): On the pathology of the morbid state commonly called chronic Bright's disease with contracted kidney (arterio-capillary fibrosis). *Trans. Med. Chir. Soc.*, 55:273–329.
16. Hall, G. H., Farson, D. A., and Bissell, M. J. (1982): Lumen formation by epithelial cell lines in response to collagen overlay. *Proc. Natl. Acad. Sci. USA*, 79:4672–4676.
17. Harrison, E. G., and McCormack, L. V. (1971): Pathologic classification of renal arterial disease in renovascular hypertension. *Mayo Clin. Proc.*, 46:161–166.
18. Hueck, W. (1920): Anatomisches untersuchungen zur Frage nach Wesen and Ursache der Arteriosclerose. *Munch. Med. Wochenschr.*, 67:835–837.
19. Johnson, G. I. (1868): On certain points in the anatomy and pathology of Bright's disease. *Trans. Med. Chir. Soc.*, 51:57–78.
20. Jones, D. B. (1974): Arterial and glomerular lesions associated with severe hypertension. *Lab. Invest.*, 31:303–313.
21. Jores, L. (1904): Uber die Arteriosklerose der kleinen Organ arterien. *Virchows Arch.*, 178:367–406.
22. Kincaid-Smith, P. (1980): Malignant hypertension: Mechanisms and management. *Pharmacol. Ther.*, 9:245–269.
23. Kleinman, H. K., Klebe, R. J., and Martin, G. R. (1981): The role of collagenous matrices in the addition and growth of cells. *J. Cell Biol.*, 88:473–479.
24. Linton, A. L. (1969): Microangiopathic hemolytic anemia and the pathogenesis of malignant hypertension. *Lancet*, 1:1277.
25. Mauer, S. M., Steftes, M. W., Azar, S., et al. (1978): The effects of Goldblatt hypertension on the development of the glomerular lesions of diabetes mellitus in the rat. *Diabetes*, 27:738–744.
26. McCormack, L. J., Poutasse, E. F., Meaney, T. F., Noto, T. J., and Duston, H. P. (1966): Arteriographic correlation of renal artery disease. *Am. Heart J.*, 72:188–198.
27. McGee, W. F., and Ashworth, C. T. (1963): Fine structure of chronic hypertensive arteriopathy in the human kidney. *Am. J. Pathol.*, 43:273–299.
28. Meyer, D., Helmchen, U., and Bohle, A. (1973): Hypertensive glomerulae. *Schaden Verh. Dtsch. Ges. Pathol.*, 57:392–393.
29. Moritz, A. R., and Oldt, M. R. (1937): Arteriolar sclerosis in hypertensive and non-hypertensive individuals. *Am. J. Pathol.*, 13:679–728.
30. Olsen, J. L., Hostetter, T. H., Rennke, H. G., et al. (1982): Altered charge and size selective properties of the glomerular wall: A response to reduced renal mass. *Kidney Int.*, 22:112–118.
31. Ooshima, A., Fuller, G. G., Cardinale, G. J., et al. (1974): Increased collagen synthesis in blood vessels of hypertensive rats and its reversal by antihypertensive agents. *Proc. Natl. Acad. Sci. USA*, 71:3019–3023.
32. Pamnani, M. B., and Overbeck, H. W. (1975): Vascular wall composition in renal hypertension (Abstr.). *Fed. Proc.*, 34:282.
33. Paronetto, F. (1965): Immunocytochemical observations on the vascular necrosis and renal glomerular lesions of malignant nephrosclerosis. *Am. J. Pathol.*, 46:901.
34. Rohrbach, D. H., Wagner, C. W., Star, V. L., et al. (1983): Reduced synthesis of basement membrane heparan sulphate proteoglycan in streptozotocin-induced diabetic mice. *J. Biol. Chem.*, 258:11672–11677.
35. Rokitansky, C. (1852): Uber einige der wichtigsten Krankheiten der Arterien. *Denkschrift Konigl. Akad. Nis.*, 4:49.
36. Schloss, G. (1948): Die Histogenese und Pathogenese der Gefassveranderungen beim experimentellen renalen Drosselung-Schochdruck der Ratte. *Schweiz. Z. Allg. Pathol.*, 11:109–113.
37. Stanley, J. C., Ernst, C. B., and Fry, W. J. (1984): *Renovascular Hypertension*. W.B. Saunders, Philadelphia.
38. Sterzel, R. B., Gao, Y., Kriz, W., Waldherr, R., Briggs, J., and Schnermann, J. (1986): Renal disease precedes hypertension in salt sensitive Dahl rats. *Kidney Int.*, 29:259.
39. Tobian, L., Olson, R., and Chesley, G. (1969): Water content of arteriolar wall in renovascular hypertension. *Am. J. Physiol.*, 216:22–24.
40. Tracy, R. E. (1981): Hypertension and arteriolar sclerosis of the kidney, pancreas, adrenal gland and liver. *Virchows Arch.*, 391:91–106.
41. Udenfreund, S., Cardinale, G., and Spector, S. (1981): Hypertension induced vascular fibrosis and its reversal

by antihypertensive drugs. In: *Frontiers in Hypertension Research,* edited by J. H. Laragh, F. R. Buhler, and D. W. Seldin, pp. 404–411. Springer, New York.

42. Valenzuela, R., Gogate, P. A., Deodar, S. D., and Gifford, R. W. (1980): Hyaline arteriolonephrosclerosis. Immunofluorescent findings in vascular lesions. *Lab. Invest.,* 43:530–534.
43. Wiener, J., Lattes, R. G., Meltzer, B. G., et al. (1969): Evidence for increased vascular permeability—The cellular pathology of experimental hypertension. *Am. J. Pathol.,* 54:187–207.
44. Wiener, J., Spiro, D., and Lattes, R. G. (1965): Arteriolar hyalinosis and fibrinoid change—The cellular pathology of experimental hypertension. II. *Am. J. Pathol.,* 47:457–485.
45. Woliasky, H. (1972): Longterm effects of hypertension on the rat aortic wall. *Circ. Res.,* 30:301–309.
46. Zollinger, H. V. (1966): Niere und ableitende Harnwege. In: *Spezielle Pathologische Anatomie, Band 3,* edited by W. Doerr and E. Uehlinger, p. 577–585. Springer Verlag, Berlin.

The Kidney in Hypertension, edited by
Norman M. Kaplan, Barry M. Brenner,
and John H. Laragh. Raven Press,
New York © 1987.

Identifying Patients with Renovascular Hypertension

E. D. Vaughan, Jr., T. G. Pickering, and J. H. Laragh

The Cardiovascular Center and Department of Medicine, and The James Buchanan Brady Foundation, Department of Surgery/Division of Urology, The New York Hospital-Cornell Medical Center, New York, New York 10021

The need to accurately identify patients with renovascular hypertension is predicated on the assumption that the natural history and the consequences of the disease differ from essential hypertension. Moreover, a cost-effective approach must be developed, since renovascular hypertension is responsible for only 5% to 10% of the total hypertensive population. Earlier the value of identifying patients with renovascular hypertension was not felt to warrant the expenses involved (34,35).

Addressing these issues, it is now apparent that this form of hypertension is difficult to control with conventional antihypertensive medications (25), and more effective agents that can control the blood pressure can lead to impairment of renal function (13,30) or renal loss secondary to renal arterial occlusion (51). In addition, most renovascular lesions are progressive with time, and there is little evidence to suggest that successful control of hypertension influences the natural history of the various pathologic entities (19, 36, 43). Hence the goals in treating patients with renovascular hypertension differ from treatment of patients with essential hypertension, mandating preservation of renal function as well as control of the hypertension.

Fortunately, the development of newer diagnostic tests, which often do not require hospitalization, to identify these patients (37,55) has reduced the previous high cost of evaluation, resulting in a more aggressive diagnostic approach. In this chapter we will review the current diagnostic strategies that are useful in identifying patients with renovascular hypertension, with emphasis on renin determinations and the utilization of angiotensin-converting enzyme inhibitors in a diagnostic fashion.

NATURAL HISTORY

There have been relatively few reports about the natural history of renal artery lesions. However, the limited data available have suggested that many patients with both atherosclerotic disease (59) and fibromuscular disease (36) will have progressive disease. However, it has been impossible from the initial renal arteriograms to predict which lesions would actually undergo progression (33,47). The important question of progression has been addressed recently by Schreiber and co-workers, and more precise information is now available (43).

Serial angiographic studies over a mean interval of 52 months in 85 patients with atherosclerotic disease revealed progressive vascular obstruction in 37 patients (44%). Total arterial occlusion occurred in 14 patients and occurred most commonly in patients with a greater than 75% stenosis on the initial arteriogram. As would be expected, decline in renal function was more common in those patients with progressive disease. Accordingly, the authors suggested that renal revascularization might be indicated for preservation of renal function in patients whose advanced atherosclerotic disease was a major threat to overall renal function. These patients are characterized by azotemia and high-grade renal artery stenosis (greater than 75%), bilateral high-grade stenosis, and stenosis involving a solitary kidney (43).

Sixty patients with medial fibroplasia were also followed for a mean interval of 45 months. Progressive renal arterial obstruction was observed in 22 of 66 patients (33%); however, there were no cases of progression to total occlusion. Of particular interest was the similar development of progressive disease in patients greater than 40 years of age (15 of 46). Previously it was felt that the disease was stable in this age group (36). Despite the angiographic progression, demonstrated increases in serum creatinine or reduction in renal size seldom occurred. Accordingly, the authors did not suggest renal revascularization for preservation of renal function in this group.

IDENTIFYING THE PATIENT WITH RENOVASCULAR HYPERTENSION

Clinical means by which patients with functionally significant renal artery stenosis can be identified have proven to be more elusive than might have been predicted. Certainly there are no pathognomonic clinical characteristics that lead to a reliable diagnosis (45). There are, however, a number of clinical features which should arouse suspicion that renovascular hypertension may be present. These are summarized in Table 1.

The only laboratory finding of importance is hypokalemia. The low potassium is due to secondary hyperaldosteronism. However, a low serum K^+ is found in less than 20% of patients with renovascular hypertension.

In many patients, however, none of the usual clinical clues are present to prompt a definitive evaluation. Thus, the unreliability of clinical information led to the development of a variety of approaches to screen for the patient with renovascular hypertension.

Differential Renal Function Studies

The observation in animals that partial occlusion of the renal artery resulted in increased fractional reabsorption of sodium and water (2) and increased urinary concentration of nonreabsorbable solute led to the development of differential renal function studies (24). The initial criterion for a positive test was a 50% decrease in urine flow and a 15% or greater decrease in sodium concentration from the affected kidney. The test underwent numerous modifications (47), with the most popular including the infusion of inulin, *p*-aminohippuric acid (PAH), and antidiuretic hormone during a urea-saline diuresis to accentuate the disparity in salt and water reabsorption between the two kidneys (48).

However, the complexity involved in performing differential split renal function studies coupled with the development of more accurate methods to measure activity of the renin-angiotensin system has almost eliminated the use of this technique. Generally, at this time differential renal function studies are performed only if renin studies are equivocal or the patient has unilateral parenchymal disease. In contrast, the Vanderbilt group still feels that in many cases renin studies and split renal function studies are complementary and that the omission of either will increase the false negative rate (14). In the setting of unilateral parenchymal disease, differential function studies are most useful. The treatment choices are nephrectomy or antihypertensive medical management, and the latter is preferable if the affected kidney is contributing substantially to the total renal function. Hence the technique is utilized to measure the glomerular filtration rate of the involved kidney. If the kidney has sufficient function to sustain life, then medical treatment should be the first management strategy.

Intravenous Urogram, Radionuclide Renography, and Digital Subtraction Angiography

The rapid sequence intravenous urogram (IVP) is actually a radiographic differential renal func-

Table 1. *Clinical clues suggestive of renovascular hypertension*[a]

Historical clues	Comment
Hypertension in the absence of any family history of hypertensive disease	Suspect if family history negative; however, about 1/3 of patients with renovascular hypertension will have a positive family history
Age of onset of hypertension: less than 25 years or greater than 45 years	The average age of onset for essential hypertension is 31 ± 10 (SD) years. Children and young adults usually will have fibromuscular disease whereas adults over 45 years are more likely to have atherosclerotic narrowing of arteries
Abrupt onset of moderate to severe hypertension	Whereas essential hypertension usually begins with a "labile" phase before mild hypertension becomes established, renovascular hypertension usually has a more telescoped natural history, often first appearing as moderate hypertension of recent onset
Development of severe or malignant hypertension	Renovascular hypertension often becomes moderately severe and is prone to produce acceleration or malignant phase hypertension; both forms of hypertension involve markedly increased renin release
Headaches	Essential hypertension is usually asymptomatic. There seem to be more headaches with renovascular hypertension, possibly related to its severity, or high levels of angiotensin II, a potent cerebrovascular vasoconstrictor
Cigarette smoking	In a recent survey, 74% of patients with fibromuscular renal artery stenosis were smokers; 88% of those with atherosclerotic disease smoke (38)
White race	Renovascular hypertension is uncommon in the black population
Resistance to or escape from blood pressure control with standard diuretic therapy or antiadrenergic	Probably the most typical feature of renovascular hypertension is that it responds poorly to diuretics and often only transiently to antiadrenergic drugs
Excellent antihypertensive response to converting enzyme inhibitors, e.g., captopril	Converting enzyme inhibitors block the renin-angiotensin system most effectively and are therefore highly specified agents
Clues from examination and routine laboratory	
Retinopathy	Hemorrhages, exudates, or papilledema indicate acceleration or malignant phase
Abdominal or flank bruit	A helpful clue, but commonly present in elderly individuals, and occasionally present in younger patients who have no apparent vascular stenosis
Carotid bruits or other evidence of large vessel disease	Commonly the vascular pathology is not limited to the renal bed
Hypokalemia in the untreated state or in response to a thiazide diuretic	Increased aldosterone stimulation by the renin-angiotensin system tends to reduce the serum potassium level. In untreated essential hypertension this does not occur. Thiazide diuretics accentuate this phenomenon in renovascular hypertension

[a]From ref. 58.

tion study utilizing the contrast material as the indicator. Reduced renal blood flow is indicated by decreased renal mass or size, decreased glomerular filtration rate by delayed calyceal appearance time of contrast, and hyperreabsorption of water by delayed hyperconcentration of nonreabsorbable solute, the iodinated contrast material. The most reliable abnormality seen in patients with proven unilateral renovascular hypertension is delayed calyceal appearance time of the side of the offending lesion (3). Accordingly the rapid sequence series of 1- to 4-min films after injection is critical if this test is to be utilized.

The accuracy of the urogram depends on the population under study. Hence if the urograms of a group of patients with proven renovascular hypertension are reviewed, 80% to 90% will show positive criteria (31). However, when populations of hypertensive patients have been screened, the false positive rate (a positive study in a patient with essential hypertension) of approximately 10% has also been found. Since over 90% of the overall hypertensive population is composed of patients with essential hypertension, this false positive rate is translated into an unacceptably high number of patients falsely identified as having potential renovascular disease (31).

The accuracy of cooperative study of renovascular hypertension, and the later analysis of the data (53) as to the interpretation of the value of the IVP for screening, have recently been challenged in a comprehensive review of the published data (20). The authors tabulated the sensitivity and specificity of the rapid sequence IVP in studies in which the renal artery architecture was proven by arteriography. They concluded that for a total of 2,040 cases there was a 74.5% sensitivity and an 86.2% specificity. This specificity is considerably better than the 60% figure reported in the cooperative study (3). They concluded that the rapid sequence IVP still played a major role in the diagnosis of renovascular hypertension.

They continued to review the current literature giving the results of digital subtraction angiography (DSA) utilizing the same criteria. DSA is a technique utilizing image enhancement and computer assistance to extract venous images to allow visualization of the aorta and renal arteries following intravenous injection of contrast (21). Their conclusion was that DSA was no more specific than the IVP, although it was more sensitive. However, since 7.4% of all DSA studies were uninterpretable, there was little advantage to this more invasive and more expensive test. Disadvantages of the intravenous DSA are shown in Table 2.

Table 2. *Disadvantages of intravenous renal digital subtraction angiography*

Low spatial resolution
Small field size
Increased irradiation dose
Nonselective contrast injection
High contrast load
Misregulation artifact

The authors continued to apply Bayes' theorem to the two tests but failed to include a potential 2% or 5% incidence of renovascular hypertension to their analysis. A revised analysis is shown in Table 3. Thus it is clear that at the most likely prevalence estimates the predictive value of a positive test to identify renal arterial disease is unacceptably low.

In addition there is a major flaw in the analysis, which assumes that the renal arterial lesion found on arteriography can be equated with renovascular hypertension. The development of arteriography gave us an accurate means of identifying renal arterial disease (17). However, it soon became apparent that normotensive patients undergoing arteriography for other reasons often had renal arterial disease (15), and autopsy figures subsequently confirmed the radiologic findings (22). Accordingly, the finding of renal arterial disease alone is not sufficient justification to warrant correction in a hypertensive patient. The true definition of renovascular hypertension demands that the hypertension resulting from the renal arterial lesion is relieved following correction of the renal arterial lesion.

Moreover, the presence of a positive urogram in a patient with renal arterial disease does not predict the blood pressure response to surgery. In the Cooperative Study of Renovascular Hypertension abnormal urograms were found in 80% of both the cured patients and those patients whose blood pressure failed to respond to surgical repair (3).

Similarly, the radionuclide renogram, despite numerous modifications, has been plagued with variability, which has led to even less specificity. In fact, review of a variety of techniques found a false positive rate of 25% (32), whereas a later study utilizing a refined technique reduced the false negative rate to 10%, still no better than the urogram (16). In summary, the intravenous urogram, the DSA, and nuclide

Table 3. *Predictive value of screening tests for renovascular hypertension*[a]

	IVP[b]	DIVA[b]	PRA[c,d]	Single dose[e] captopril
Sensitivity (%)	75	88	80	100
Specificity (%)	86	89	84	95
False + (%)	14	11	16	5
False − (%)	25	12	20	0
Predictive value[f] (%)				
Prevalence 2%	9.9	14.6	9.3	29
5%	22.1	30.5	20.8	51.3
10%	37.5	48.1	35.7	69
Exclusion value[f] (%)				
Prevalence 2%	99.4	99.7	99.5	100
5%	98.5	99.3	98.8	100
10%	96.7	98.5	97.4	100

Calculations:

$$\text{Predictive value} = \frac{\text{Sensitivity} \times \text{prevalence}}{(\text{Sens.} \times \text{prev.}) + \text{false pos. rate} \times (100 - \text{prev.})} \times 100$$

$$\text{Exclusion value} = \frac{\text{Specificity} \times (100 - \text{prevalence})}{[\text{Specif.} \times (100 - \text{prev.}) + \text{false neg. rate}] \times \text{prev.}} \times 100$$

[a]Abbreviations: (IVP) intravenous urogram; (DIVA) digital angiography; (PRA) plasma renin activity.
References: [b]20; [c]41; [d]4; [e]37; [f]27.

studies have failed to achieve suitable sensitivity and specificity to serve as reliable screening tests for renovascular hypertension.

Accordingly a diagnostic strategy should include tests which identify both the functional significance of a renal arterial lesion as well as its mere presence (55).

Increased Renin Secretion—The Peripheral Plasma Renin

After the initial work of Dr. Harry Goldblatt (18), it was assumed that excess renin secretion, leading to excess angiotensin II (AII) formation, was the underlying derangement in renovascular hypertension. Unfortunately this possibility was soon challenged when circulating plasma renin activity (PRA) was found to be normal in both animal models (1) and a fraction of patients with renovascular hypertension (29). This latter review of the literature found the peripheral PRA to be elevated in only 109 of 196 patients (56%) with verified cases of correctable renovascular hypertension. However, upon careful review of the primary papers it is apparent that these samples were often obtained under conditions that are now recognized to invalidate or limit accurate interpretation of the values obtained. For example, it is now recognized that PRA is inversely related to sodium intake and must be indexed in some fashion to the state of sodium balance (Fig. 1). Moreover, all antihypertensive drugs influence PRA and must be stopped 2 weeks before blood sampling for PRA. Aids to increase the accuracy of determinations of peripheral PRA are shown in Table 4.

The rationale for emphasis on the peripheral PRA is that it represents an index of renin secretion (44). There exists a common misconception that increased renin secretion is determined from differential renal vein renin measurements. Actual renin secretion (renal vein renin concentration minus arterial renin concentration multiplied by renal blood flow) is rarely determined. Accordingly, a high renal venous renin concentration may reflect increased secretion with normal renal blood flow or, alternatively, a normal amount of renin secreted into reduced renal blood flow (i.e., secretion = concentration × flow).

Increased secretion of renin should be characteristic of renovascular hypertension and should

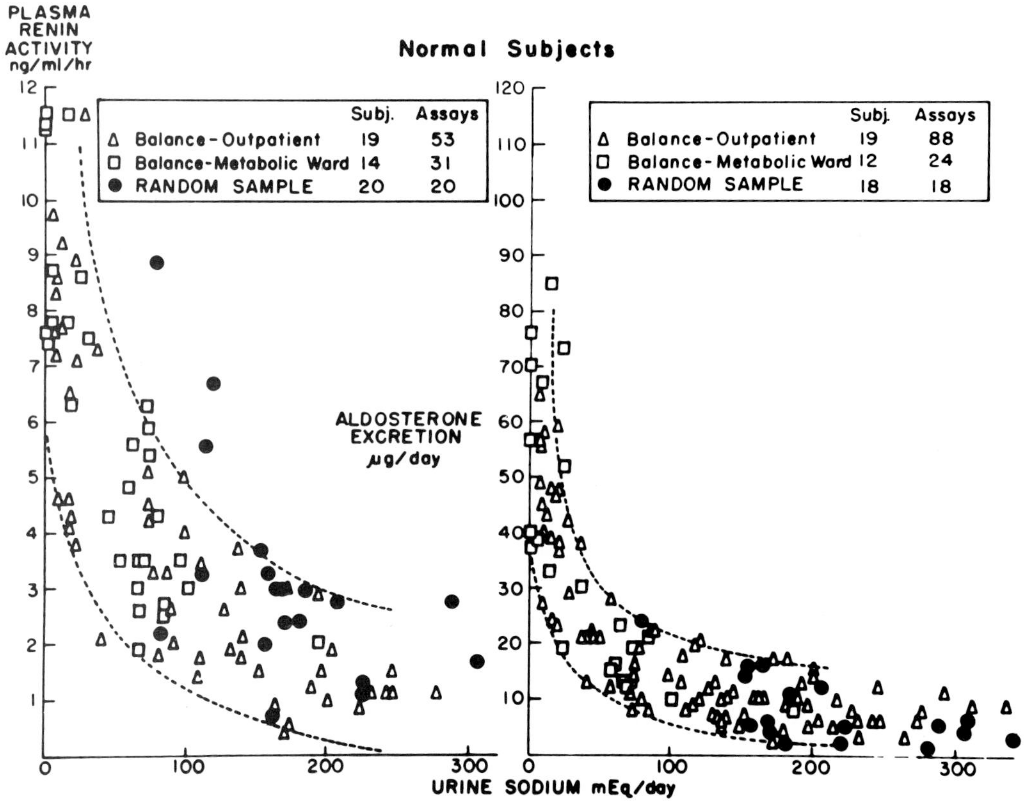

FIG. 1. Relation of both renin activity in plasma samples obtained at noon and of the corresponding 24-hour urinary excretion of aldosterone to the concurrent daily rate of sodium excretion. For these normal subjects, the data describe a similar dynamic hyperbolic relationship between each hormone and sodium excretion. Of note is the fact that subjects studied on random diets outside the hospital exhibited similar relationships, a finding which validates the use of this nomogram in studying outpatients or subjects not receiving constant diets. (From ref. 27a.)

therefore be reflected by elevated peripheral PRA as compared with PRA values obtained from normotensive controls when collected and analyzed under exactly the same conditions. Peripheral PRA (determined in blood collected at noon after 4 hr of patient ambulation), when indexed against the rate of urinary sodium excretion, is an excellent tool in identifying abnormally high renin secretion. In a recent study of patients who subsequently had successful transluminal angioplasty, the peripheral PRA was elevated in 80% of those studied (Fig. 2). Moreover, the PRA always decreased and often returned to normal following successful renal angioplasty, thereby confirming the hypothesis that the peripheral PRA is an indicator of increased renin secretion, which is corrected following relief of the offending stenotic lesion (41).

Measurement of PRA in this manner as a screening test for renovascular hypertension has certain limitations. In addition to a 20% false negative rate (i.e., a normal PRA indexed against sodium excretion) in patients with proven renovascular hypertension, there is a technical problem. Many patients with renovascular hypertension have severe life-threatening hypertension or coexistent heart disease, which precludes cessation of antihypertensive medication prior to collecting blood for peripheral PRA determinations. Thus, sampling blood while patients are on drugs invalidates the accuracy of peripheral PRA as a practical screening tool. In

Table 4. *Aids to increase the accuracy of determinations of peripheral plasma renin activity (PRA)*[a]

Problem	Solution
The "normal" value for PRA varies from laboratory to laboratory	Clearly understand the factors that affect "normal" values in your laboratory: time of sampling, state of ambulation (upright posture influences PRA), state of sodium intake
The method of collection of blood samples from patients may vary from that used to collect samples designed to establish normal range	Utilize identical conditions for sampling
All antihypertensive and diuretic drugs after PRA	Stop all treatment 2 weeks prior to blood sampling for PRA
PRA is inversely related to sodium intake/excretion	Collect a 24-hr urine for sodium determinations at the time that you collect blood for PRA; use the sodium intake level that your laboratory uses to define their normal range[b]
Inferior vena cava renin used as "peripheral"	Obtain a peripheral blood for PRA as described on a day separate from renal vein sampling

[a]From ref. 54.
[b]If a new methodology is being established, suggest the development of a renal/sodium index.

addition, 16% of patients with essential hypertension also have high PRA (5). Taken altogether, these problems have led to the search for an additional test to screen for renovascular hypertension (Table 3).

Enhanced Accuracy of Peripheral Plasma Renin Activity by Stimulation with Angiotensin-Blocking Drugs

The first angiotensin-blocking agent used for testing in human hypertension was saralasin. The initial results demonstrated that the compound did, as predicted, lower blood pressure in high-renin forms of hypertension, including renovascular (4). In a second generation of human studies with saralasin, the partial agonist activity of the drug was exposed (6, 11). Thus, in clinical settings where PRA was low, the drug actually increased blood pressure. Moreover, the blood pressure lowering effect of the drug was found to be inversely proportional to the sodium intake. Accordingly, although reasonably accurate in identifying patients with renovascular hypertension (23), the usefulness of the test is limited because of the need for intravenous in-

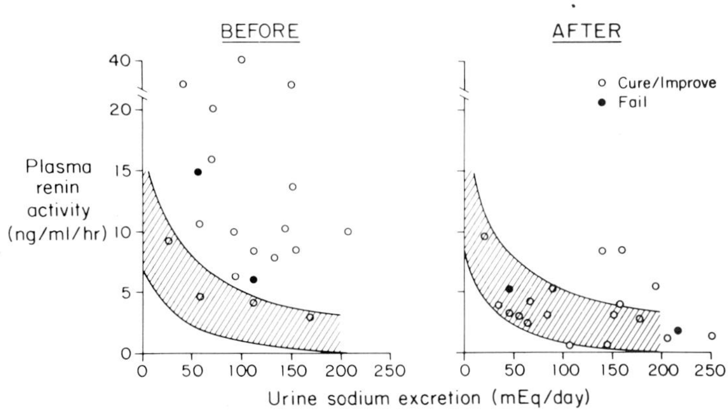

FIG. 2. Effect of angioplasty on peripheral plasma renin activity indexed against 24-hour sodium excretion. Left panel: before angioplasty. Right panel: 6 months after angioplasty. Hatched area shows normal range. (From ref. 41.)

fusion, the agonist effect of the drug, and the influence of sodium balance on the blood pressure response to the agent.

A second approach to the use of angiotensin blockade to expose renovascular hypertension came from experience following the development of converting enzyme inhibitors that block angiotensin II formation. One of the peptides obtained from the venom of the *Bothrops jararaca* viper, teprotide or SQ-20881, was shown to block the vasopressor effect of angiotensin I, and it was possible to demonstrate a close direct correlation between the pretreatment level of PRA and the magnitude of the depressor response (12). Moreover, in untreated hypertensive patients on the same normal sodium intake, intravenous teprotide lowered blood pressure to the greatest extent in the group profiled as high-renin by the renin-sodium index, but did not lower blood pressure significantly in the low-renin subgroup. From these studies, it was possible to predict that inhibition of converting enzyme might be a useful diagnostic approach for detecting angiotensin-dependent forms of hypertension.

The success of this intravenous nonapeptide converting enzyme inhibitor was a potent stimulus to the development of an orally active form, the first of which to be used in humans being captopril (SQ-14225). Captopril has the potential for being used as a diagnostic probe, like teprotide, since it has a rapid onset of action (10–15 min) reaching a peak effect by 90 min (9). Initial studies showed a close relationship between the pretreatment PRA and the magnitude of the depressor response induced after the first dose of captopril (9).

With the availability of the oral converting enzyme inhibitor captopril, we began using single oral test doses instead of intravenous infu-

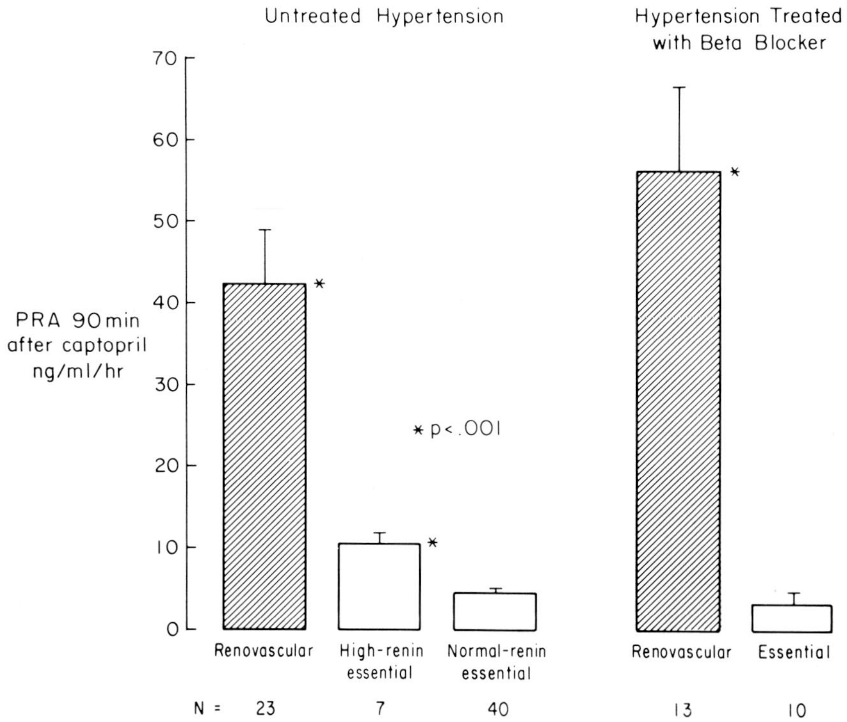

FIG. 3. Levels of plasma renin activity in renovascular and essential hypertension 90 minutes after a single dose of captopril. A marked reactive hyperreninemia was found in the group with renovascular hypertension whether or not they were already receiving beta-blocker therapy. (From ref. 8.)

Table 5. *Single dose captopril test*[a]

Drugs

The patient should be off all antihypertensive medicines for at least 2 weeks if possible. Otherwise, leave on a β-blocker but avoid diuretics, converting enzyme inhibitors, and nonsteroidal antiinflammatory drugs for at least 1 week, ideally 2 weeks

Diet

A diet with normal or high-sodium content is necessary. Too low a sodium intake will produce false positive results. If there is a question about diet, a 24-hr urine collection for sodium will closely reflect the intake

Procedure

The patient is seated comfortably for 20 to 30 min prior to testing and is maintained in this position for the duration of the test

Blood pressure is measured at 20, 25, and 30 min (three stable baseline measurements should be obtained), then blood is sampled for plasma renin activity (PRA) (in a lavender top vacutainer kept at room temperature)

A 25-mg captopril tablet is crushed (to insure that it dissolves) and 30 ml of water are added to prepare a suspension. The patient is instructed to drink the suspension, wash the contents out twice, and drink those also

Blood pressure and PRA are remeasured after 30 and 60 min

From ref. 37.

sions. Results very similar to those obtained using the intravenous competitive antagonist saralasin or the converting enzyme inhibitor teprotide were found, including a marked rise in PRA (7, 10). An additional advantage was the observation that renovascular hypertensive patients being treated with a β-adrenergic blocker still responded to oral administration of captopril with a fall in blood pressure and a rise in PRA (Fig. 3) (8).

The protocol for using single oral doses of captopril to screen for renovascular hypertension is shown in Table 5 and current criteria for interpretation are summarized in Table 6, with modifications for other methods in Table 7. In a recent study of 246 hypertensive patients, the test was highly accurate in patients without renal insufficiency. The test identified all 56 patients with proven renovascular disease among 200 hypertensive patients without renal dysfunction. In this group false positive results occurred in only two of 112 patients with essential hypertension and six with secondary hypertension (37).

Table 6. *Single dose captopril test: criteria that distinguish patients with renovascular hypertension from those with essential hypertension*[a]

Stimulated PRA[b] ≥ 12 ng/ml/hr *and*

Absolute increase in PRA of ≥ 10 ng/ml/hr *and*

Percent increase in PRA ≥ 150%, or 400% *if* the baseline PRA < 3 ng/ml/hr

[a]From ref. 37.

[b]Plasma renin activity.

In summary, the single dose captopril appears to accurately separate patients with renovascular or renal hypertension from essential hypertensives. In addition, a 24-hr urine collection is not necessary and the patient can remain on β-blockade. Hence the test is complementary to the renin-sodium index to identify renin hypersecretion (Table 3).

Contralateral Suppression of Renin Secretion and an Elevated Renal Vein to Arterial Renin Relationship—Use of Differential Renal Vein Renin Determinations

Since the development of the technique (26), differential renal vein renin determinations have emerged as the most useful tool in identifying correctable renovascular hypertension. The most common approach has been to calculate the renal vein renin ratio, that is, stenotic divided by normal side PRA values with some arbitrary "positive" ratio (usually 1.5:1). The major limitation in this method is in selecting a ratio that has the accuracy to divide precisely patients with renovascular hypertension from those with essential hypertension (29). Generally, a positive renal vein ratio predicts a fall in blood pressure following correction of the vascular lesion in over 90% of cases. However, a negative ratio does

Table 7. *Three renin criteria for positive captopril test result using renin values from kits or clinical laboratories*[a]

Source	Stimulated PRA[b] (ng/ml/hr)	Absolute increase in PRA (ng/ml/hr)	Plasma renin cutoff point[c] for percent increase in PRA
Laragh	≥12	≥10	3.0
Biotech kit[d]	≥9.2	≥7.7	2.3
Nichols Institute Roche Biochemical Lab Metpath Labs	≥7.3	≥6.1	1.8
Smith-Kline Clinical Labs Mayo Medical Labs	≥5.7	≥4.7	1.4

[a]From ref. 37.
[b]Plasma renin activity.
[c]Percent increase in PRA of 150% or more if baseline PRA is above or equal to this value; percent increase in PRA of 400% or more if baseline PRA is below this value.
[d]Previously Squibb kit.

not preclude a successful response to revascularization. In the review of Marks and Maxwell, 49% of patients with negative ratio were cured by appropriate surgical intervention (29). However, these patients were a minority of the total patients studied, and the actual false negative rate was 15% (62/412 patients).

In addition, the collection of renal vein blood alone for PRA is subject to the risk of a sampling error due to either incorrect catheter placement or sampling from a renal vein that does not subtend the renal area supplied by the stenotic artery. Sampling from the inferior vena cava below the renal veins is a safeguard against this source of error, and the absence of a 50% renin increment from both kidneys together identifies an inadequate differential renal vein renin study (56).

Finally, a positive renal vein ratio does not exclude bilateral renin secretion, albeit asymmetric, which would indicate bilateral renal disease. In this setting correction of a unilateral lesion might not totally correct the underlying pathology, with subsequent failure of total blood pressure control.

In view of these limitations of the traditional renal vein ratio analysis, another method for analysis of renin values has been devised and is based on the characteristics of experimental one-clip, two-kidney Goldblatt hypertension, as detailed in Table 8 and Fig. 4.

Hypersecretion of renin, as determined by the renin-sodium index or captopril stimulation, serves as the primary criterion for the diagnosis of renovascular hypertension. A second criterion is the demonstration of the absence of renin secretion from the contralateral (or noninvolved) kidney. Suppression of renin secretion from this kidney can be determined by subtracting the renal arterial PRA (A) from the renal venous PRA (V). Since the inferior vena caval (IVC) renin and aortic renin are the same, the IVC renin value can be substituted for (A) in this equation (44). Hence, patients with curable renovascular hypertension exhibit an absence of renin secretion from the opposite kidney, i.e., $(V - A) = 0$, also termed "contralateral suppression" of renin (50,56). Contralateral suppression of renin indicates that the noninvolved kidney is responding in an appropriate, "normal" fashion to the elevated blood pressure, increased circulating AII levels, and/or increased sodium chloride at the macula densa by shutting off renin secretion. This phenomenon is at times present not only in patients with unilateral renal arterial lesions but also in patients with bilateral disease, demonstrated by arteriograms, who have a dominant lesion on one side (40).

A third criterion is based on studies of renal vein and arterial renin relationships in patients with essential hypertension. The mean renal ve-

Table 8. *Renin values for predicting curability of renovascular hypertension*[a]

Collection of samples (moderate sodium intake ± 100 mEq/day)		
Ambulatory peripheral renin and 24-hr urine sodium excretion under steady-state conditions (i.e., not on day of arteriography)		
Collection of blood for PRA[b] before and after converting enzyme blockade		
Collection of supine		
Renal vein renin from suspect kidney (*V1*) and inferior vena cava renin (*A1*)		
Renal vein renin from contralateral kidney (*V2*) and inferior vena cava renin (*A2*)		
Enhancement of renin secretion by converting enzyme blockade if initial renin sampling is inconclusive		
Criteria for predicting cure		
High PRA in relation to 24-hour urinary sodium		Measurement of hypersecretion of renin
Contralateral kidney:	$(V2 - A2) = 0$	An indicator of absent renin secretion from the contralateral kidney
Suspect kidney:	$(V1 - A1)/A1 = 0.50$	An indicator of unilateral renin secretion
	$(V1 - A1)/A1 > 0.50$	Measurement of reduced renal blood flow
$\frac{(V - A)^c}{A} + \frac{(V - A)}{A} < 0.50$ in patients with high PRA		
Means (a) Incorrect sampling		
(b) Segmental disease		Repeat with segmental sampling

[a]From ref. 57.
[b]Plasma renin activity.
[c](*V*) Venous PRA; (*A*) arterial PRA.

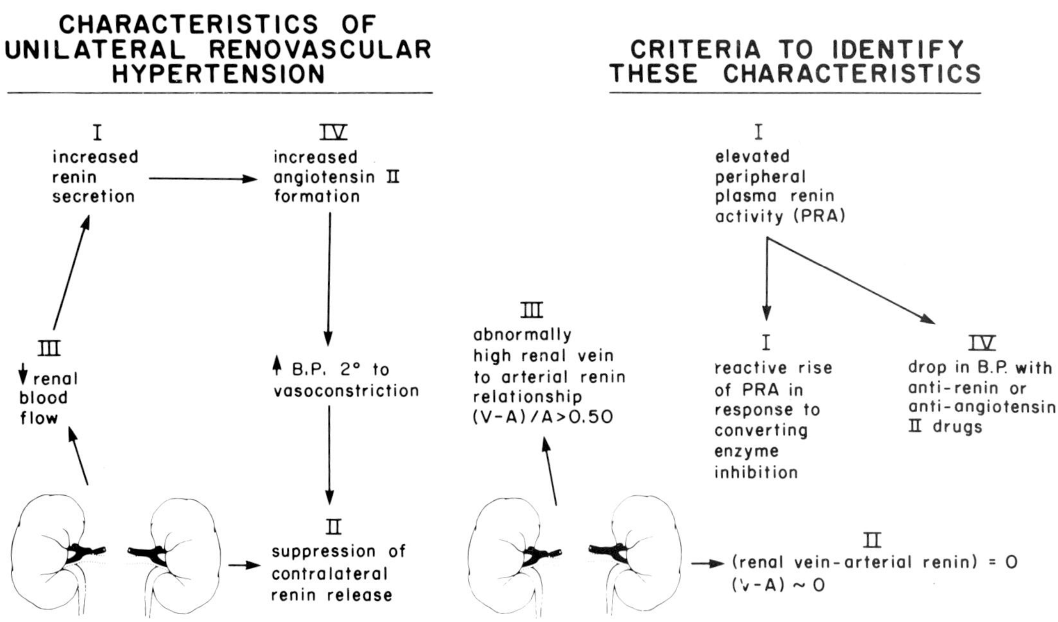

FIG. 4. Characteristics of the early phase of two-kidney, one-clip Goldblatt hypertension in the rat (left) and the criteria derived from the animal model that identify the patient with correctable renal hypertension. (From ref. 55.)

nous renin level has been determined to be approximately 25% higher than arterial PRA (Fig. 5) (44). Hence, a total renin increment (both kidneys) of approximately 50% is necessary to maintain a given peripheral renin level $(V - A)/A = 50\%$. However, a reduction in renal blood flow also influences the renal venous renin level. In this setting, the renal venous renin concentration will be misleadingly high, shifting the renal vein to arterial renin relationships upwards. Hence, the elevation of the increment above approximately 50% becomes an index of the severity of the reduction in blood flow consequent to the obstructing vascular lesion (Fig. 5). The combination of these criteria found in

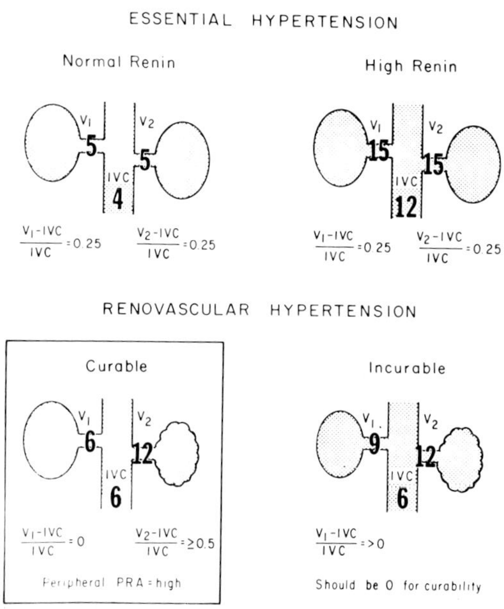

FIG. 5. Renal vein renin diagnostic patterns. In essential hypertension (*top*), at all levels of renin secretion, the renin level in each renal vein is about 25% greater than either the peripheral arterial or venous levels. In the setting of unilateral renin secretion (curable renovascular hypertension), the active kidney is solely responsible for maintaining the peripheral renin levels. Hence, the increment is 50% (0.5) and becomes progressively greater as the renal blood flow is reduced. Unequal bilateral renin secretion (*bottom right*) indicates bilateral disease and decreases the chance of cure following corrective unilateral surgery. (From ref. 27b.)

a group of patients managed by renal revascularization is shown in Fig. 6 (56).

In a group of 46 hypertensive patients with arteriographically proven unilateral renal artery stenosis who underwent successful angioplasty, 34 patients had technically successful sampling (41). Twelve patients had studies that were judged to be unsuccessful; nine sets of values were rejected because the combined increment from the two sides was less than 0.50. It is of interest that six of nine patients were taking captopril chronically and exhibited high systemic levels of PRA (between 14 and 99 ng/ml/hr) at the time of sampling. These data suggest that chronic converting enzyme blockade with captopril may invalidate renal vein renin analysis by a mechanism that is presently unclear. At the other extreme, three patients had extremely low peripheral PRA (<1 ng/ml/hr) at the time of sampling, two of whom were taking β-blockers. This latter situation is potentially clarified by captopril stimulation (see below).

Of the 34 patients with technically acceptable values, there were 23 true positives, no false positives, three true negatives, and eight false negatives. Of the eight false negatives, four had a $(V - A)/A$ between 0.40 and 0.48, and six showed contralateral suppression. Only two patients had symmetrical renal vein renins (41). Hence, the present approach gave a sensitivity of 74% and specificity of 100%, better indices than those found in renin ratio analysis.

Converting Enzyme Inhibition to Enhance the Accuracy of Renal Vein Renin Analysis

Following the initial report of renin stimulation by angiotensin blockade (42), several groups of investigators have reported increased renin release from the ischemic kidney with converting enzyme inhibition (28,52). The magnitudes of these induced changes are shown in Fig. 7. These data were determined from 26 patients with unilateral renovascular hypertension. Not shown in this illustration is the observation that the inferior vena cava levels (systemic or peripheral levels) were comparable to those values measured from the normal side,

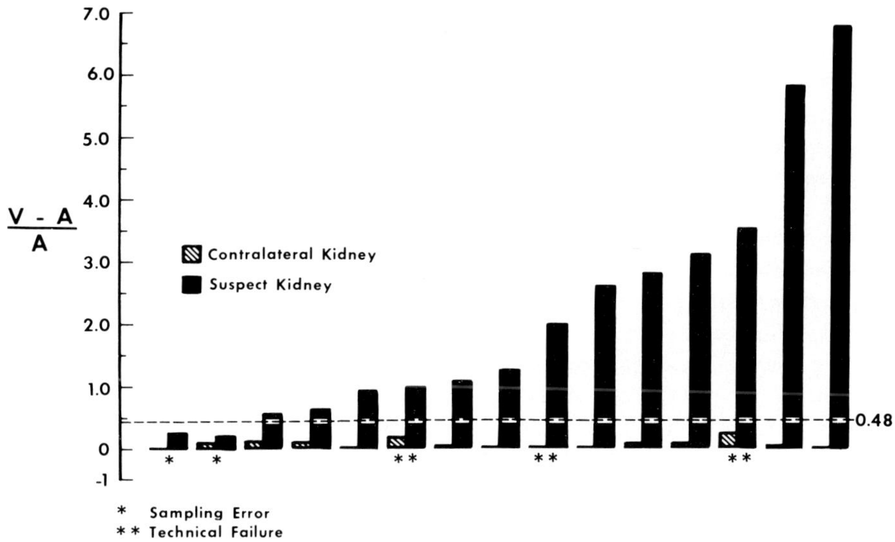

FIG. 6. Of 15 patients with renovascular hypertension, 13 exhibited (V-A)/A in excess of 48% from the suspect kidney and a suppressed value from the contralateral kidney. V is renal venous PRA: A is arterial or infrarenal inferior vena cava PRA. Asterisks denote the 3 patients who had values suggesting surgical curability yet who had residual or recurrent hypertension due to technical failure. The other patients were cured. (From ref. 56a.)

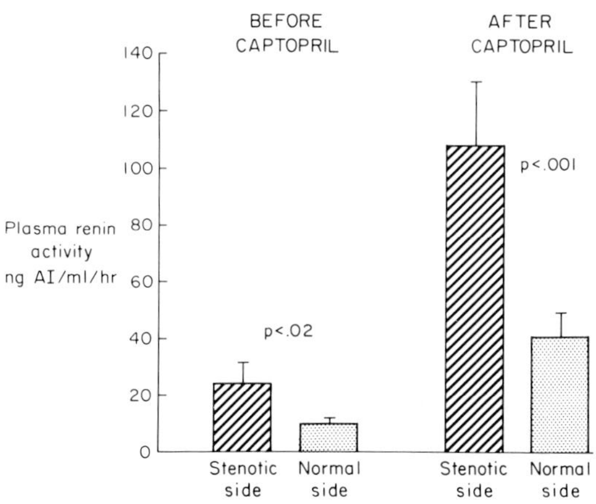

FIG. 7. Renal vein renin determinations (renal vein levels only) in patients with documented renovascular hypertension before and after captopril stimulation. Captopril accentuates renin secretion from the ischemic kidney. Not shown are the inferior vena cava levels which are the same as the levels measured from the normal side both before and after captopril stimulation. (From ref. 58.)

revealing the continued suppression of renin secretion from that kidney even after stimulation. Although more information is required to distinguish the subtleties (i.e., bilateral renovascular disease, branch lesions, total occlusions, coexistent renal parenchymal disease, etc.), it is clear that stimulation adds to the analysis in certain specific situations: (a) when patients are already on drug therapy, e.g., β-blockers, and the renin levels are generally reduced; (b) when there is a question about the reliability of the PRA measurements, particularly of low levels; (c) where experience performing renal vein renins is limited and subject to sampling errors; and (d) where there already exist equivocal values.

In summary, renal vein renin sampling after captopril stimulation accentuates renin release from ischemic renal tissue, which is particularly useful when values are equivocal, branch stenoses are present, or renovascular disease is superimposed on coexisting hypertension or renal disease. We anticipate that the addition of converting enzyme inhibition during renal venous sampling for renin will virtually eliminate the false negative analyses that have previously limited the accuracy of the studies.

ANATOMIC CONFIRMATION OF THE FOUR CRITERIA

It should be noted that virtually the entire evaluation of the hypertensive patient can now be accomplished without hospitalization, thus avoiding much of the expense previously felt to be too excessive to warrant evaluation (34, 35). We have performed over 300 renal vein renin samplings in outpatients, with 100 of them accompanied by digital angiography (DIVA), which is approximately 90% accurate in identifying renal arterial lesions (39). We utilize a central injection for the DIVA, which gives better definition of the renal vasculature. The major error arises with branch or segmental disease involving the smaller renal vessels.

Accordingly, DIVA can be utilized both to accompany renal vein sampling for renin to give anatomic definition of the renal vasculature, and to follow patients following correction of a renovascular lesion (46). The only caveat is to remember that the DIVA only demonstrates anatomical vascular disease and the functional significance of the lesion must still be demonstrated.

Taken altogether, screening criteria have been identified that provide great assurance that the patient with renovascular disease will be both physiologically and anatomically characterized and the success of a corrective procedure can be predicted. When these criteria have been identified, then the patient is admitted to the hospital for definitive management of the offending lesion.

VALIDATION OF THE CRITERIA

In addition to a favorable clinical response to renal angioplasty, we have also had the unique opportunity to study the effect of restoration of blood flow on renal vein renin concentration and renin secretion (41,57). To accomplish this goal, we have monitored the immediate effect of successful angioplasty on renal renin secretion. Thirty minutes following angioplasty, there was a marked reduction in the renal vein renin from the previously stenotic side (Fig. 8). The residual ipsilateral increment of renal vein renin was approximately 50% above the peripheral level, whereas contralateral renin suppression persisted. This 50% increment has been predicted previously to occur in the setting of unilateral renin secretion and normal renal blood flow (44).

Several months after angioplasty, there was marked fall in peripheral PRA with a return to normal in most patients, indicating a reduction in renin secretion (Fig. 2). Of equal interest is the restoration of bilateral renin increment of about 25% above the inferior vena cava renin level (Fig. 8). Hence, contralateral renin suppression reversed following successful angioplasty. This 25% increment from both kidneys is characteristic of the renin secretory pattern found in patients with essential hypertension (41).

The finding that the renal renin secretory char-

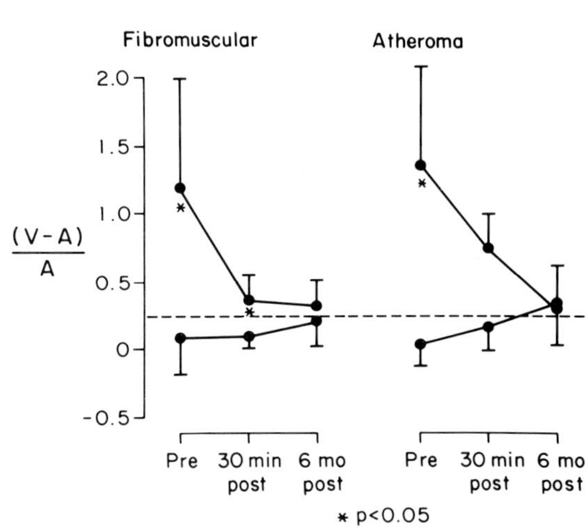

FIG. 8. Effect of angioplasty on renal vein renins. Samples were taken immediately before angioplasty, 30 minutes after, and 6 months after. The higher values correspond to the ischemic kidney, the lower to the contralateral kidney. Asterisk indicates significant difference between the 2 kidneys, and the dotted line is the normal level of (V-A)/A (0.24). (From ref. 41.)

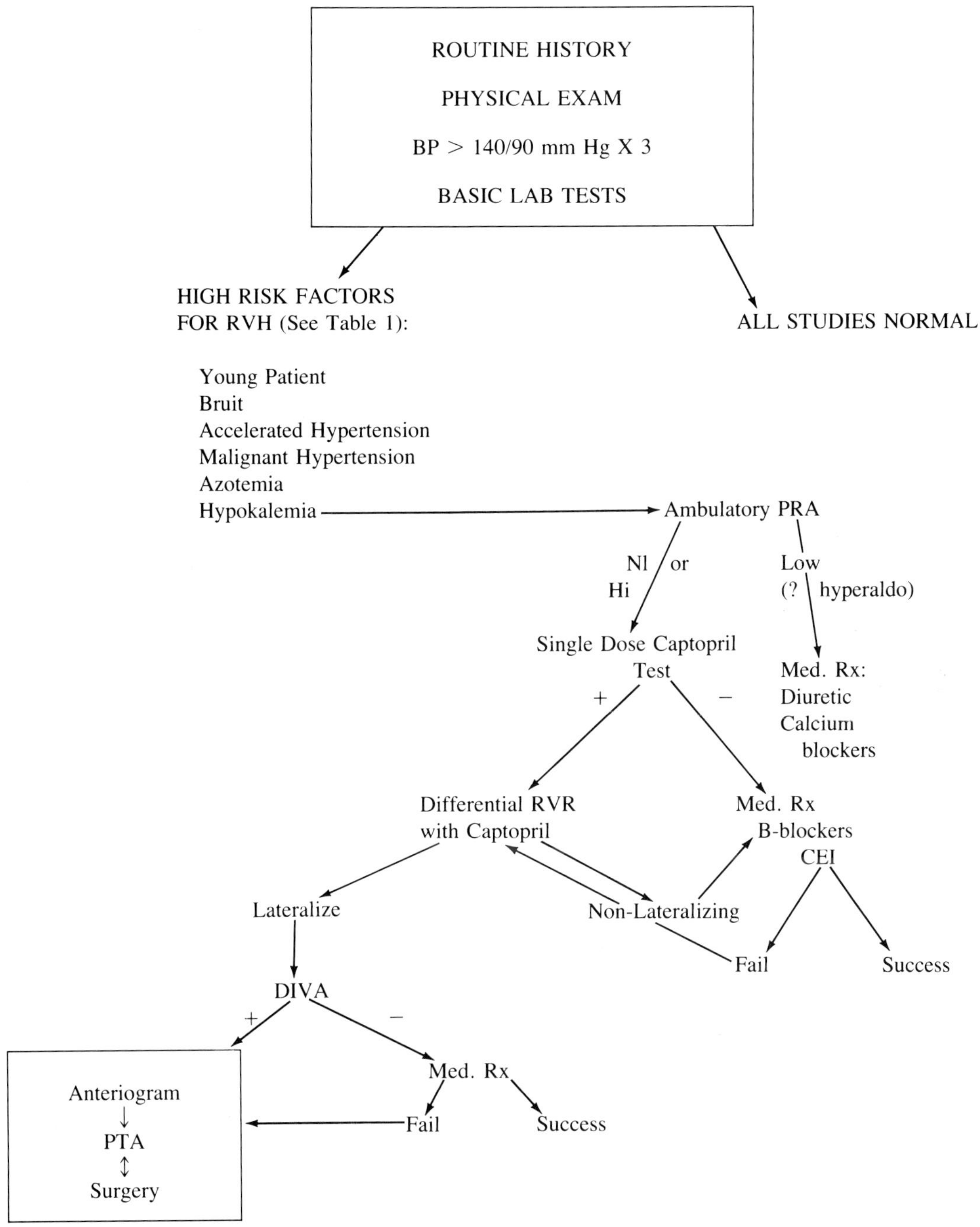

FIG 9. Evaluation for renovascular hypertension. (From ref. 46a.)

acteristics of renovascular hypertension reverse following successful angioplasty with correction of the hypertension is strong support that they truly reflect the abnormal secretory behavior of renin in curable renovascular hypertension.

IDENTIFYING THE POTENTIALLY CURABLE PATIENT: A COST-EFFECTIVE APPROACH

Our current approach is outlined in Fig. 9. All patients with fixed hypertension are potential candidates for this protocol, since we believe that nearly all patients with renovascular hypertension when identified can be best managed by angioplasty or revascularization. With respect to this empirical protocol, it could be argued that highly suspected patients could be screened initially with a digital angiogram. However, the functional significance of an anatomic lesion with respect to ischemia-induced renin release still must be established, so we routinely begin with a peripheral PRA.

In our experience, a low PRA is rarely found in untreated patients with nonazotemic renal arterial disease, and we therefore do not usually continue this evaluation in these patients unless they demonstrate refractoriness to treatment. Patients with high or normal PRA undergo a peripheral captopril test. The test cannot be performed if the patient is taking captopril chronically. If the test is positive, then the differential renal vein sampling and digital angiography are performed together. The sampling procedure is ideally done first, and then the catheter is advanced into the superior vena cava for injection of contrast material. This combined study is performed in the radiology suite, following which the patient lies quietly in the hypertension unit for 2 to 4 hr before returning home.

After the diagnostic criteria have been established, the patient is briefly hospitalized for selective arteriography and percutaneous transluminal angioplasty.

We continue to believe that the functional significance of a renal artery lesion must be identified before the therapeutic decision is directed toward intervention.

ACKNOWLEDGMENTS

This work was supported by the National Heart, Lung, and Blood Institute (HL 18323 SCR) of the National Institutes of Health.

REFERENCES

1. Ayers, C. R., Harris, R. H., and Lefer, L. G. (1969): Control of renin release in experimental hypertension. *Circ. Res.* (*Suppl.* 1), 24/25:103–112.
2. Blake, W. D., Wegria, R., Ward, H. P., and Frank, C. W. (1950): Effect of renal arterial constriction on excretion of sodium and water. *Am. J. Physiol.*, 163:422–429.
3. Bookstein, J. J., Abrams, H. L., Buenger, R. E., Lecky, J., Franklin, S. S., Reiss, N. D., Bleifer, K. H., Klatte, E. C., Varady, P. D., and Maxwell, M. H. (1972): Radiologic aspects of renovascular hypertension. Part II. The role of urography in unilateral renovascular disease. *JAMA*, 220:1225.
4. Brunner, H. R., Gavras, H., Laragh, J. H., and Keenan, R. (1973): Angiotensin II blockade in man by SAR1-Ala8-angiotensin II for understanding and treatment of high blood pressure. *Lancet*, 2:1045–1048.
5. Brunner, H. R., Laragh, J. H., Baer, L., Newton, M. A., Goodwin, F. T., Krakoff, L. R., Bard, R. M., and Buhler, F. R. (1972): Essential hypertension: Renin and aldosterone, heart attack, and stroke. *N. Engl. J. Med.*, 286:441–449.
6. Carey, R. M., Vaughan, E. D., Jr., Ackerly, J. A., Peach, M. J., and Ayers, C. R. (1978): The immediate pressor effect of saralasin in man. *J. Clin. Endocrinol. Metab.*, 46:36–43.
7. Case, D. B., Atlas, S. A., and Laragh, J. H. (1979): Reactive hyperreninemia to angiotensin blockade identified renovascular hypertension. *Clin. Sci.*, 57:313s–316s.
8. Case, D. B., Atlas, S. A., and Laragh, J. H. (1982): Physiologic effects and blockade. In: *Frontiers in Hypertension Research,* edited by J. H. Laragh, F. R. Buhler, and D. W. Seldin, pp. 541–550. Springer-Verlag, New York.
9. Case, D. B., Atlas, S. A., Laragh, J. H., Sealey, J. E., Sullivan, P. A., and McKinstry, D. N. (1978): Clinical experience with blockade of the renin-angiotensin-aldosterone system by an oral converting enzyme inhibitor (SQ 14225, captopril) in hypertensive patients. *Prog. Cardiovasc. Dis.*, 21:195–206.
10. Case, D. B., and Laragh, J. H. (1979): Reactive hyperreninemia following angiotensin blockade with either saralasin or converting enzyme inhibitor: A new approach to screen for renovascular hypertension. *Ann. Intern. Med.*, 91:153–160.
11. Case, D. B., Wallace, J. M., Keim, H. J., Sealey, J. E., and Laragh, J. H. (1976): Usefulness and limitations of saralasin, a weak competitive agonist for angiotensin II, for evaluating the renin and sodium factors in hypertensive patients. *Am. J. Med.*, 60:825–836.
12. Case, D. B., Wallace, J. M., Keim, H. J., Weber, M. A., Drayer, J. I. M., White, R. P., Sealey, J. E.,

and Laragh, J. H. (1976): Estimating renin participation in hypertension: Superiority of converting enzyme inhibitor over saralasin. *Am. J. Med.*, 61:790–796.
13. Chrysant, S. G., Dunn, M., and Marples, D. (1983): Severe reversible azotemia from captopril therapy. *Arch. Intern. Med.*, 143:437–441.
14. Dean, R. H. (1984): Renovascular hypertension: An overview. In: *Vascular Surgery,* Chapter 107, edited by R. B. Rutherford. W. B. Saunders, Philadelphia.
15. Eyler, W. R., Clark, M. D., Garman, J. E., Rian, R. L., and Meininger, D. E. (1962): Angiography of the renal areas including a comparative study of renal arterial stenosis in patients with and without hypertension. *Radiology,* 78:879–891.
16. Franklin, S. S., and Maxwell, M. H. (1975): Clinical workshop for renovascular hypertension. *Urol. Clin. North Am.*, 2:301.
17. Freeman, N. E., Leeds, F. M., and Elliot, W. (1954): Thromboendarterectomy for hypertension due to renal artery occlusion. *JAMA,* 156:1077.
18. Goldblatt, H., Lynch, J., Hanzel, R. F., and Summerville, W. W. (1934): Studies on experimental hypertension. I. The production of persistent elevation of systolic blood pressure by means of renal ischemia. *J. Exp. Med.*, 59:347.
19. Goncharenko, V., Gerlock, A. J., Shaff, M. I., and Hollifield, S. W. (1981): Progression of renal artery fibromuscular dysplasia in 42 patients as seen on angiography. *Radiology,* 139:45–51.
20. Harvey, R. J., Krumlovsky, F., delGroco, F., and Martin, H. G. (1985): Screening for renovascular hypertension: Is renal digital-subtraction angiography the preferred noninvasive test? *JAMA,* 254:388–393.
21. Hillman, B. J., Smith, J. R. L., Pond, G. D., Ovitt, T. W., and Capp, M. P. (1983): Photoelectric radiology. In: *Radiology, Vol. 4,* edited by W. N. Hanafec and G. H. Wilson. John Wiley and Sons, New York.
22. Holley, K. E., Hunt, J. C., Brown, A. L., Kincaid, O. W., and Sheps, S. G. (1964): Renal artery stenosis: A clinical-pathologic study in normotensive patients. *Am. J. Med.*, 37:14–22.
23. Horn, M. L., Conklin, V. M., Keenan, R. E., Varady, P. D., and Dinardo, J. (1979): Angiotensin II profiling with saralasin: Summary of the Eaton Collaborative Study. *Kidney Int. Suppl.* 9:S115–S122.
24. Howard, J. E., and Conner, T. B. (1954): Use of differential renal function studies in the diagnosis of renovascular hypertension. *Am. J. Surg.*, 107:58.
25. Hunt, J. C., and Strong, C. S. (1973): Renovascular hypertension: Mechanisms, natural history and treatment. *Am. J. Cardiol.*, 32:562–574.
26. Judson, W. E., and Helmer, O. M. (1965): Diagnostic and prognostic values of renin activity in renal venous plasma in renovascular hypertension. *Hypertension,* 13:79–89.
27. Krakoff, L. R. and Perla, C. (1983): Screening for renovascular hypertension. *J. Cardiovasc. Med.*, p. 555.
27a. Laragh, J. H., Baer, L., Brunner, H. R., Buhler, F. R., Sealey, J. E., and Vaughan, E. D., Jr. (1974): The renin-angiotensin-aldosterone system in pathogenesis and management of hypertensive vascular disease. *Hypertension Manual*, edited by John H. Laragh, pp. 313–351. Dun-Donnelley Publishing Corp., New York.
27b. Laragh, J. H., and Sealey, J. E. (1977): Renin-sodium profiling: Why, how, and when in clinical practice. *Cardiovasc. Med.*, 2:1053–1075.
28. Lyons, D. F., Streck, W. F., Kem, D. C., et al. (1983): Captopril stimulation of differential renins in renovascular hypertension. *Hypertension,* 5:615.
29. Marks, L. S., and Maxwell, M. H. (1975): Renal vein renin value and limitations in the prediction of operative results. *Urol. Clin. North Am.*, 2:311–325.
30. Mason, J. C., and Hilton, P. J. (1983): Reversible renal failure due to captopril in a patient with transplant artery stenosis. *Hypertension,* 5:623.
31. Maxwell, M. H., and Lupu, A. N. (1968): Excretory urogram in renal arterial hypertension. *J. Urol.*, 100:395–406.
32. Maxwell, M. H., Lupu, A. N., and Taplin, G. V. (1968): Radioisotope renogram in renal arterial hypertension. *J. Urol.*, 100:376–383.
33. McCormack, L. J., Poutasse, E. F., Meaney, T. F., Noto, T. J., and Dustan, H. P. (1966): A pathologic arteriographic correlation of renal arterial disease. *Am. Heart J.*, 72:188–198.
34. McNeil, B. J., and Adelstein, S. J. (1975): Measures of clinical efficacy: The value of case finding in hypertensive renovascular disease. *N. Engl. J. Med.*, 293:221–226.
35. McNeil, B. J., Varady, P. D., and Burrows, B. A. (1975): Measures of clinical efficacy: Cost-effectiveness calculations in the diagnosis and treatment of hypertensive renovascular disease. *N. Engl. J. Med.*, 293:216–221.
36. Meaney, T. F., Dustan, H. P., and McCormack, L. J. (1968): Natural history of renal arterial disease. *Radiology,* 9:877–887.
37. Muller, F. B., Sealey, J. E., Case, D. B., Atlas, S. A., Pickering, T. G., Pecker, M. S., Preibisz, J. J., and Laragh, J. H. (1986): The captopril test for identifying renovascular disease in hypertensive patients. *Am. J. Med.*, 80:633.
38. Nicholson, J. P., Alderman, M. H., Pickering, T. G., Teishman, S. L., Sos, T. A., and Laragh, J. H. (1983): Cigarette smoking in renovascular hypertension. *Lancet,* 2:765–766.
39. Osborne, R. W., Jr., Goldstone, J., Hillman, B. J., et al. (1981): Digital video subtraction angiography: Screening technique for renovascular hypertension. *Surgery,* 90:932–939.
40. Pickering, T. G., Sos, T. A., Vaughan, E. D., Jr., and Laragh, J. H. (1986): Differing patterns of renal vein renin secretion in patients with renovascular hypertension, and their role in predicting the response to angioplasty. *Nephron.*, 44:8–11.
41. Pickering, T. G., Sos, T. A., Vaughan, E. D., Jr., Case, D. B., Sealey, J. E., Harshfield, G. A., and Laragh, J. H. (1984): Predictive value and changes of renin secretion in hypertensive patients with unilateral renovascular disease undergoing successful renal angioplasty. *Am. J. Med.*, 76:398–404.
42. Re, R., Noveline, R., Escourrou, M.-T., Athanasoulis, C., Burton, J., and Haber, E. (1978): Inhibition of angiotensin-converting enzyme for diagnosis of renal-artery stenosis. *N. Engl. J. Med.*, 298:582–586.

43. Schreiber, M. J., Pohl, M. A., and Novick, A. C. (1984): The natural history of atherosclerotic and fibrous renal artery disease. *Urol. Clin. North Am.*, 11:383–392.
44. Sealey, J. E., Buhler, F. R., Laragh, J. H., and Vaughan, E. D., Jr. (1973): The physiology of renin secretion in essential hypertension: Estimation of renin secretion rate and renal plasma flow from peripheral and renal vein renin levels. *Am. J. Med.*, 55:391–401.
45. Simon, N., Franklin, S. S., Bleifer, K. H., and Maxwell, M. H. (1972): Clinical characteristics of renovascular hypertension. *JAMA*, 220:1209–1218.
46. Sos, T. A., Sniderman, K. W., Pickering, T. G., et al. (1983): Percutaneous transluminal renal angioplasty in renovascular hypertension due to atheroma or fibromuscular dysplasia. *N. Engl. J. Med.*, 309:274.
46a. Sosa, R. E., and Vaughan, E. D., Jr. (1983): Evaluation of surgically curable hypertension. AUA Update Series, Vol. II, Lesson 31.
47. Stamey, T. A. (1963): In: *Renovascular Hypertension*.Williams and Wilkins, Baltimore. MD.
48. Stamey, T. A., Nudelman, I. J., Good, T. H., Schwentker, E. N., and Hendricks, F. (1961): Functional characteristics of renovascular hypertension. *Medicine*, 40:347.
49. Stewart, B. H., Dustan, H. P., Kiser, W. S., Meaney, T. F., Straffon, R. A., and McCormack, L. J. (1970): Correlation of angiography and natural history in evaluation of patients with renovascular hypertension. *J. Urol.*, 104:231–238.
50. Stockigt, J. R., Noakes, C. A., Collins, R. D., Schambelan, M., and Biglieri, E. G. (1972): Renal-vein renin in various forms of renal hypertension. *Lancet*, 1:1194–1198.
51. Textor S. C., Novick, A. C., Tarazi, R. C., et al. (1985): Critical perfusion pressure for renal function in patients with bilateral atherosclerotic renal vascular disease. *Ann. Intern. Med.*, 102:308–314.
52. Thibonnier, M., Joseph, A., Sassano, P., Guyenne, T. T., Corvol, P., Raynaud, A., Seurot, M., and Gaux, J. C. (1984): Improved diagnosis of unilateral renal artery lesions after captopril administration. *JAMA*, 251:56–60.
53. Thornbury, J. R., Stanley, J. C., and Fryback, D. G. (1982): Hypertensive urogram: A nondiscriminatory test for renovascular hypertension. *AJR*, 138:43–49.
54. Vaughan, E. D., Jr. (1979): Laboratory test in the evaluation of renal hypertension. *Urol. Clin. North Am.*, 6:485–502.
55. Vaughan, E. D., Jr. (1985): Renovascular hypertension. *Kidney Int.*, 27:811–827.
56. Vaughan, E. D., Jr., Buhler, F. R., Laragh, J. H., Sealey, J. E., Baer, L., and Bard, R. H. (1973): Renovascular hypertension; renin measurements to indicate hypersecretion and contralateral suppression, estimate renal plasma flow and score for surgical curability. *Am. J. Med.*, 55:402–414.
56a. Vaughan, E. D., Jr., Carey, R. M., Ayers, C. R., Peach, M. J., Tegtmeyer, C. J., and Wellons, H. A., Jr. (1979): Physiologic definition of blood pressure response to renal revascularization in patients with renovascular hypertension. *Kid. Int.*, 15:S83–S92.
57. Vaughan, E. D., Jr., Sos, T. A., Sniderman, K. W., Pickering, T. G., Case, D. B., Sealey, J. E., and Laragh, J. H. (1981): Renal vein renin secretory patterns before and after transluminal angioplasty in patients with renovascular hypertension: Verification of analytic criteria. In: *Frontiers in Hypertension Research*, edited by J. H. Laragh, pp. 173–179. Springer-Verlag, New York.
58. Vaughan, E. D., Jr., Case, D. B,. Pickering, T. G., Sosa, R. E., Sos, T. A., Laragh, J. H. (1984): Clinical evaluation of renovascular hypertension and therapeutic decision. *Urol. Clin. North Am.*, 11:393–408.
59. Wollenweber, J., Sheps, S. G., and David, D. G. (1968): Clinical course of atherosclerotic renovascular disease. *Am. J. Cardiol.*, 21:60–71.

The Kidney in Hypertension, edited by
Norman M. Kaplan, Barry M. Brenner,
and John H. Laragh. Raven Press,
New York © 1987.

Imaging Evaluation of the Hypertensive Patient

Bruce J. Hillman

Department of Radiology, University of Arizona College of Medicine, Tucson, Arizona 85724

During the past decade, there have developed new imaging technologies applicable to the diagnosis and treatment of renal hypertension. Most notable among these have been ultrasonography, computed axial tomography (CT), digital subtraction angiography (DSA), and percutaneous transluminal angioplasty (PTA) and embolization. In general, these advances have made it easier, safer, and less costly to evaluate and treat patients with renal disease causing hypertension. Their availability also has raised questions concerning the conventional philosophy of indiscriminant medical therapy for hypertension.

Indeed, considering the potential of these technologies, and in view of data indicating prolonged lifespan and fewer target organ complications accruing to patients with renal hypertension undergoing definitive treatment (22,23,33,35), it is likely that too few patients are being evaluated for a renal etiology of their blood pressure elevation. In large measure, this is simply a reflection of physicians' reliance on habitual practices and unfamiliarity with new technologies. However, it also is related to uncertainty over the prevalence of treatable renal hypertension, and hence the cost effectiveness of evaluating greater numbers of patients.

This presentation will review the contributions of new imaging technologies to the diagnosis and treatment of hypertension, indicate how they might alter the preferred approach to assessing patients for possible renal hypertension, and discuss an alternative approach to hypertensive patients that may be more appropriate in view of the technological changes. It should be noted, however, that the evaluation of patients for renal hypertension remains a controversial area, and that the views presented are to some extent subjective.

DIAGNOSING RENAL DISEASE, ASSESSING ITS RELATIONSHIP TO HYPERTENSION, AND IMAGING-GUIDED TREATMENT

Renal disorders that may cause hypertension are divisible into three broad categories:

Disorders of the major vasculature
Arteritides
Parenchymal diseases secondarily affecting the circulation

In each case, the pathogenesis of hypertension is related, at least initially, to the hypersecretion of renin in response to altered hemodynamics. Later in the course of disease, renal failure with salt and water retention may become a more important pathogenetic mechanism. Space limitations prevent a thorough discussion of the entities encompassed by each of these disease categories. General characteristics are described in this section; for more specific discussion of imaging methods and findings, the interested reader is referred to specialized reference works (1,33).

Diseases of the Major Vasculature

This category of conditions is further divisible into those resulting in stenotic and nonstenotic lesions. Of these two groups, stenotic renovascular disease is by far the more common etiology of renovascular hypertension, and is almost certainly the most common cause of treatable hypertension in adults (9,36).

Renal Artery Stenosis

According to the Cooperative Study on Renovascular Hypertension, approximately two-thirds of renal artery stenoses are caused by atherosclerosis, with most of the remainder being secondary to fibrodysplastic disease (9). Trauma, complications of surgical or radiological treatment, some pharmacologic agents, and a number of unusual conditions, such as neurofibromatosis and Takayasu's arteritis, are less common causes of renal artery stenoses.

Atherosclerotic renal artery stenosis either derives from aortic plaques or manifests as primary renal arterial stenosis in the proximal third of the main renal artery. Lesions are usually eccentric and extend variably down the length of the renal artery (9,57,69). A poststenotic dilatation (Fig. 1) may be present, reflecting either the effect of a "jet" of blood hitting the arterial wall, or a response to nonlaminar flow. Bilateral involvement is common. Lesions often progress on sequential evaluation (57,69).

There are a number of fibrodysplastic variants that result in renal artery stenosis. The one that accounts for the majority of encountered lesions is medial fibroplasia. Though frequently termed "fibromuscular hyperplasia," this is a misnomer; the media is replaced by disordered fibrosis, rather than being hypertrophied. Angiographically, this abnormality is described as resembling a "string of beads" (Fig. 2) (29,69). Point narrowings alternate with dilated segments that are of greater diameter than the normal renal artery. As with all of the fibrodysplastic variants, lesions usually are discovered in the mid- and distal main renal artery and in branch vessels. Intimal dysplasia is the most common ste-

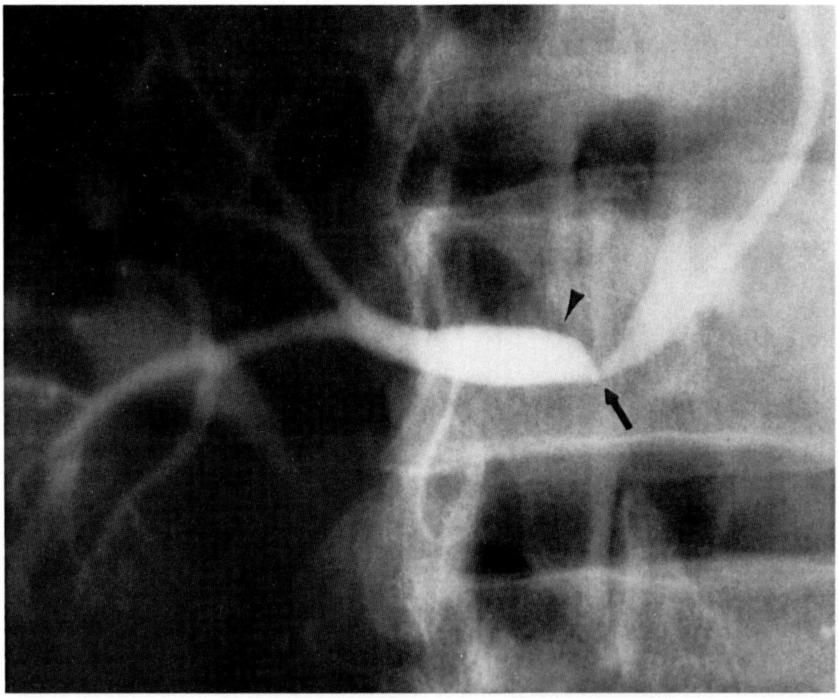

FIG. 1. Selective injection of the right renal artery demonstrates an eccentric focal stenosis secondary to atherosclerosis (*arrow*). There is poststenotic dilatation (*arrowhead*).

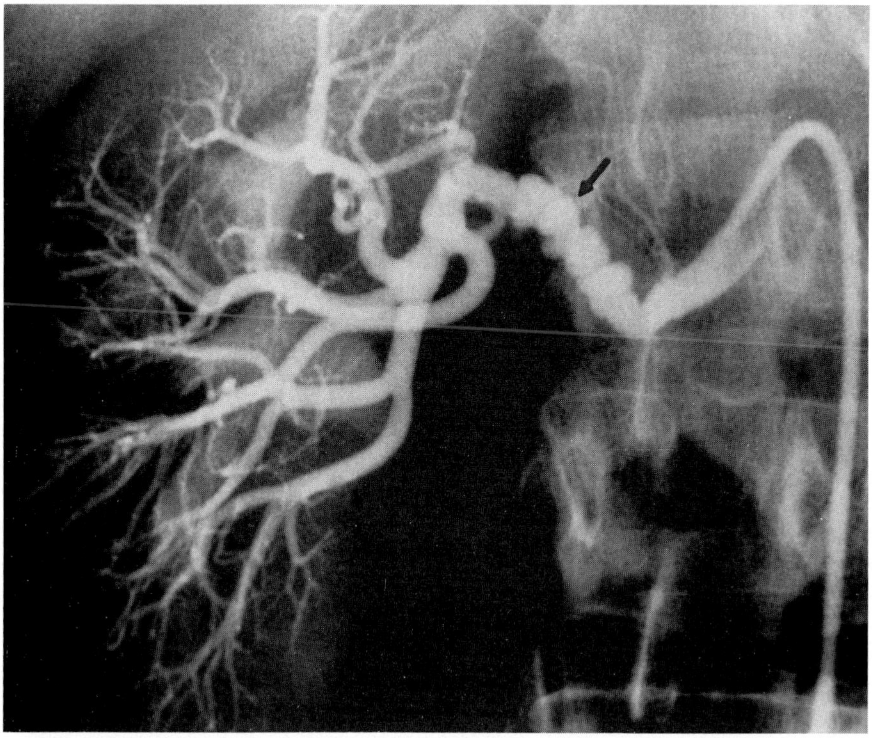

FIG. 2. A complex stenosis representing medial fibroplasia is demonstrated by selective right renal artery injection (*arrow*). The lesion is composed of alternating dilated segments and constricting bands.

notic lesion of childhood (18). This disorder produces circumferential lesions that may involve any focus of the major renal arterial circulation (Fig. 3), including isolated branch vessel lesions (68). That this is the case has important implications for renal vein renin sampling, since subselective venous sampling may be necessary to elicit an abnormality (39,42,62). Fibromuscular hyperplasia, perimedial fibroplasia, and adventitial fibroplasia are less common variants. The importance of determining which disorder is the cause of the lesion has been placed in doubt by recent work that depicts arteriography as less successful in differentiating among them, and between atherosclerosis and fibrodysplasia, than previously thought (69). Similarly, it may be less important to do so, if, as this investigation purports, all of the variants have a similarly significant propensity to progress over time (30).

In the past, the initial imaging study requested for evaluating suspected major vascular lesions causing hypertension was excretory urography (Fig. 4), radionuclide imaging, or a combination of the two. However, relatively low sensitivity and specificity associated with these studies (10,73)—particularly in view of the acknowledged low prevalence of renal hypertension—led to questioning of the efficacy of this approach. In addition a positive result did not actually depict the responsible lesion. Most notably, McNeil and co-workers demonstrated the high monetary and health costs of screening hypertensive patients using these modalities, definitive diagnosis by conventional arteriography, and treating discovered cases by available surgical techniques (49,50). This work set the tone for further recommendations that evaluation for renal hypertension should be reserved for patients with particularly suspicious presen-

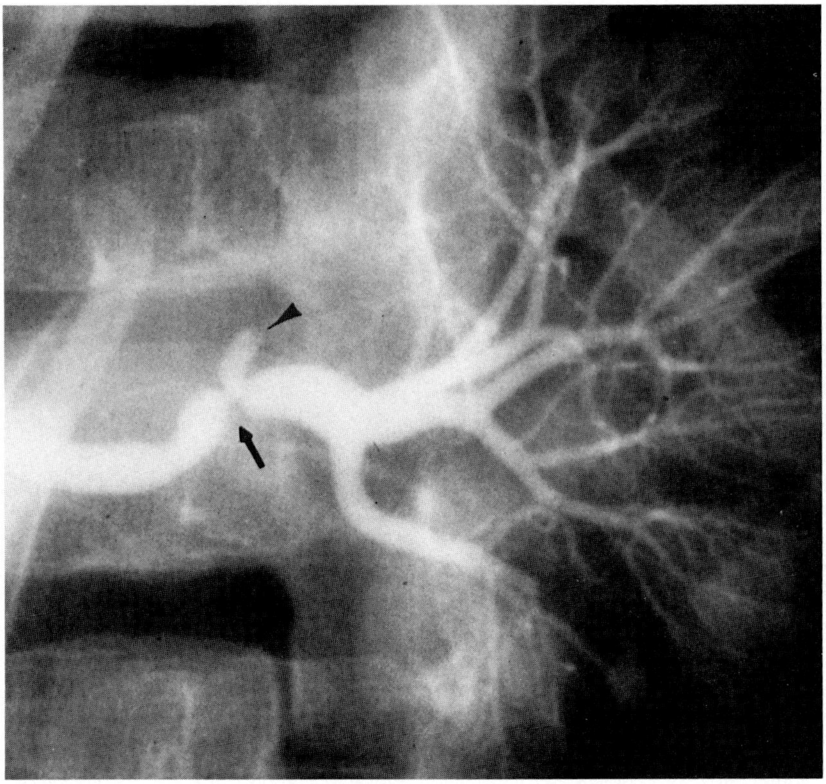

FIG. 3. Left renal arteriography depicts a severe renal artery stenosis in a child (*arrow*). The lesion represents intimal dysplasia; there is an associated aneurysm (*arrowhead*).

tations or who had failed a trial of medical therapy (33). Few authorities any longer apply excretory urography or radionuclide scanning to the investigation of renovascular hypertension.

More recently, some have advocated initial evaluation by intravenous DSA (IV-DSA) (32). They argued that the technique—involving peripheral venous or right atrial contrast administration and digital photoelectronic, rather than film-screen, imaging—offered safer and less expensive screening and definitive diagnosis (Fig. 5). It also proffered the opportunity for simultaneous renal vein renin analysis. However, the success experienced by advocates was not shared universally, probably because of early technological differences among equipment and differences in the skill and interest of practitioners. As a result, interest has waned in applying IV-DSA to evaluating patients for renovascular hypertension, though it still may be a useful initial examination in cooperative patients with good cardiac function.

Advancements in digital technology are increasingly promoting the use of intraarterial DSA (IA-DSA) as the most suitable initial examination for possible renovascular hypertension (Fig. 6). This represents nothing more than a return to the position often stated in the past that it is most cost effective to perform the definitive test first (8,40). Moreover, certain qualities of IA-DSA represent safety and expense improvements over conventional film-screen angiography. Among these are that the higher contrast resolution of digital technology permits the use of smaller catheters and smaller contrast doses. That images are displayed immediately on a CRT screen avoids the time and expense of film processing, making the examination faster, easier,

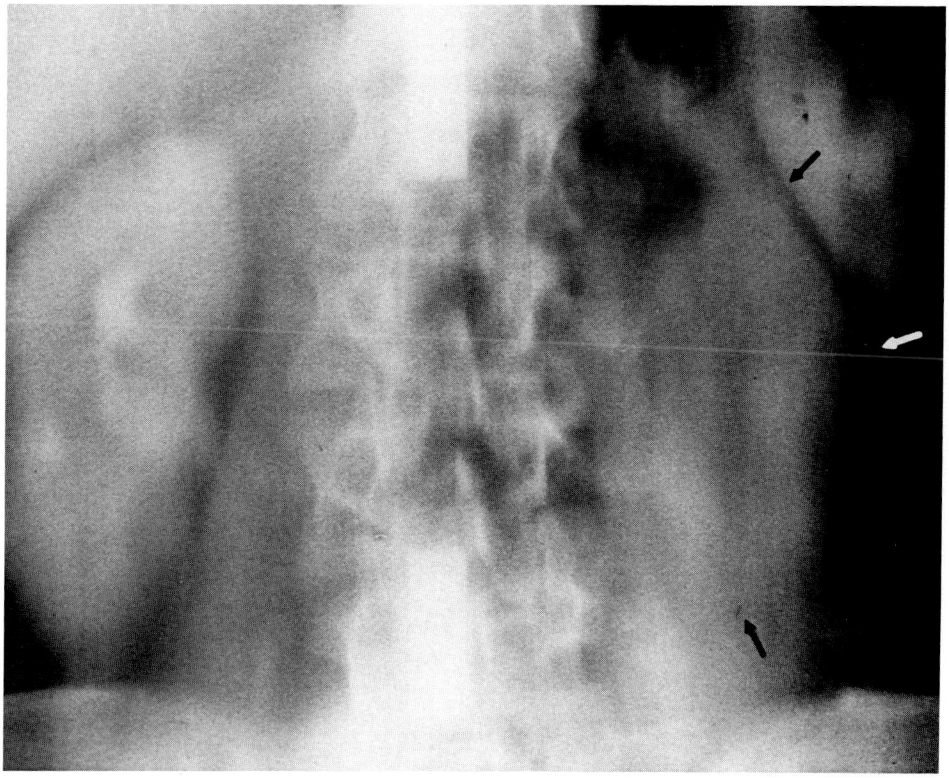

FIG. 4. The image is an exposure performed 3 min after intravenously injecting contrast material for hypertensive urography. Contrast material has reached the collecting system of the normal right kidney. That the left kidney (*arrow*) is smaller and no contrast material is seen in the collecting system implies reduced blood flow secondary to renal artery stenosis.

and less expensive (56). The combination of these virtues has made IA-DSA an outpatient procedure in most patients, despite the need for arterial puncture and catheterization. Finally, at the time of the procedure, a discovered lesion can be evaluated for angiographic signs of hemodynamic significance: severity of narrowing and the presence of a collateral circulation (Fig. 7). When appropriate, percutaneous transluminal treatment can be attempted immediately for definitive amelioration of hypertension. This approach eliminates the possibility of assessment by renal vein renin analysis unless it is performed well in advance of arteriography. Still, many practitioners have become disenchanted with the false negative rate of renal vein sampling and are increasingly relying on the cited radiographic evidences of significance to arrive at treatment determinations. Particularly as economic considerations become more pronounced, IA-DSA is likely to become the preferred approach to screening and diagnosis of renovascular hypertension. Still unknown is the role that magnetic resonance imaging (MRI) may play in vascular diagnosis and quantitation of blood flow. Preliminary results are promising; however, much technological development will be necessary before the potential of MRI for noninvasive diagnosis of renovascular hypertension might be realized.

Regardless of the angiographic modality employed, the goal of the procedure is to depict major vascular abnormalities that might be causing hypertension, define their severity and extent, and evaluate the parenchymal circulation for evidence of associated disease that might

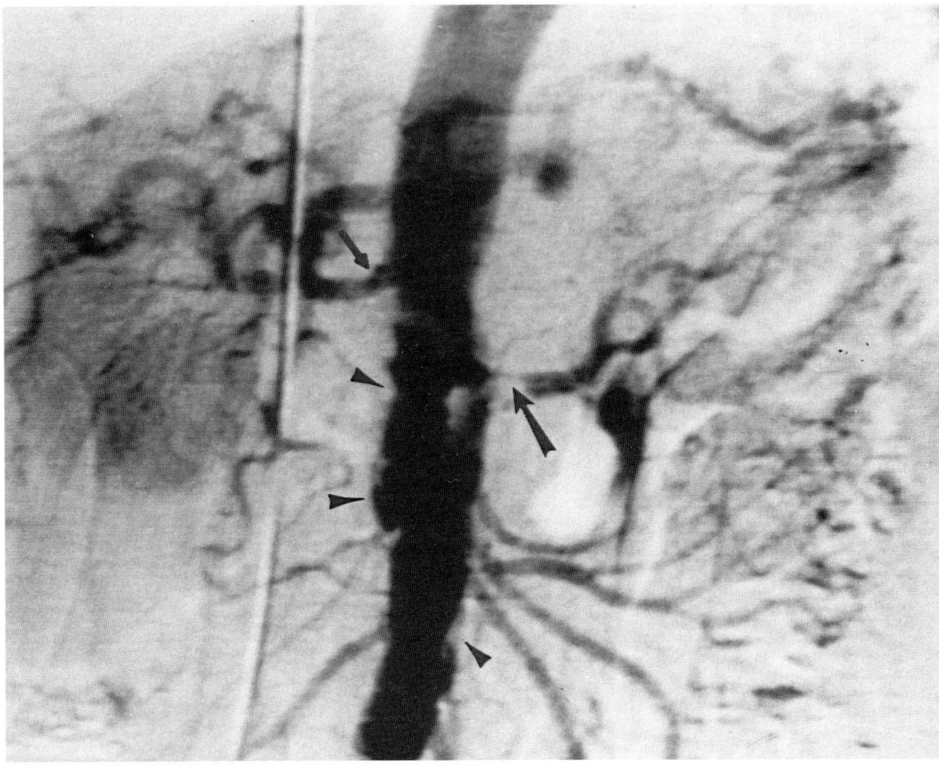

FIG. 5. A hypertensive middle-aged male underwent IV-DSA examination for evaluation of possible renovascular disease. There is diffuse infrarenal aortic atherosclerosis (*arrowheads*). The right renal artery is irregular proximally (*small arrow*), but no stenosis is present. There is a severe postostial stenosis of the left renal artery (*large arrow*).

predict a poor result for interventional therapy. As noted above, the arteriogram should be evaluated for a collateral circulation that might imply that the renovascular disease discovered is, indeed, the cause of the hypertension.

Imaging-guided transluminal treatment for renovascular hypertension is discussed in detail elsewhere in this volume. For stenotic lesions, success with PTA has improved dramatically since its advent, such that its efficacy now approximates that of surgery (16,19,47,52,67,72). As with surgery, PTA is more successful in treating fibrodysplastic lesions than atherosclerosis, unilateral, and/or limited disease, and is better applied to primary renal artery than osteal lesions (16,19,52,67). The technique is applicable to completely occluded arteries and branch vessel stenoses (16). This latter virtue promotes conservation of renal tissue. Finally, PTA is associated with lower morbidity and mortality than traditional surgical treatment for renovascular hypertension. A failed attempt at PTA or recurrent stenoses precludes neither repeat PTA nor surgical therapy. Because of its relative benignity, some have suggested a trial of PTA as the initial treatment for all stenotic lesions suspected of causing hypertension (67).

Nonstenotic Major Vascular Lesions

The diagnostic process for discovering nonstenotic major vessel abnormalities that might be causing hypertension is similar to that described for renal artery stenosis. Again, definitive diagnosis is by some form of arteriography. The most common such abnormality that has

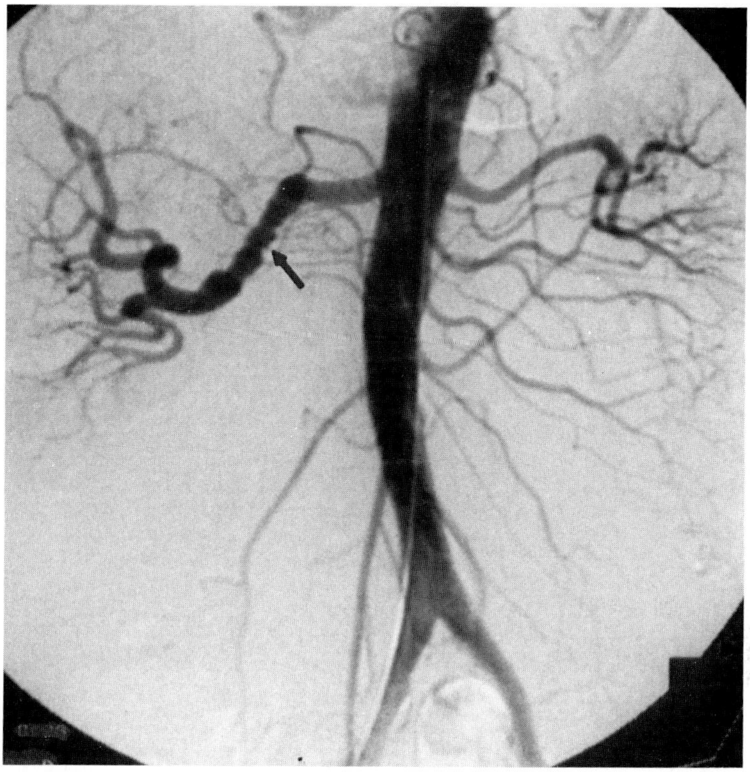

FIG. 6. IA-DSA was performed to evaluate a hypertensive young woman for a renovascular etiology. Medial fibroplasia invests the middle and distal thirds of the right renal artery (*arrow*).

been associated with blood pressure elevation is renal artery aneurysm. Though most renal artery aneurysms are discovered incidentally during angiograms on normotensive patients, certainly numerous cases have been reported where aneurysmectomy has ameliorated hypertension (21,34). Presumably, in these cases, the aneurysm was either compressing a major vessel or in some other manner resulting in disordered hemodynamics. Arteriovenous communications—most of which are traumatic but a minority congenital (70)—cause hypertension by shunting blood away from normal renal tissue. The result is ischemia and abnormally high renin secretion. Traumatic fistulae generally involve only one or a few feeding arteries, a pseudoaneurysm, and one or several veins (Fig. 8). Congenital aneurysms usually present as a tangle of small vessels. For both disorders, the pathognomonic arteriographic finding is the near simultaneous contrast opacification of renal artery and vein.

Renal artery aneurysms and arteriovenous communications also may be treated transluminally, but by embolization (Fig. 9) (13,17,44, 53,54). Many of the advantages cited for PTA hold for transluminal embolization therapy of amenable lesions. Particularly important is that directable catheters permit treatment to be directed specifically at the lesion, with relatively little damage being incurred by adjacent normal renal tissue.

Arteritides

This category of diseases primarily affects the peripheral intraparenchymal circulation; however, more proximal vessels, including the main

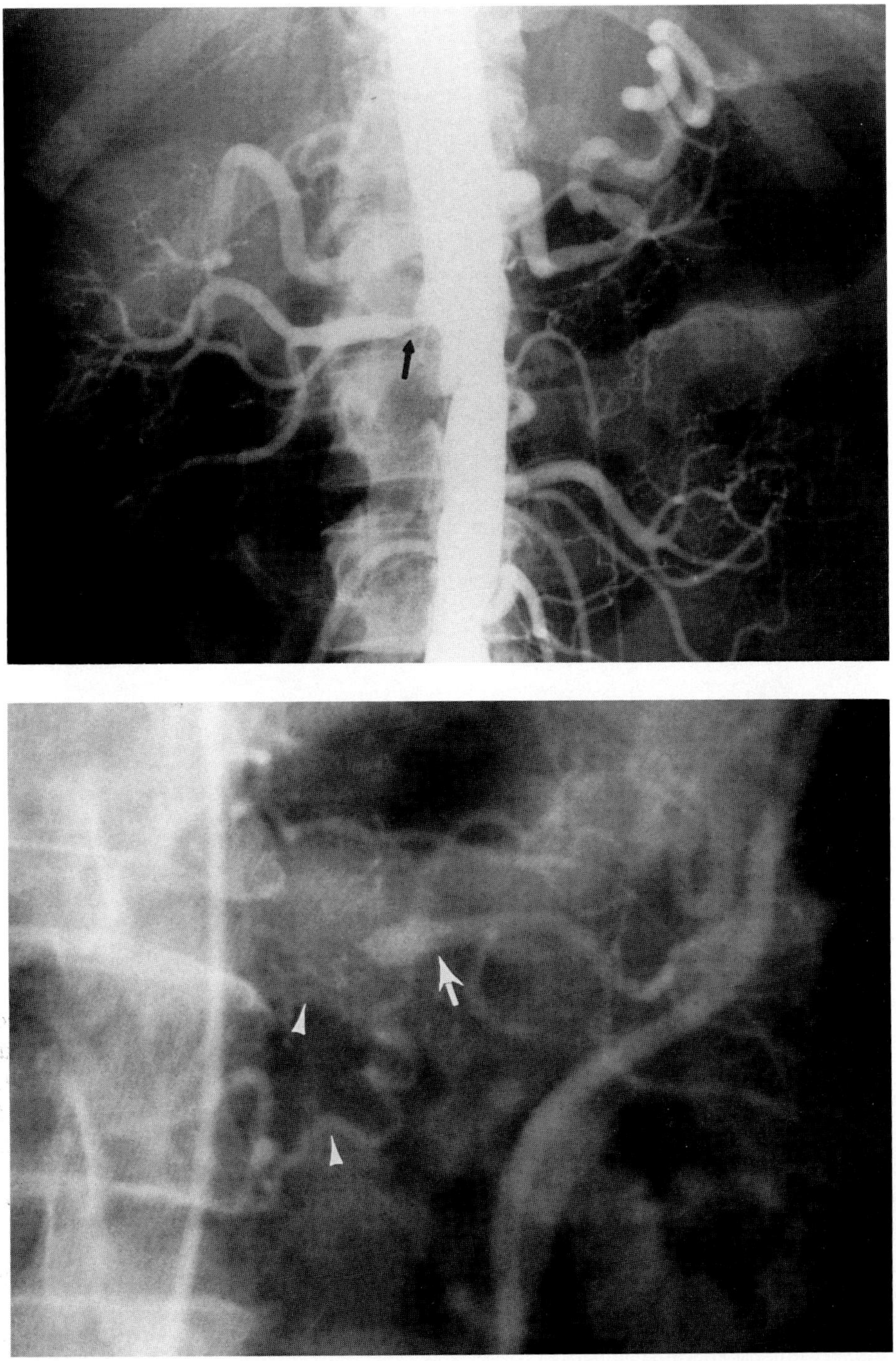

A

B

FIG. 7. A. Aortography demonstrates aortic atherosclerosis and a moderate right renal artery stenosis (*arrow*). There is apparent occlusion of the left renal artery. **B.** Coned down view of the region demonstrates late filling of the left renal artery (*arrow*) by collateral vessels (*arrowheads*).

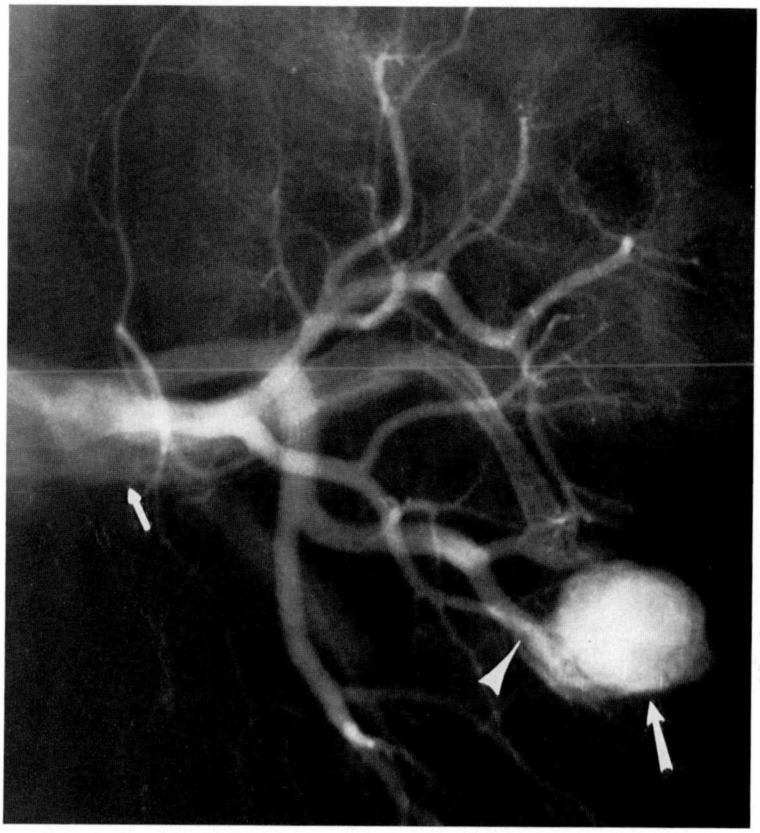

FIG. 8. There is a traumatic arteriovenous fistula. An artery (*arrowhead*) feeds a pseudoaneurysm (*large arrow*); there is simultaneous opacification of the renal vein (*small arrow*).

renal artery, sometimes manifest evidence of involvement. Entities included among the arteritides (angiitides) are polyarteritis nodosa; arteritis related to abusing multiple illicit drugs, especially amphetamine; scleroderma and lupus erythematosis; acute glomerulonephritis; renal allograft rejection; and radiation nephritis.

Clinical presentation often will suggest the diagnosis and precipitate renal biopsy. In other cases, an imaging evaluation may be undertaken. Excretory urography or renal ultrasonography will most often result in nonspecific findings. Kidneys may be large, normal, or small, depending on the stage of the process; contrast material density in the parenchyma and its concentration in the collecting system usually will be diminished. Definitive diagnosis of an arteritis is by arteriography (Fig. 10). Though it previously was believed that such findings as microaneurysms, a "spotted" capillary phase, or reduced corticomedullary differentiation had histologic significance, it is now generally accepted that there is considerable overlap in the angiographic findings among arteritides. Usually, the small vessels will be irregular and truncated. The peripheral circulation will have a generally sparser than normal appearance. Small and large aneurysms may appear with any of the arteritides, and may appear and disappear in the same patient on sequential angiograms (12,24,27,31,43,45,60,75). The capillary phase images will demonstrate inhomogeneous opa-

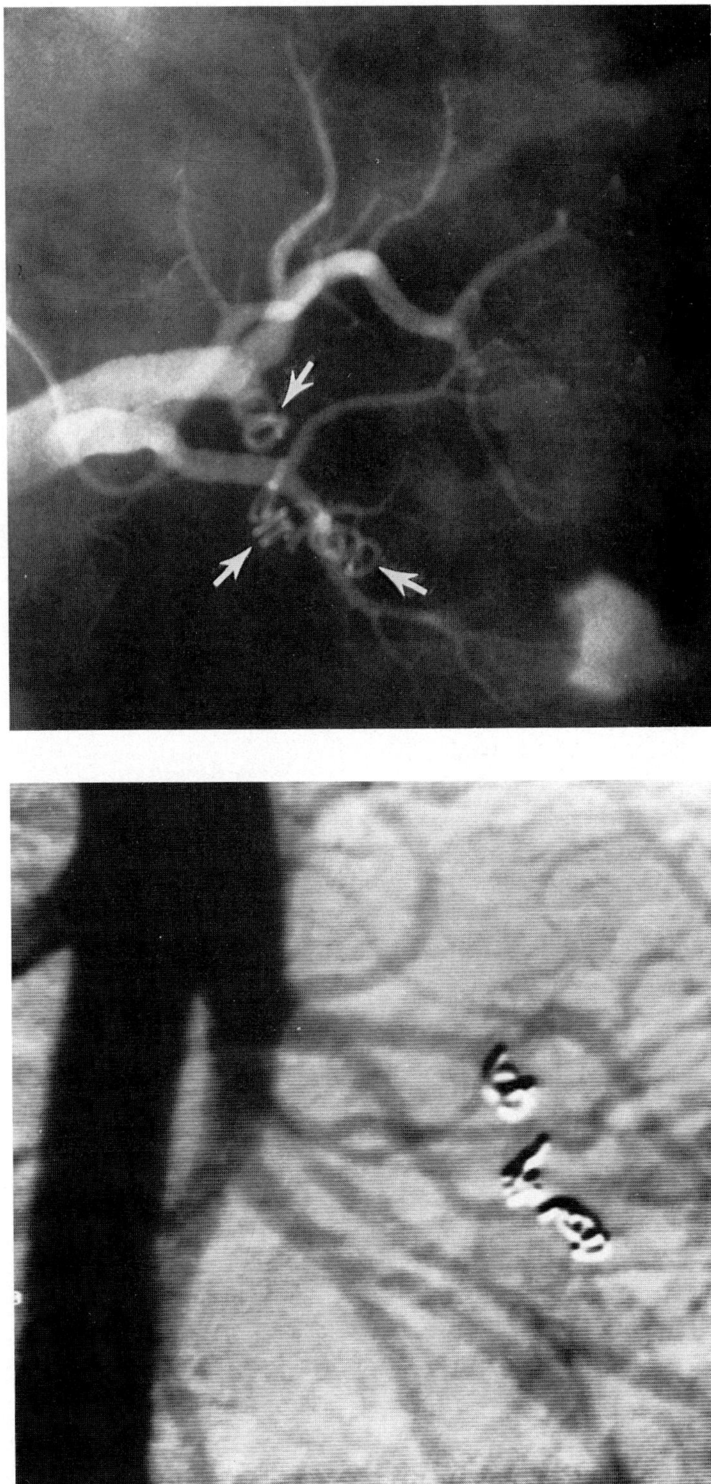

A

B

FIG. 9. A. The arteriovenous fistula depicted in Fig. 8 was embolized using Gianturco coils (*arrows*). **B.** One month following the embolization procedure, an IV-DSA examination demonstrates complete occlusion of the fistula, with no recurrence.

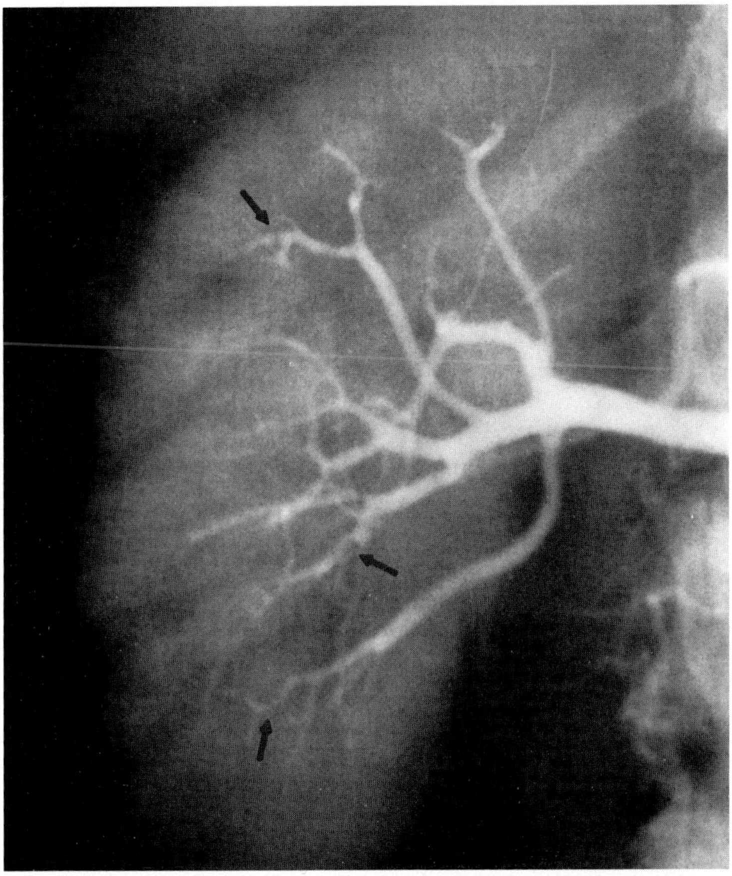

A

FIG. 10. A. Severe polyarteritis nodosa involves the right kidney. The arterial phase of the arteriogram depicts severe truncation of the renal vascular arborization, with nonopacification of distal vessels. There are many irregular-appearing vascular lumina (*arrows*). **B.** The capillary phase of the arteriogram is inhomogeneous. The more lucent regions represent foci of reduced blood flow to the microcirculation and resultant ischemia.

cification of the parenchyma. The more lucent foci are believed to represent ischemic regions that may be the source of the renin hypersecretion (24,31,58). Because of the sporadic nature of these processes, diagnosis by arteriography is felt by many to be more reliable than needle biopsy (33). There is some debate concerning the potential role of IA-DSA in diagnosing arteritides. Digital imaging results in decreased spatial resolution relative to film-screen technique. Some authorities believe that only high-quality, magnification film-screen angiography is suitable for diagnosis of subtle cases.

The acute phase of arteritis may, with any of the cited conditions, progress to an "end-stage kidney." In these cases, arteriography will depict a greatly diminished renal arterial arborization. Proximal arteries will involute, consistent with the reduced metabolic demands of the remaining renal tissue. There will be little corticomedullary differentiation and both components of the parenchyma will be reduced (Fig. 11) (7,51). It usually is not possible to determine what was the responsible pathological process. Whereas there is no role for radiological treatment in the acute phase, transcatheter embolization may be most suitable for infarcting non-

B
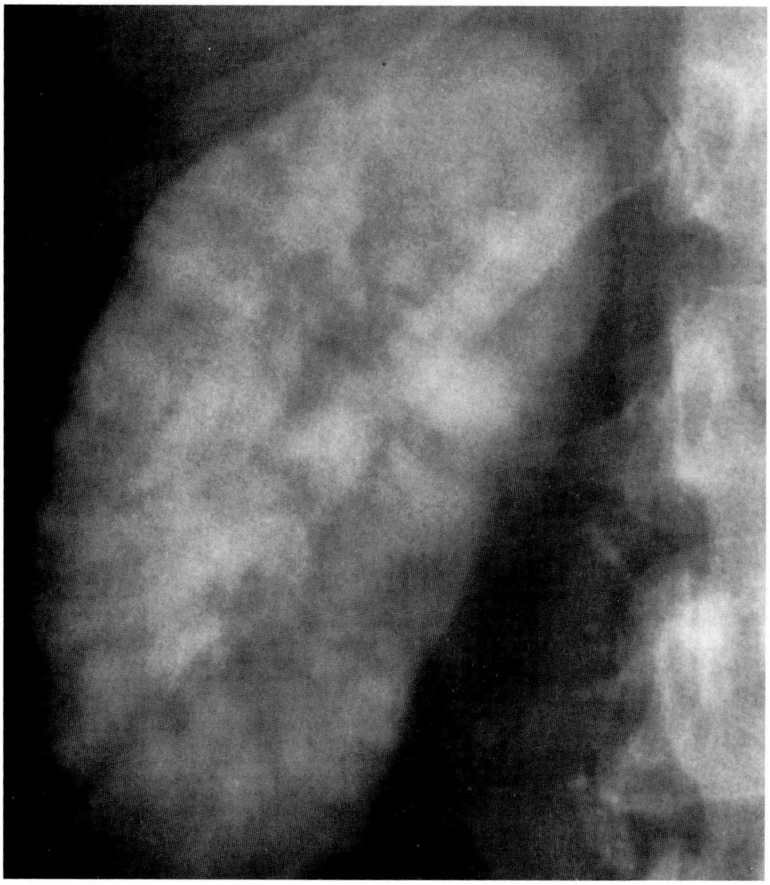

FIG. 10. *Continued*

or minimally functioning kidneys that are causing uncontrollable hypertension (2,44,48,55). This procedure is relatively safe in skilled hands and may obviate the need for surgical nephrectomy. Particulate agents that have been employed include gelfoam, often in combination with coils, and native blood clot. More recently, alcohol, heated contrast material, and quick-hardening polymers have been used successfully to infarct the renal parenchyma.

Parenchymal Diseases Secondarily Affecting the Circulation

A long list of conditions that are not primarily related to the renal circulation secondarily may affect renal hemodynamics and result in hypertension. In broad categories, these include parenchymal processes, such as chronic atrophic pyelonephritis; trauma, resulting in intraparenchymal or subcapsular hemorrhage; cysts and neoplasms; complications of partial nephrectomy or angiography; and hydronephrosis.

The event precipitating the patient's presentation for care or the patient's history, signs, and symptoms will help to determine whether and in what manner the patient ought to be evaluated. For example, in cases where there is suspicion of significant urinary tract trauma, the first examination will be either urography or CT, depending on whether there is believed to be multiorgan injury (26). Depending on the severity of renal injury, the patient either will be taken to surgery or managed conservatively.

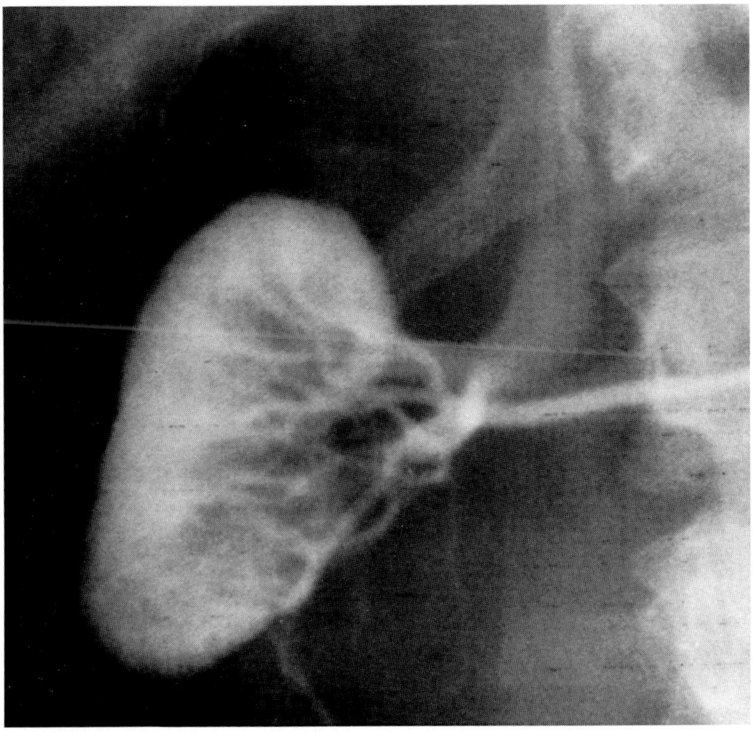

FIG. 11. A selective right renal arteriogram was performed on this patient with a history of glomerulonephritis. The involuted renal circulation, small renal size, poor corticomedullary differentiation, and reduced flow—manifested in this case by contrast material being present in arterial, capillary, and venous structures simultaneously—are typical of "end-stage" kidney.

Hypertension is a late sequela. In cases of parenchymal infarction, tissue surrounding the infarcted focus may become ischemic. Excretory urography will manifest a region of lucency.

Subcapsular hematomas produce hypertension by extrinsic compression of the renal parenchyma. Excretory urography and angiography may be interpreted as normal. However, ultrasonography or CT will demonstrate the characteristic lenticular-shaped fluid collection adjacent to renal tissue (3,14,20). If this condition, often referred to as Page kidney, is identified early, treatment by percutaneous drainage is often successful (20,71). Once a subcapsular hematoma becomes encapsulated by fibrosis, surgical treatment usually is required.

Renal neoplasms cause hypertension by secreting renin-like substances, by compressing normal parenchyma, or by producing arteriovenous shunts that result in normal tissue ischemia (59,66). Initial diagnosis of a mass is most often by excretory urography. Ultrasound and CT are useful for characterizing lesions as either simple cysts or solid. CT also is the most efficacious means of staging malignant neoplasms to determine appropriate therapy. Angiography is employed considerably less frequently than it was prior to the advent of these modalities, and is most often reserved for preoperative planning in cases where other than total nephrectomy is contemplated.

Hypertension is very frequently associated with autosomal dominant polycystic kidney disease. Early diagnosis of this condition is best accomplished employing ultrasonography or CT and facilitates genetic counseling. In addition, ultrasound or CT occasionally can distinguish a cyst into which there has been recent bleeding or that has become infected, permitting percutaneous relief of acute symptoms. MRI bears an important potential in this regard.

Finally, simple cysts suspected of causing hypertension—an unusual but not unreported event—may be treated by percutaneous puncture under ultrasound or CT guidance. Even if fluid recurs, the blood pressure response can be documented to determine whether further treatment might be beneficial. Nonsurgical neoplasms may be treated by transcatheter embolization for amelioration of symptoms.

HYPERTENSION IN CHILDHOOD AND ADOLESCENCE

Perhaps the most important point to be made concerning hypertension in children and adolescence is that, unlike adults, the majority of patients have a definable, often curable etiology for their elevated blood pressure (15,25,28). The incidence of secondary hypertension, relative to idiopathic hypertension, declines with age (37). However, the discovery of hypertension even into young adulthood should mandate an investigation for a treatable etiology because of the difficulties of enforcing a lifetime pharmacologic regimen, the potential for target organ complications, and the greatly increased risks of a shortened lifespan.

The same categories of diseases cited for adult hypertension also engender hypertension in minors. However, different pathological entities are usually responsible. As noted above, atherosclerosis is extremely rare in children. Thus, renal artery stenosis is usually the result of intimal dysplasia. Renal parenchymal disease, particularly chronic atrophic pyelonephritis, is a particularly prevalent etiology of hypertension, and is usually discovered by ultrasonography or excretory urography after several episodes of urinary tract infection. Glomerulonephritis is another frequently encountered etiology. Tumor-associated hypertension is rare, but has been described in association with virtually all pediatric abdominal tumors, including Wilms' tumors, neuroblastoma, and reninomas.

One category of disorders is far more frequently encountered in children than adults: coarctation. Coarctation may be typical—occurring in the region immediately surrounding the ductus arteriosus—or atypical. Atypical coarctations are often abdominal. They may be engendered idiopathically, or be attributable to such conditions as Takayasu's arteritis, neurofibromatosis, or the ingestion of ergotrates (5,38,41,74). Associated stenoses may affect branch vessels; among these the renal arteries are most frequently involved. As might be expected, definitive diagnosis and characterization of the extent of abnormalities is by one form or another of arteriography. IA-DSA may be particularly suitable for diagnosing childhood abnormalities because of the rapidity of its performance. The same imaging-guided interventional procedures described for adults are applicable to childhood lesions.

APPROACH TO THE HYPERTENSIVE PATIENT

A central disagreement over whether screening large numbers of hypertensive patients will be cost effective revolves about the controversy over how often a treatable renal etiology will be discovered. Estimates for the prevalence of renal hypertension among all hypertensives range from as low as 0.3% to greater than 30% (4,11,15). An often-quoted figure is 5%, but many believe that 3% might be more realistic. Seventy-five percent of hypertension is mild, controllable by diet or diuretic alone (50). The incidence of renal hypertension in this group of hypertensives generally is believed to be negligible. For this reason, because there are fewer side effects associated with medical treatment of mild hypertension, and because the costs of their medical regimen are so low, few would suggest that these individuals undergo evaluation for renal hypertension.

However, more severe blood pressure elevation, requiring two or more drugs for blood pressure control, presents a very different situation. The rate of compliance with antihypertensive drug regimens is low (63,70) and is made worse by attendant drug-related side effects. Side effects also may affect patients' performance at their work and adversely impinge on their social functioning as well. Noncompliance bears a significant risk of eventual life-threatening complications, most prominently stroke, heart disease, and renal failure. There is evidence that this risk is more severe among patients with renal hypertension undergoing medical treatment (22,23,35). Drug regimens necessary to control patients' blood pressure frequently are expensive. Finally, if one allows that virtually all renal hypertension occurs among patients with moderate or severe hypertension, the prevalence of this group of disorders is no longer inconsequential, but approaches 10%.

This combination of considerations has led some to suggest a more aggressive attitude toward investigating moderately and severely hypertensive patients for a renal etiology of their disease, and treating discovered abnormalities (33). As indicated in the previous sections, how to embark on this process depends considerably on individual patients' presentations. However, if there are no significant history, physical, or laboratory findings to direct the investigation toward a specific abnormality, a major vascular lesion should be the primary consideration. During the early development of digital angiography, Hillman and colleagues suggested performing IV-DSA as a screening, and often diagnostic, initial procedure (32). In comparing the costs accrued by screening by IV-DSA all moderately and severely hypertensive patients, adding the costs of percutaneous and surgical treatment, and allowing for their own rates of failure by this regimen, the authors showed monetary costs comparable to that expected with indiscriminate medical therapy. Although no monetary costs were assigned, the authors noted that the more aggressive approach bore a likely lower incidence of long-term complications and expectations of greater lifespan.

Though variants of this approach have been perpetuated at some American and European institutions, IV-DSA has fallen out of favor among many for its lower reliability than intraarterial techniques. As noted above, the development of outpatient IA-DSA, and even outpatient PTA (46,61), now makes feasible the cost-effective use of these techniques for the primary investigation and treatment of renovascular hypertension. Cost savings result from the performance of both diagnosis and treatment during the same procedure. This is facilitated by the rapidity of digital angiography and of digital imaging-guided PTA.

Still, for these and the other cited imaging advances to be truly effective in improving health care for hypertension, they must be much more extensively utilized than is currently the case. Though definitive evidence of cost effectiveness is lacking, individuals requiring two or more drugs for control of their hypertension probably should be considered for evaluation by outpatient arteriography. This is only valid, however, so long as both the patient and the referring physician are in agreement that definitive therapy will be sought should a treatable lesion be discovered. In the past, this decision often was put off until after diagnostic studies had been performed. The current financial exigencies in health care demand that physicians no longer perform expensive procedures simply to gather information, but rather will be dedicated to using this information appropriately for treatment planning.

REFERENCES

1. Abrams, H. L., ed. (1983): *Abrams Angiography. Vascular and Interventional Radiology*. 3rd ed. Little, Brown and Company, Boston.
2. Adler, J., et al. (1978): Gelfoam embolization of the kidneys for treatment of malignant hypertension. *Radiology*, 128:45.
3. Amparo, E. G., and Fagan, C. J. (1982): Page kidney. *J. Comput. Assist. Tomogr.*, 6:839.
4. Bech, K., and Hilden, T. (1975): The frequency of secondary hypertension. *Acta Med. Scand.*, 197:65.
5. Beerman, L. B., et al. (1980): Coarctation of the aorta in children. *Am. J. Dis. Child.*, 134:464.
6. Berglund, G., et al. (1976): Prevalence of primary and secondary hypertension: Studies in a random population sample. *Br. Med. J.*, 2:554.
7. Bookstein, J. J., and Clark, R. L. (1980): *Renal Microvascular Disease. Angiographic-Microangiographic Correlates*. Little, Brown and Company, Boston.
8. Bookstein, J. J., and Walter, J. F. (1975): The role of abdominal radiography in hypertension secondary

to renal or adrenal disease. *Med. Clin. North Am.*, 59:169.
9. Bookstein, J. J., et al. (1972): Radiologic aspects of renovascular hypertension. Part III. Appraisal of arteriography. *JAMA*, 221:368.
10. Bookstein, J. J., et al. (1972): Radiologic aspects of renovascular hypertension. Part II: The role of urography in unilateral renovascular disease. *JAMA* 220:1225.
11. Borhani, N. O., and Borkman, T. S. (1968): *Alamata County Blood Pressure Study*. Department of Public Health, Berkeley, California.
12. Bron, K. M., et al. (1965): The diagnostic value of angiographic observations in polyarteritis nodosa. *Arch. Intern. Med.*, 116:450.
13. Cassidy, M. J. D., et al. (1982): Post-biopsy renal arteriovenous fistula: Successfully embolized with a Gianturco mini coil. *Postgrad. Med. J.*, 58:570.
14. Chamorro, H. A., et al. (1981): Multi-imaging approach in the diagnosis of Page kidney. *Am. J. Roentgenol.*, 136:620.
15. Chrispin, A. R., and Scatliff, J. H. (1973): Systemic hypertension in childhood. *Pediatr. Radiol.*, 1:75.
16. Cicuto, K. T., et al. (1981): Renal artery stenosis: Anatomic classification for percutaneous transluminal angioplasty. *Am. J. Roentgenol.*, 137:599.
17. Clark, R. A., et al. (1983): Angiographic management of traumatic arteriovenous fistulas: Clinical results. *Radiology*, 147:9.
18. Clayman, A. S., and Bookstein, J. J. (1973): The role of renal arteriography in pediatric hypertension. *Radiology*, 108:107.
19. Colapinto, R. J., et al. (1982): Percutaneous transluminal dilatation of the renal artery: Followup studies on renovascular hypertension. *Am. J. Roentgenol.*, 139:727.
20. Conrad, M. R., et al. (1976): Sonography of the Page kidney. *J. Urol.*, 116:293.
21. Cummings, K. B., et al. (1973): Renal artery aneurysms and hypertension. *J. Urol.*, 109:144.
22. Davis, B. A., et al. (1979): Prevalence of renovascular hypertension in patients with grade III or IV hypertensive retinopathy. *N. Engl. J. Med.*, 301:1273.
23. Dean, R. H., et al. (1981): Renovascular hypertension. Anatomic and renal function changes during drug therapy. *Arch. Surg.*, 116:1408.
24. Ekelund, L., and Lindholm, T. (1973): Angiography in collagenous disease of the kidney. *Acta Radiol. Diagn.*, 15:413.
25. Fay, R., and Kaufman, J. J. (1974): Renal hypertension in children. *Urology*, 3:148.
26. Federle, M. P., et al. (1981): Role of computed tomography in renal trauma. *Radiology*, 141:455.
27. Fisher, R. G. (1981): Renal artery aneurysms in polyarteritis nodosa: A multiepisodic phenomenon. *Am. J. Roentgenol.*, 136:938.
28. Fry, W. J., et al. (1973): Renovascular hypertension in the pediatric patient. *Arch. Surg.*, 107:692.
29. Gill, W. M., and Meaney, T. F. (1969): Medial fibroplasia of the renal artery. *Radiology*, 92:861.
30. Goncherenko, V., et al. (1981): Progression of renal artery fibromuscular dysplasia in 42 patients as seen on angiography. *Radiology*, 139:45.
31. Herchman, A., et al. (1970): Angiographic findings in polyarteritis nodosa. *Radiology*, 94:147.
32. Hillman, B. J., et al. (1982): The potential impact of digital subtraction angiography on screening for renovascular hypertension. *Radiology*, 142:577.
33. Hillman, B. J. (1983): *Imaging and Hypertension*. W. B. Saunders Co., Philadelphia.
34. Hubert, J. P., Jr., et al. (1980): Solitary renal artery aneurysm. *Surgery*, 87:557.
35. Hunt, J. C., and Strong, C. G. (1973): Renovascular hypertension. Mechanisms, natural history and treatment. *Am. J. Cardiol.*, 32:562.
36. Kaufman, J. J. (1979): Renovascular hypertension: The UCLA experience. *J. Urol.*, 121:139.
37. Kilcoyne, M. M. (1976): Adolescent hypertension. *NY State J. Med.*, 76:2002.
38. Klecker, R. L., and Roth, J. B. (1974): Visceral neurofibromatosis and hypertension in childhood. *Pediatrics*, 53:417.
39. Korobkin, M., et al. (1976): Segmental renal vein sampling for renin. *Radiology*, 118:307.
40. Lalli, A. F. (1981): Is the hypertensive urogram a necessary examination? *J. Can. Assoc. Radiol.*, 32:11.
41. Lande, A. (1976): Takayasu's arteritis and congenital coarctation of the descending thoracic and abdominal aorta: A critical review. *Am. J. Roentgenol.*, 127:227.
42. Lee, S. M., and Drach, G. W. (1980): Renovascular hypertension from segmental renal artery stenosis: Importance of segmental renal vein renin sampling. *J. Urol.*, 124:704.
43. Lester, P. D., and Koehler, P. R. (1971): The renal angiographic changes in scleroderma. *Radiology*, 99:517.
44. Lieberman, S. F., et al. (1983): Percutaneous vasoocclusion for nonmalignant renal lesions. *J. Urol.*, 129:805.
45. Longstreth, P. L., et al. (1974): Renal microaneurysms in a patient with systemic lupus erythematosus. *Radiology*, 113:65.
46. Manashil, G. D., et al. (1983): Outpatient transluminal angioplasty. *Radiology*, 147:7.
47. Martin, L. G., et al. (1985): Percutaneous angioplasty in clinical management of renovascular hypertension: Initial and long-term results. *Radiology*, 155:629.
48. McCarron, D. A., et al. (1976): Therapeutic bilateral renal infarction in end-stage renal disease. *N. Engl. J. Med.*, 294:652.
49. McNeil, B. J., and Adelstein, S. J. (1975): The value of case finding in hypertensive renovascular disease. *N. Engl. J. Med.*, 293:211.
50. McNeil, B. J., et al. (1975): Cost-effectiveness calculations in the diagnosis and treatment of hypertensive renovascular disease. *N. Engl. J. Med.*, 293:216.
51. Mena, E., et al. (1973): Angiographic diagnosis of renal parenchymal disease. *Radiology*, 108:523.
52. Miller, G. A., et al. (1985): Percutaneous transluminal angioplasty vs. surgery for renovascular hypertension. *Am. J. Roentgenol.*, 144:447.
53. Moreau, J. F., et al. (1982): Post-biopsy false arterial aneurysm of a transplanted kidney: Treatment by bucrylate transcatheter embolization. *J. Urol.*, 128:116.

54. Morris, D. C., et al. (1983): Subselective embolization for non-neoplastic conditions of the kidney. *Can. Radiol. Assoc. J.*, 34:103.
55. Nanni, G. S., et al. (1983): Control of hypertension by ethanol renal ablation. *Radiology*, 148:51.
56. Norman, D., et al. (1985): Intraarterial digital subtraction imaging cost considerations. *Radiology*, 156:33.
57. Novick, A. C. (1981): Atherosclerotic renovascular disease. *J. Urol.*, 126:567.
58. Pope, T. L., Jr., et al. (1981): CT features of renal polyarteritis nodosa. *Am. J. Roentgenol.*, 136:986.
59. Reeve, H. R., et al. (1979): Hypertensive crisis associated with renal cell carcinoma. *Urology*, 14:378.
60. Robins, J. M., and Bookstein, J. J. (1972): Regressing aneurysms in periarteritis nodosa. *Radiology*, 104:39.
61. Saint-Georges, G., and Aube, M. (1985): Safety of outpatient angiography. A prospective study. *Am. J. Roentgenol.*, 14:235.
62. Schambelan, M., et al. (1974): Selective renal vein renin sampling in hypertensive patients with segmental renal lesions. *N. Engl. J. Med.*, 290:1153.
63. Schoenberger, J. A., et al. (1972): Current status of hypertension control in an industrial population. *JAMA*, 222:559.
64. Scott, J. A., et al. (1983): Angiographic assessment of renal artery pathology. *Am. J. Roentgenol.*, 141:1299.
65. Sechas, M. N., et al. (1974): Post-traumatic renovascular hypertension. *Surgery*, 76:666.
66. Sonda, L. P., III, et al. (1982): Clinical aspects of non-vascular renal causes of hypertension. *Urol. Radiol.*, 3:257.
67. Sos, T. A., et al. (1983): Percutaneous transluminal renal angioplasty in renovascular hypertension due to atheroma or fibromuscular dysplasia. *N. Engl. J. Med.*, 309:274.
68. Stanley, J. C., et al. (1981): Pediatric renal artery occlusive disease and renovascular hypertension. *Arch. Surg.*, 116:669.
69. Stewart, B. H., et al. (1970): Correlation of angiography and natural history in the evaluation of patients with renovascular hypertension. *J. Urol.*, 104:231.
70. Stokes, J. B., II, et al. (1973): Hypertension control: The challenge of patient education. *N. Engl. J. Med.*, 289:1369.
71. Sufrin, G. (1975): The Page kidney: A correctable form of arterial hypertension. *J. Urol.*, 113:450.
72. Tegtmeyer, C. J., et al. (1984): Renal angioplasty: Current status. *Am. J. Roentgenol.*, 142:17.
73. Webb, J. A., and Talner, L. B. (1979): The role of intravenous urography in hypertension. *Radiol. Clin. North Am.*, 17:187.
74. Wiggelinkhuizen, J., and Cremin, D. J. (1978): Takayasu's arteritis and renovascular hypertension in childhood. *Pediatrics*, 62:209.
75. Winograd, J., et al. (1976): The spotted nephrogram of renal scleroderma. *Am. J. Roentgenol.*, 126:734.

The Kidney in Hypertension, edited by Norman M. Kaplan, Barry M. Brenner, and John H. Laragh. Raven Press, New York © 1987.

Principles of Antihypertensive Drug Therapy: An Overview

Norman M. Kaplan

Professor of Internal Medicine, University of Texas Health Science Center at Dallas, Dallas, Texas 75235

The preceding chapters examined the role of the kidney in the pathogenesis and clinical features of hypertension; the ones that follow will examine the therapy of hypertension, with emphasis on the effects of various antihypertensive drugs on the kidney and the therapy of renal forms of hypertension.

This chapter will broadly view the principles of antihypertensive drug therapy, providing both general guidelines applicable to all hypertensives and specific features relative to those with renal forms. Hopefully, I will ease the way into the subsequent chapters without contradicting or repeating their content.

WHOM TO TREAT

Current Practice and Future Projections

The numbers of patients being treated for hypertension have been rapidly expanding, partly because of greater recognition of those with elevated blood pressure, but even more because of the increased acceptance of the need for therapy among the larger portion who have minimally elevated blood pressure. As seen in Fig. 1, 80% of all those with an elevated blood pressure have "mild" hypertension, defined as a diastolic blood pressure (DBP) between 90 and 104 mm Hg (1).

As a result of the increasing use of active therapy among more and more patients with milder degrees of hypertension, hypertension is now the most common indication for office visits to physicians in the United States, the number of visits for hypertension having increased from 19.6 million in 1960 to 55.4 million in 1983 and being projected to increase to 111.9 million visits by 1995 (J. U. Cohen, Pharmaceutical Prospects, Healthcare Forecasting, Inc., Glastonbury, CT; *personal communication*). When seen for hypertension, most of these patients are given one or more prescriptions for antihypertensive drugs, at a rate significantly higher than for other medical diagnoses (2). Physicians in the United States tend to treat patients with lesser degrees of hypertension, often all of those with DBP readings above 90 mm Hg (3), compared to the usual practice in England (4) and Canada (5) of beginning drug therapy only when the DBP is above 100 mm Hg.

The number of patients being treated will almost certainly continue to expand: The number of hypertensives in the United States has been estimated to be as high as 57.7 million, only one-third of whom are being treated (6); even minimally elevated blood pressure is increasingly being considered to be a risk for premature cardiovascular disease, with people having DBP between 80 and 89 mm Hg categorized as being at "intermediate risk" (7); more antihypertensive drugs that are easier to take and more widely advertised are being made available.

The Consequences of Current Practice

This continued expansion of the active drug therapy of millions of people with mild hyper-

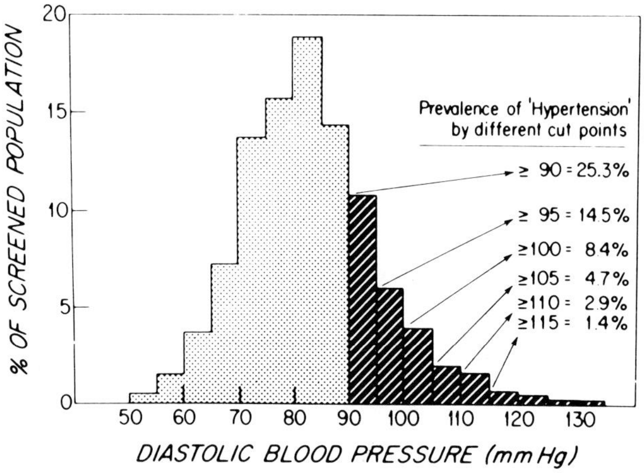

FIG. 1. Frequency distribution of diastolic blood pressure at home screen of 158,906 persons, 30–69 years of age, Hypertension Detection and Follow-Up Program, 1974. (From ref. 1.)

tension has been justified by the attribution to the broader therapy of hypertension of a major role in the falling rates of both morbidity and mortality from stroke and heart attacks that have occurred since 1968 in the United States (8). However, the broader therapy of hypertension likely has played only a minor role in the falling rates, estimated to be in the order of less than 10%, compared to larger roles for the cessation of smoking and for lowering of serum cholesterol levels by changes in the diet (9).

Moreover, it appears that the therapy of hypertension as it has been practiced has not provided the degree of protection that might be expected from the lowering of blood pressure levels. Data from England show that treated hypertensives under the age of 50 still had a threefold increase in mortality compared with the general population (10). Among a smaller group of patients treated for 6 years, the incidence of coronary disease remained higher than that predicted by posttreatment blood pressure levels (11). Among 7,610 Japanese men in Hawaii, those who received antihypertensive therapy had a higher subsequent 10-year mortality from cardiovascular diseases, including heart attacks and strokes, as compared with untreated men at every level of blood pressure (12).

Evidence from Controlled Trials

These reports suggest a lesser benefit from currently practiced antihypertensive therapy than should have been seen, questioning both the value of therapy *per se* and, even more so, the mode of therapy. Even more definitive evidence, however, is available from six controlled large-scale trials of the therapy of mild hypertension published over the past few years (13–18) (Table 1). All of these trials used a diuretic as the first and often only drug, with the exception of the MRC trial, which used either a diuretic or a beta-blocker.

The trials uniformly showed protection from stroke among those whose blood pressure was lowered but overall protection from heart attacks was not demonstrated, with higher rates of coronary mortality observed in three of the six. Numerous reasons may be responsible for this disparity. Stroke may be more directly related to the presence of high blood pressure, whereas coronary disease is caused by multiple factors; it may, therefore, take longer than 5 years and the correction of more than just hypertension to show protection from coronary disease. On the other hand, the therapy used in these trials may have produced risks for coronary disease while reducing the risks for stroke and other cardiovascular complications that are more directly related to the high blood pressure.

The concluding statement in the report of the MRC trial, the largest and most recent of them all, is worth noting: "The trial has shown that if 850 mildly hypertensive patients are given active hypertensive drugs for one year about one stroke will be prevented. This is an important

Table 1. *Trials of drug therapy of mild hypertension*

Trials (ref.)	Mortality rates per 1,000 person-years					
	Cerebrovascular disease			Coronary heart disease		
Drugs vs placebo	No Rx	Rx	Difference	No Rx	Rx	Difference
Australian (13)	0.9	0.4	−56%	1.6	0.7	−56%
Oslo (14)	1.0	0	−100%	1.0	2.7	+170%
Elderly (10)	16.0	11.0	−32%	24.0	15.0	−38%
MRC[a] (9)	0.6	0.4	−33%	2.3	2.5	+9%
More vs less drugs	Less	More		Less	More	
HDFP[b] (17)	1.6	0.9	−41%	5.6	4.5	−20%
MRFIT[c] (18)						
Normal ECG		Not reported		3.4	2.6	−24%
Abnormal ECG		Not reported		2.9	4.9	+70%

[a](MRC) medical research council.
[b](HDFP) Hypertension detection and follow-up program.
[c](MRFIT) Multiple risk factor intervention tiral.

but an infrequent benefit. Its achievement subjected a substantial percentage of the patients to chronic side effects, mostly but not all minor. Treatment did not appear to save lives or substantially alter the overall risk of coronary heart disease. More than 95% of the control patients remained free of any cardiovascular event during the trial" (16).

In conclusion, the evidence from both uncontrolled observations and from controlled trials leaves considerable uncertainty about the value of antihypertensive therapy, as it has been provided, in reducing the risks for coronary disease, although the risks for stroke clearly are reduced. I will come back to the issue of the apparent failure of prior and current modes of therapy to provide protection from the major complication of untreated hypertension, coronary disease.

Current Recommendation

As noted before, most American physicians have assumed that most patients with diastolic blood pressures above 95 mm Hg, and many with diastolics above 90 mm Hg, should be given antihypertensive drug therapy. Elsewhere, higher levels of pressure are taken as indication of the need for therapy.

From the available evidence, these general guidelines seem appropriate in deciding whom to treat:

- The majority of patients who have relatively mild hypertension should have repeated measurements of their blood pressure for at least 3 to 6 months before entering active drug therapy. In many, the initial high readings will fall, likely reflecting dampening of the anxiety associated with the initial screening as well as the tendency for regression toward the mean (19). Home blood pressures are useful and 24-hr ambulatory readings may provide even better delineation of the range of the blood pressures (20) and the long-term prognosis (21). In Perloff and colleagues' (21) comparison between multiple sets of office readings and the average of a set of 24-hr ambulatory readings, the long-term prognosis was clearly better among those whose ambulatory readings were considerably lower than the office readings, as was noted in almost 80% of the entire group of 1,076 patients.
- During the period of observation, various nondrug modalities should be utilized that may bring and keep the pressure down. More about these will be covered later in this chapter.
- The decision to treat should not be based on the blood pressure alone but on the entire cardiovascular risk status. The data from the Framingham study provide the clearest indication of the additive—and even more than additive—roles of the other known risk factors, as shown in Fig. 2 for a 40-year-old

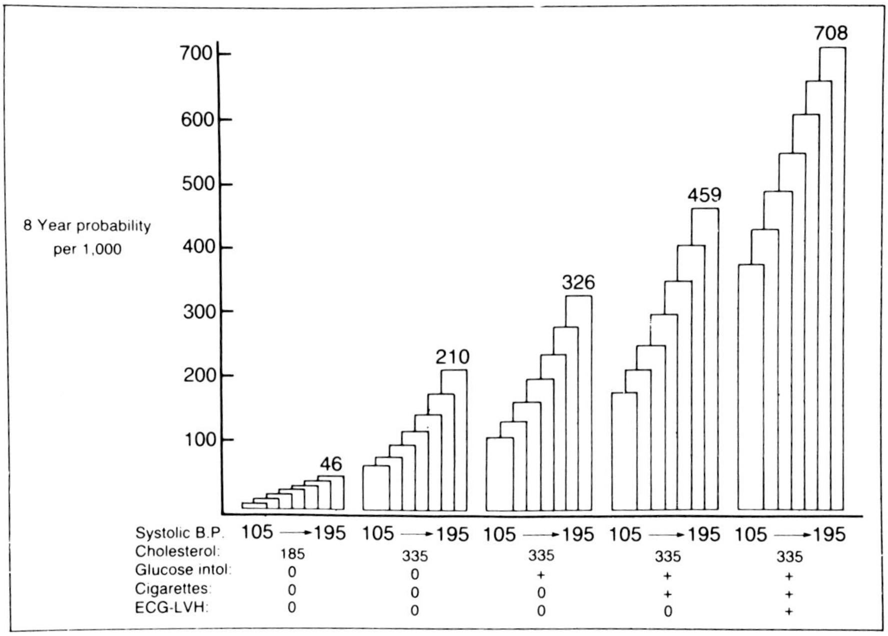

FIG. 2. Risk of cardiovascular disease according to systolic blood pressure at specified levels of other risk factors. Men aged 40 years, Framingham study, 18-year follow-up. (From ref. 22.)

male (22). The individual sets of bars in Fig. 2 indicate the increasing risk for the appearance of a serious cardiovascular event in the next 8 years with increasing levels of systolic blood pressure (SBP), first in the absence of the other major risk factors, on the left, and with the addition of more and more of the others, going across the figure to the right. Without other risk factors, the likelihood of a cardiovascular complication with a SBP of 195 mm Hg is 4.6%; with all of the other risk factors, the likelihood rises to 70.8%.

- In the future, additional ways beyond the Framingham criteria may be used to predict with more certainty the long-term prognosis for cardiovascular complications. As noted earlier, 24-hr ambulatory blood pressure recordings may be one such way; echocardiography for assessment of left ventricular size and function may be another.
- Note that the Framingham data use the systolic blood pressure, which has been found to provide better prognostic information than did the diastolic level. Systolic elevations are particularly common among the elderly and they pose a distinct risk for stroke as well as other cardiovascular complications (23). Based on such evidence, it is probably justifiable to attempt gentle and gradual reduction of systolic levels above 170 mm Hg at any age, assuming the patient has a reasonable life expectancy. A controlled trial to document the efficacy of therapy of isolated systolic hypertension in the elderly, the SHEP trial, has recently been started. Although it will be 7 to 10 years before the evidence about efficacy is available, preliminary data show that the systolic elevations can be successfully reduced in about 80% of such people by relatively small doses of a diuretic (24).
- Based on the overall risk profile and the response to a 3- to 6-month trial of nondrug therapies, antihypertensive drugs should probably be started in most whose DBP remains above 95 mm Hg. Those at higher risk should be given antihypertensive drugs at lower levels. One group, in particular, who are at inordinately high risk if left untreated are di-

abetics with nephropathy, i.e., glomerulosclerosis, as described in Chapter 5. They have been shown to be protected by antihypertensive therapy (25), and such therapy should probably be given if the DBP is above 85 mm Hg. In the absence of adequate clinical data, we are not certain at which level to begin treatment, but it seems certain that they need even tighter control than nondiabetic hypertensives to protect them against progressive renal damage.

Criteria for the institution of active drug therapy in other groups are provided elsewhere (26). These include children, pregnant women, and patients with other cardiovascular disorders. Special needs for patients with underlying renal disease will be covered in Chapter 17.

HOW TO TREAT

Once having decided to treat, the issue turns to the choice of therapy. I believe that various nondrug modalities should always be included, with or without drugs. The evidence for their efficacy and acceptance continues to mount (27), although proof that, by themselves, they will reduce cardiovascular complications likely will never be obtained.

Nondrug Therapies

Nondrug therapies (Table 2) can be effective in reducing the blood pressure in a sizable portion of the hypertensive population. For those with mild hypertension, by far the majority, a 5 to 10 mm Hg fall in blood pressure may be enough to lower them below the level considered in need of drug therapy, often well below 140/90 mm Hg. Even if not adequate by themselves, the nondrug therapies will likely improve the efficacy of drug therapies and reduce some of their side effects. Used in a reasonable manner, they pose no risks and little interference with the quality of life. Even if they do not lower the blood pressure, they may reduce other risk factors for cardiovascular disease.

Table 2. *Nondrugs for therapy of hypertension*

If obese, weight reduction
Dietary sodium restricted to 2 g (88 mmol) per day
More fiber and less saturated fat
Supplemental potassium, magnesium, and calcium if deficiency exists
Alcohol limited to 2 ounces per day
Regular isotonic exercise
Relaxation therapy

Surveys indicate that an enlarging portion, now a majority, of physicians recommend nondrug therapy alone for those with DBP below 95 mm Hg (3). Physicians attach the greatest importance to sodium reduction and weight reduction.

Thus, despite occasional disclaimers that such nondrug approaches are seldom effective, rarely accepted, and infrequently maintained, there is nothing to be lost from their use. If advocated enthusiastically and implemented by frequent follow-up and continued motivation, a sizable number of patients will benefit from them.

Weight Reduction

Obesity commonly accompanies hypertension and the two may be causally connected, perhaps via insulin resistance (28). The association is mainly seen in people with centrally deposited body fat ("apples") rather than in those with peripheral obesity ("pears") (29). Although some find that the severity of the hypertension and the long-term risks for cardiovascular disease among obese people are less than for normal-weight people with the same blood pressures (30), others find the risks for coronary disease to be equal among hypertensives with varying amounts of excess body weight (31).

Whether they are at more or less risk, obese hypertensives will usually have a fall in blood pressure if they lose weight and this is often accompanied by other favorable changes, particularly when compared to the effects of antihypertensive drugs (27). In two carefully controlled studies, a group of young obese hypertensives were randomly allocated to a placebo, caloric restriction, or metoprolol for 21 weeks (32,33) (Table 3). Compared to the beta-

Table 3. *Effects of 21 weeks of therapy in three groups of obese hypertensives*[a]

	Weight reduction	Metoprolol	Placebo
Weight (kg)	−8.3	+2.5	+0.5
Systolic blood pressure (mm Hg)	−14.2	−12.4	−8.9
Diastolic blood pressure (mm Hg)	−12.7	−7.5	−4.4
Left ventricular mass index (g/m^2)	−14.8	−1.3	−1.5
Total cholesterol (% change)	−6%	+4%	+3%
HDL[b]-cholesterol (% change)	+6%	−10%	+2%

[a]Data from ref. 32 and 33.
[b](HDL) High-density lipoprotein.

blocker, weight reduction of an average of 8.3 kg resulted in a greater fall in blood pressure, a reduction in left ventricular hypertrophy, and an improvement in the lipid profile.

The fall in blood pressure with weight loss may be enhanced (or dependent upon) a decrease in sodium intake. In a study of 18 moderately obese men, the 10 who kept sodium intake unchanged did not have a fall in blood pressure, despite a 9.1 kg decrease in weight, whereas the eight who reduced sodium intake by 95 mmol/day had a 4 to 19 mm Hg fall in blood pressure with a similar 9.3 kg weight loss (34). The investigators found a fall in plasma norepinephrine with weight loss and sodium restriction, whereas those who kept sodium intake unchanged had no fall in plasma norepinephrine and a heightened pressor response to norepinephrine infusion.

Sodium Restriction

Most, but not all (35), authorities agree that moderate sodium restriction, to a level of 2 g a day (equal to 5 g of sodium chloride or 88 mmol), will lower the blood pressure in most hypertensives. As with all therapies, drug or nondrug, the degree of fall in blood pressure is directly correlated with the pretreatment level (36) (Fig. 3). As with all therapies, only some will respond to sodium restriction. Varying degrees of sodium sensitivity have been identified in small-scale studies (37). It may be possible to neatly subdivide hypertensives into sodium-sensitive and -insensitive groups, but it is more likely that the response covers a continuous spectrum, some more, others less responsive. Regardless, all can be advised to reduce dietary sodium, since there are no dangers to such moderate restriction. Those whose blood pressure responds well should be encouraged to continue; the remainder will likely also achieve an additional benefit of moderate sodium restriction if they are given diuretics: The degree of diuretic-induced potassium wastage will be reduced if less sodium reaches the distal exchange site (38).

As with all good things, it is possible to overdo sodium restriction. Very low sodium intake, in the range of 10 to 20 mmol/day, besides being almost impossible to achieve, may so stimulate the renin-angiotensin-aldosterone mechanism as to both raise the blood pressure and increase potassium excretion (39).

Potassium Supplementation

The dietary changes needed to reduce sodium by half will likely double potassium intake. In fact, the benefits of sodium restriction may be largely attributable to the concomitant increase in potassium intake (40). Most dietary sodium has been put into foods during the processing, originally as a way to preserve, now as a way to enhance taste. With the processing, potassium is leached out. Natural foods are, with virtually no exceptions, low in sodium and high in potassium. Processed foods are almost always higher in sodium and lower in potassium than the natural forms.

The extra potassium from larger quantities of natural foods should be enough to provide whatever benefits extra potassium can achieve. Only

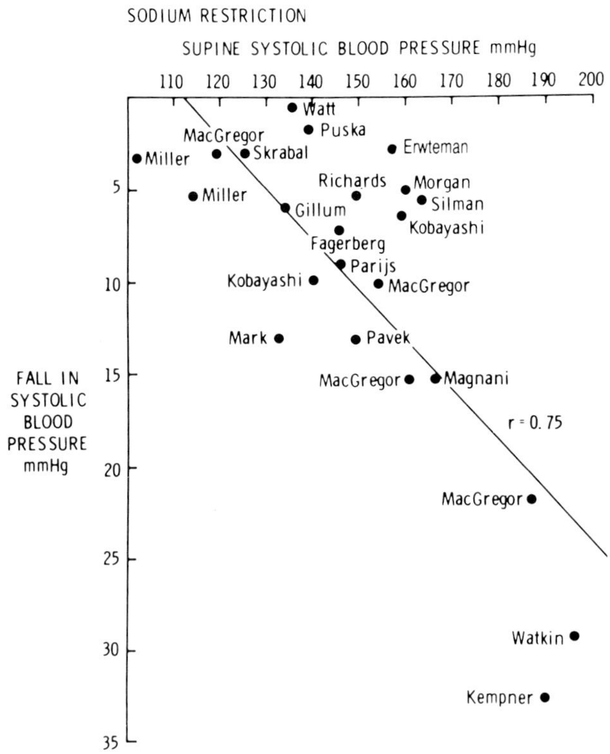

FIG. 3. Fall in supine systolic blood pressure with sodium restriction plotted against pretreatment supine systolic blood pressure in data from published studies whose first author is shown. (From ref. 36.)

those who are potassium depleted, usually by long-term diuretic therapy, may need potassium supplements, and they may achieve a fall in blood pressure as a consequence of correction of hypokalemia (41). The combination of a potassium-sparing agent with the diuretic is a rational and widely practiced way to reduce the degree of diuretic-induced potassium wastage.

Magnesium Supplementation

It seems unlikely that magnesium supplements will lower the blood pressure (42), but hypomagnesemia may be a cause of arrhythmias and the use of magnesium supplements may protect against them. In a randomized study, the administration of i.v. magnesium started on the day of admission in half of 130 patients with an acute myocardial infarction was associated with a decrease in 4-week mortality from 19% (placebo) to 7% (magnesium), related to a reduction of serious arrhythmias from 47% to 21% (43).

Calcium Supplementation

Hypertension has been claimed to be associated with dietary calcium deficiency, and calcium supplements have been found to reduce blood pressure in some patients (44). The data on calcium supplements remain preliminary and inconsistent. We (45), McCarron and Morris (46), and Resnick et al. (47) find that some hypertensives have a pronounced fall in blood pressure when given calcium carbonate or citrate, but other patients have just as pronounced a rise in blood pressure, and there is nothing now known that can separate those who respond favorably from those who respond adversely.

For now, I suggest that calcium supplements not be given to treat hypertension and, if calcium is used for osteoporosis, the blood pressure be checked to ensure that it does not rise. On the other hand, there seems good reason to encourage higher dietary calcium intake, particularly among thin white women, and there is no need to reduce calcium intake while reducing sodium intake.

Moderation of Alcohol

More than 2 ounces of ethanol per day will likely raise the blood pressure (48), but less than 2 ounces of ethanol per day may lower the blood pressure (49) and will likely protect against coronary disease. (An ounce of alcohol is found in two standard drinks: two beers, two 4-ounce glasses of wine, or two shots of whiskey.) Therefore, hypertensives should be encouraged to limit their daily intake to less than 2 ounces of ethanol but they need not be advised to abstain completely. Regular alcohol consumption at a level of 1 to 2 ounces per day has been found to be associated with lesser rates of coronary disease (50).

Exercise

Regular isotonic exercise has been found frequently to lead to a fall in blood pressure. In one study, a fall in mean blood pressure from 117 mm Hg to 97 mm Hg was seen among 105 hypertensives after 3 months of daily walking or running for 2 miles (51). The falls in blood pressure were not correlated with changes in body weight. Further, when 15 of these patients became sedentary for 3 months, the blood pressure rose in 10.

More tightly controlled studies have also shown a reduction of blood pressure in the range of 10 mm Hg after regular isotonic exercise for 1 to 3 months (52,53). These falls in blood pressure are accompanied by and probably related to falls in plasma catechols (52), with a reduction in both peripheral resistance and heart rate (53).

Long-Term Effects of Nondrug Therapies

The preceding evidence, and a great deal more, documents the short-term efficacy of various nondrug therapies. The question remains as to whether they will work over the long term in ordinary clinical practice. Few data are available but long-term trials are in process and preliminary evidence suggests that nondrug therapy may keep the blood pressure down in many patients. The evidence includes two studies involving patients who successfully completed 5 years of drug therapy in the Hypertension Detection and Follow-Up Program and whose drugs were then discontinued (54,55). In both, the number of patients whose diastolic blood pressures remained below 90 mm Hg for the next 1 to 3 years was significantly higher if they used lower sodium and/or lower calorie diets than if they did not.

The Choice of Initial Drug Therapy

Even if the various nondrug therapies are successful, many patients will remain with systolic levels above 160 and diastolic levels above 95, which will usually indicate the need for antihypertensive drug therapy. As noted earlier, some patients at high risk, such as diabetics with nephropathy, should be treated at lower levels of pressure; others, such as older women who have no other risk factors, may best be left off drugs. All should remain under surveillance, since the pressure may rise to levels clearly mandating therapy.

For patients whose pressures are above the level indicating the need for therapy, the clinician must make a major decision: which drug to use. The decision is important for two interrelated reasons: First, if that initial drug is successful, as it likely will be, it may be taken for the rest of the patient's life, for as long as 40 years or more; second, the long-term side effects of antihypertensive drugs may not be easily recognized, either because we are not aware of them or because our patients do not call them to our attention. Remember that the cholesterol-raising effect of diuretics was not identified until these drugs were widely used for almost 20 years.

Diuretic As First Choice

Diuretics are now chosen by about 90% of practitioners as the first drug in the therapy of mild hypertension (3). The practice rose empirically: Diuretics were among the earliest orally effective drugs made available, they were effective, relatively well accepted by patients, and capable of sustaining their antihypertensive action indefinitely. Other drugs, such as methyldopa and guanethidine, were tried as initial agents but a tendency for fluid retention to blunt their effectiveness was often noted. The increase in plasma volume reflects a tendency by the kidneys of hypertensive patients to retain sodium and water whenever the blood pressure is lowered by nondiuretic agents. Such reactive fluid retention is a natural reaction to the lowering of the blood pressure by the kidneys of hypertensive patients, which have their pressure-sodium excretion relationship reset at a higher level. With direct vasodilators, an additional mechanism is involved, the activation of the renin-angiotensin system with secondary increases in aldosterone. However more recently introduced drugs, including beta-blockers, converting enzyme inhibitors (CEIs), and calcium blockers, less commonly cause sodium retention, either because they inhibit the renin-aldosterone mechanism or because they increase renal blood flow. They may, then, be chronically used without the need for diuretics.

Until recently, then, there was an apparent logic of the choice of a diuretic as initial therapy, since about half of patients could be controlled on it alone and, if another drug was needed, the diuretic was often required to obtain maximal effectiveness. However, concerns about the widespread use of diuretics as the initial choice of therapy have increasingly been voiced in the past few years.

These concerns involve some of the side effects of diuretics (Fig. 4). Although they will also be addressed in Chapter 12, a brief overview will indicate why they have caused concern. Some, such as postural hypotension, hyponatremia, and prerenal azotemia, are usually of little consequence. Others, such as hyperuricemia and hypercalcemia, are common but seldom harmful. But others may increase the risk for cardiovascular complications, reducing or blunting the protection provided by the lowering of the blood pressure. These include hypokalemia, worsening of glucose tolerance, and

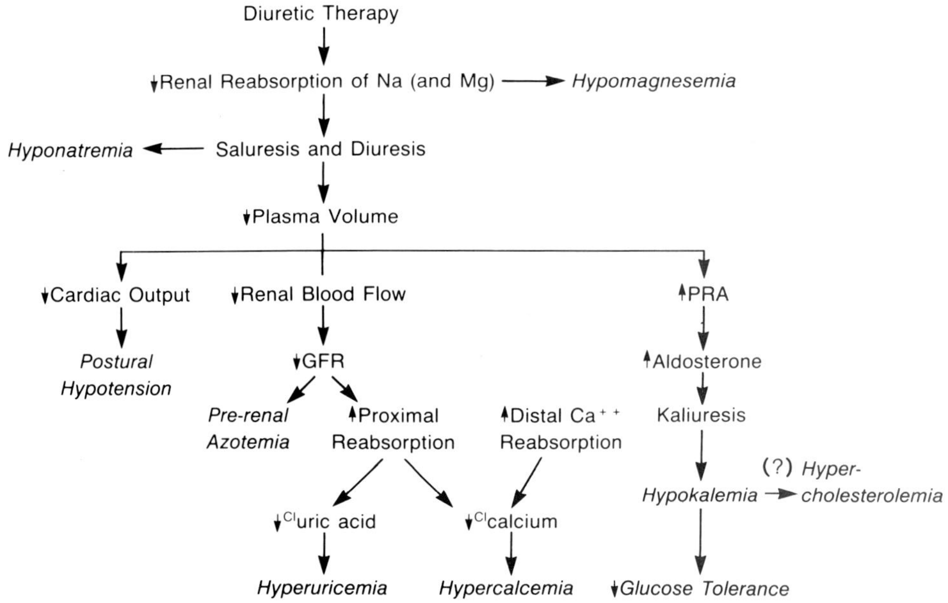

FIG. 4. Mechanisms by which chronic diuretic therapy may lead to various complications. (GFR) Glomerular filtration rate; (PRA) plasma renin activity. (From ref. 26.)

rises in plasma cholesterol, a complication that is shown in Fig. 4 with a question mark as to its mechanism, since its relationship to hypokalemia has not been proved. In one small study, diuretics caused a 20 mg/dl rise in serum cholesterol despite prevention of hypokalemia by either potassium-sparing agents or potassium supplements (56).

Hypokalemia

The average fall in plasma potassium with sustained use of diuretics is approximately 0.7 mmol/liter, inducing hypokalemia in approximately 30% of patients (57). The primary hazard of diuretic-induced hypokalemia is the tendency to increase myocardial irritability, inciting ventricular ectopic activity, particularly in hypertensives who have a higher incidence of coronary artery disease and left ventricular hypertrophy, which in itself increases the likelihood for sudden death (58).

The arrhythmogenic potential of diuretic-induced hypokalemia may only be exposed after acute stress such as with acute myocardial ischemia. With such stress, plasma catecholamine levels rise to concentrations that have been shown themselves to reduce plasma potassium levels by 0.5 to 1.0 mmol/liter by accelerating the movement of potassium into cells (59). When added to the effects of stress, the usual diuretic-induced fall in plasma potassium concentration of 0.7 mmol/liter may be more hazardous than previously assumed. At the least, these potential risks should justify steps to reduce diuretic wastage of potassium: the use of the smallest effective dose of diuretic, a reduced dietary sodium intake, and the concomitant use of potassium-sparing agents.

Glucose Intolerance

Glucose intolerance may accompany prolonged diuretic therapy (60). The atherogenic potential of such changes in glucose tolerance is unknown, but it poses another concern about the long-term safety of diuretic therapy, since glucose intolerance was found to be an independent risk factor for cardiovascular disease in the Framingham population (22).

Plasma Cholesterol

Elevations of plasma cholesterol of 10 to 20 mg/dl usually occur with diuretic therapy (61). The atherogenic potential of a 20 mg/dl rise in plasma cholesterol can be shown by use of the Framingham data to completely reverse the reduction in risk provided by the 10 to 15 mm Hg fall in systolic blood pressure that might be expected with chronic diuretic therapy. The issue is highlighted further by the recent revelation that hypertensives tend to have more hypercholesterolemia, with or without antihypertensive therapy, than do normotensives (62) (Fig. 5).

Separately or collectively, these three biochemical changes accompanying diuretic use may be involved in the failure to find protection from coronary artery disease in three of the six trials of therapy of hypertension, all of which used a diuretic as the first step in treatment (Table 1). In the European Trial in the Elderly, wherein hypokalemia was effectively prevented by concomitant use of a potassium-sparing agent, protection against coronary disease was equal to that against stroke (15). These findings suggest that diuretics provide less protection from the progression of coronary artery disease than their antihypertensive potency should offer. Since the antihypertensive potency of diuretics is comparable to that of beta-blockers or other adrenergic inhibitors, the biochemical aberrations that accompany the diuretic may reduce or ablate the protection they provide by their reduction in blood pressure.

Despite these concerns about diuretics, their use has been defended by their proven antihypertensive efficacy and the overall protection from cardiovascular diseases they provided along with other antihypertensive drugs in patients with DBP above 100 mm Hg. But as more and more patients with less elevated pressures, including a larger portion of those with a diastolic blood pressure in the 90 to 100 mm Hg range, are being treated, concerns about risks of therapy become more critical. Such patients are at less

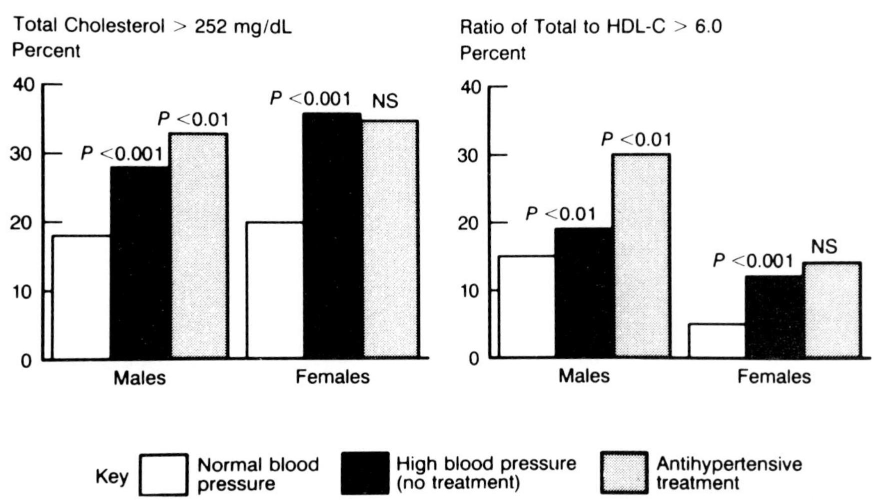

FIG. 5. Prevalence of elevated total cholesterol level and ratio of total cholesterol to high-density lipoprotein cholesterol (HDL-C) in normotensive and hypertensive groups among a random selection of 5,603 Australian men and women. In all instances, *p* values or NS designations refer to the significance between one bar and the next bar. (Data from ref. 62.)

risk from their hypertension; therefore they can be provided less protection from a reduction of their blood pressure than patients with higher pressures. Therefore, any additional risk, be it ever so small, from the therapy used to lower their blood pressure must be weighed on a balance with correspondingly less counterweight. The use of therapy that removes the large excess risk that accompanies more severe hypertension while in itself adding a small risk can easily be defended as beneficial. But for those with a milder hypertension that in itself increases risk only minimally, the use of such therapy cannot be defended.

Alternative Choices

Therefore, other drugs now available that pose fewer potential risks need to be considered as alternative choices for the initial therapy of hypertension. One point should be reiterated: There is little to choose among the various antihypertensive drugs as to their *efficacy* in lowering the blood pressure in the majority of hypertensives. Therefore, the choice of initial drug should be based mainly on side effects and long-term safety (Table 4). Unfortunately, few data are available to help make the choice. There is only one controlled study, the MRC trial, that compared two choices, a diuretic and a beta-blocker. Among the patients in the MRC trial, overall mortality was similar with the two drugs, with only nonsmoking men showing a lower rate of coronary mortality if they were given a beta-blocker than if they were given a diuretic (16).

Centrally Acting Agents

Reserpine is inexpensive, once-a-day, and relatively free of side effects if used in the small doses, 0.05 to 0.25 mg per day, shown to be as effective as larger doses (63). However, it has a bad reputation for causing severe depression and cancer, neither likely true but hard to dispel.

Methyldopa, clonidine, and guanabenz share many features as centrally acting alpha-agonists. Clonidine may cause more sedation and dry mouth, but neither it nor guanabenz is associated with the multiple "autoimmune" reactions reported with methyldopa (64). Both clonidine and guanabenz may not cause as much fluid retention as other nondiuretic antihypertensive agents. Guanabenz has been found to lower total

Table 4. *Characteristics of nondiuretic antihypertensive drugs for initial therapy*

	Advantages	Disadvantages
Central agonists	Little decrease in cardiac output Reduce lipids (guanabenz)	Sedation Dry mouth "Auto-Immune" reactions (methyldopa)
Alpha-blockers	Vasodilate Reduce lipids	Hypotension
Beta-blockers		
Non-ISA[a]	Relieve concomitant problems (e.g., migraine, angina) Cardioprotection after myocardial infarction	$Beta_2$ blockade (bronchospasm, etc.) Vasoconstrict (cold extremities) Reduce cardiac output (fatigue, loss of exercise ability) Raise triglycerides, lower HDL-cholesterol CNS effects: depression, sleep disturbances
ISA	No decrease in cardiac output No alteration of lipids	Less cardioprotection
Converting enzyme inhibitors	Vasodilate No cns effects No decrease in cardiac output	Rare but serious toxicity (renal, neutropenia) Rash, loss of taste (All likely less with enalapril)
Calcium antagonists	Vasodilate No cns effects Relieve angina	Variable bothersome but rarely serious side effects

[a](ISA) Intrinsic sympathomimetic activity.

serum cholesterol levels (65). Clonidine may be used in a transdermal patch with the hope of a smoother antihypertensive effect and fewer side effects (66).

Alpha-Blockers

Unlike diuretics and beta-blockers, which may induce adverse effects on lipids, alpha-blockers appear to be either neutral or beneficial (67). Beyond the beneficial effects on lipids, alpha-blockers lower the blood pressure in a hemodynamically more favorable manner than do diuretics or beta-blockers. Whereas much of the antihypertensive effect of beta-blockers resides in their reduction of cardiac output, alpha-blockers primarily reduce peripheral resistance and tend to have little effect on cardiac output (68). This may translate clinically into little beyond a lesser frequency of fatigue and cold extremities, but since the hemodynamic abnormality of established hypertension is an increased peripheral resistance, drugs that lower resistance should provide even more "physiologic" reduction in the blood pressure.

Beta-Blockers

The alternative approach recommended by the Third Joint National Committee (69) is to start therapy with a beta-blocker. There are now seven available in the United States and likely more on the way. As described in Chapter 10, these drugs, as a class, offer numerous advantages.

On the other hand, beta-blockers also pose numerous disadvantages. Some, such as bronchospasm, are immediate and obvious and therefore not much of a long-term problem. However, beta-blockers, like diuretics, may cause clinically inapparent but potentially hazardous effects on blood lipids (61) and glucose tolerance (60), although the mechanisms and patterns of these changes differ with the two types of drug. In multiple studies with beta-blockers, rises in triglycerides and falls in cardioprotective high-density lipoprotein (HDL)-cholesterol levels have been observed. Though these may not be induced by beta-blockers having high intrinsic sympathomimetic activity (ISA) (61), lipid levels should be monitored in all patients given any beta-blocker. For various reasons, including their lesser disturbance of lipid levels, those with

ISA (pindolol and acebutolol) seem to be more attractive than those without ISA for the treatment of uncomplicated hypertension.

Converting Enzyme Inhibitors

As described in Chapter 11, both captopril and enalapril have been approved for treatment of mild hypertension. With captopril, smaller doses of the drug than initially used to treat more severe hypertension cause relatively few side effects, particularly the more common problems that interfere with the quality of life, such as sedation and fatigue (70). Enalapril may provide all of the advantages of CEIs with even fewer side effects (71).

Studies by Drs. Norman Hollenberg, Gordon Williams, and their colleagues suggest that as many as 40% of all hypertensive patients will be particularly responsive to CEI therapy (72). These patients appear unable to modulate their adrenal or vascular responses to variations in sodium intake, apparently because of high, fixed levels of angiotensin II within the target tissues. These "nonmodulators," therefore, are unable to increase aldosterone secretion normally in response to sodium restriction, which, in turn, decreases the degree of sodium retention and fails to dampen the further release of renin. Thereby, more angiotensin II is generated when sodium intake is low, leading to more vasoconstriction and hypertension.

On the other hand, under the more usual circumstance of high sodium intake, these "nonmodulators" fail to increase renal blood flow and therefore do no excrete the sodium load as well. Body fluid volume expands and the blood pressure rises.

In addition to demonstrating that about half of hypertensive patients with normal to high plasma renin levels are "nonmodulators," these investigators have shown that even short-term therapy with CEI corrects the problems within both the adrenals and the renal vasculature. As a result, the majority of such patients have a significant fall in blood pressure with CEI monotherapy (72).

These data support the use of a CEI to correct an underlying defect that is responsible for hypertension in a considerable portion of the population. The prospect of using such specific therapy, rather than the empirical approaches that lower blood pressure because they happen to alter one or another mechanism that sustain the blood pressure, is an exciting one. Even if the relationship turns out to be less common or if it is impractical to identify the individual patients who have it, a CEI will likely be increasingly used as initial therapy. When one is used in unselected populations, about half of patients have a significant fall in blood pressure, and side effects noted frequently with other antihypertensives are uncommon. Moreover, as noted in Chapter 5, CEIs may offer a particular advantage in reducing renal vascular resistance by vasodilating the renal circulation, thereby protecting the kidneys more than other vasodilators.

Calcium Antagonists

These drugs lower the level of free calcium within vascular smooth muscle cells, mainly by blocking its entry from the extracellular fluid. These drugs, even more so than CEIs, may correct a fundamental mechanism responsible for hypertension (73). Increased concentrations of free intracellular calcium have been measured within tissues of hypertensive animals and people, perhaps as a consequence of defects in cell membrane transport mechanisms. The use of calcium antagonists may, then, correct the cause for increased vascular tone and resistance.

Whether or not they, too, are specific "corrective" therapies, calcium antagonists are potent antihypertensive agents (73). All three currently available in the United States, diltiazem, nifedipine, and verapamil, have been shown to lower blood pressure comparably to other antihypertensive drugs and with relatively few side effects. Now that they are approved for use in hypertension and with longer-lasting formulations available so that they may be given on a once- or twice-a-day basis, they will likely be used widely and early in the therapy of all degrees of hypertension. They may be particularly effective in the elderly (74).

Substitution Versus Stepped Care

It is obvious that a number of choices are available for initial (and often only) therapy for patients with mild hypertension. In addition to using one of these rather than a diuretic, another change in the present common practice of stepped care seems likely: Rather than adding a second drug if the first is not enough, stopping the first and substituting another as sole therapy.

The substitution approach is based on the premise that some patients respond better to one class of drugs than to another. Despite the generalization made earlier that all antihypertensive drugs have comparable potency, there are some patients who respond better to one or another. Elderly people and blacks seem to respond less well to beta-blockers (74) and, perhaps, to CEIs (75), and better to diuretics (76) and calcium antagonists (74,77).

Beyond such differences as may be seen in patients of different age and race, responses may be caused by differences in adherence to therapy with one or another drug. If a patient develops such intolerable side effects as to stop therapy, the problem is usually obvious and a second agent would routinely be substituted. However, patients may not volunteer or admit problems with their drugs, but instead just not take them. For whatever reason, if a patient does not have the desired effect from the initial drug, a logical next step might be to stop it and try a drug from another category. Thereby, the patient may be more successfully treated with fewer medications.

This approach is similar in principle to that advocated for many years by Dr. John Laragh (78). His approach is based on a renin profile, with an adrenergic blocker or CEI to be given to those with high or normal renins and a diuretic or calcium antagonist to those with low renin. However, the decision as to which drug to choose first can be made simply on the basis of age, race, and the presence of other cardiovascular problems.

In the future, the choice may be made on the basis of the potential for reversal of cardiac and arterial smooth muscle hypertrophy. Most, if not all, of the adrenergic inhibitors and both CEIs and calcium antagonists have been shown experimentally to reverse left ventricular hypertrophy (79). Whether that will be included in the decision to treat and the choice of therapy remains to be seen.

Beyond the First Drug

If one drug is well tolerated but is only partially effective, the addition of a second of another class is rational. Half or more of the patients in various trials involving people with DBP between 90 and 109 mm Hg require a second drug, and about 10% require three.

There is little comparative evidence on which to decide which drugs should be chosen as second or third. The tradition has been to include a diuretic if there are two and to include a direct vasodilator if there are three. Other combinations may work as well. The best study was done on 238 patients whose DBP remained above 95 mm Hg on a full dose of a diuretic and a beta-blocker (80). Prazosin and hydralazine were best tolerated, whereas minoxidil was most effective. Neither CEIs nor calcium antagonists were included in that study. CEIs or calcium antagonists may increasingly be chosen as the vasodilator rather than the "direct" acting hydralazine or minoxidil (81). Since they do not induce as much reflex sympathetic activity as the direct vasodilators, CEIs or calcium antagonists can likely be used as first, second, or third choices, as can the various adrenergic inhibitors.

Management of More Severe Hypertension

The more severe the hypertension, the more likely the need for additional drugs and larger doses of each. Therapy of severe hypertension has become increasingly more successful. Nonetheless, 5-year survival for those who progress into accelerated-malignant hypertension remains only around 50% (82), although the addition of kidney dialysis to drug therapy may allow for sustained recovery of renal function even after renal shutdown from accelerated hypertension (83). Interestingly, the survival rates for 95 patients with malignant hypertension, i.e., papilledema, was the same as for the 105 with accelerated hypertension, i.e., hemorrhages and exudates, suggesting "that malignant and accelerated hypertension are one and the same disease" (82).

The therapy for some patients with severe hypertension may require parenteral medications, as described in Chapter 13. Most will be controlled with oral medications, although three or more may be needed. Those will usually include a diuretic, particularly since many of these patients have significant renal damage causing a greater tendency for sodium retention. An adrenergic inhibitor will likely be the second drug, with the combined alpha- and beta-blocker labetalol being a rational choice. For many, a vasodilator will also be needed. As noted above, either a CEI or a calcium antagonist or a combination of the two will increasingly be chosen rather than the prior standbys, hydralazine and minoxidil. The latter drug, however, may continue to be needed for those with resistant hypertension associated with renal insufficiency.

General Guidelines for Drug Therapy

As many as half of patients begun on antihypertensive therapy will not be taking it 1 year later, most of them simply stopping the medication because of inadequate follow-up, lack of perceived benefit, or side effects. Care must be taken to prescribe drugs in a way that can easily be remembered by asymptomatic people, that will interfere little with various activities, and that will cause few side effects. These guidelines should help improve patient compliance to therapy:

- Establish the goal of therapy: to reduce blood pressure to normotensive levels with minimal or no side effects
- Educate the patient about his disease and its treatment
- Maintain contact with the patient
  - Encourage visits and calls to allied health personnel
  - Allow the pharmacist to monitor therapy
  - Make contact with patients who do not return
- Keep care inexpensive and simple
  - Do the least workup needed to rule out secondary causes
  - Obtain follow-up laboratory data only yearly unless indicated more often
  - Use home blood pressure readings
  - Use nondrug, no-cost therapies
  - Use the fewest daily doses of drugs needed
  - If appropriate, use combination tablets
- Prescribe according to pharmacological principles
  - Add one drug at a time
  - Start with small doses, aiming for 5 to 10 mm Hg reductions at each step
  - Prevent volume overload with moderate sodium restriction and, if needed, adequate diuretic
  - Stop unsuccessful therapy and try a different approach
  - If therapy is only partially successful, additional drugs of different classes may be added, preferably one at a time, in sufficient doses to achieve the goal of therapy
  - Anticipate side effects
  - Adjust therapy to ameliorate side effects that do not spontaneously disappear
- Be aware of the problem and be alert to signs of patient nonadherence. Have the patient bring medications to the office so that pill counts and checks on numbers of refills can be done if the blood pressure has not responded
- Be prepared to step down the number and doses of medications if the blood pressure remains well controlled. Some patients may be able to stop therapy completely, but they should remain under careful surveillance for return of hypertension

ACKNOWLEDGMENTS

I wish to acknowledge the secretarial assistance of Susan Beaubien and Sharon Washington in the preparation of this manuscript.

REFERENCES

1. Hypertension Detection and Follow-Up Program Cooperative Group (1977): The hypertension detection and follow-up program: A progress report. *Circ. Res.*, 40(*Suppl.* 1):I106–I109.
2. National Center for Health Statistics (B. K. Cypress) (1982): *Medication Therapy in Office Visits for Hypertension*. National Ambulatory Medical Care Survey, 1980. Advance Data from Vital and Health Statistics, No. 80, DHHS Pub. No (PHS) 82-1250. Public Health Service, Hyattsville, MD.
3. Cloher, T. P., and Whelton, P. K. (1986): Physician approach to the recognition and initial management of hypertension. *Arch. Intern. Med.*, 146:529–533.
4. Bannan, L. T., Beevers, D. G., and Wright, N. (1980): ABC of blood pressure reduction: The size of the problem. *Br. Med. J.*, 281:921–923.
5. Logan, A. G. (1984): Report of the Canadian hypertension society's consensus conference on the management of mild hypertension. *Can. Med. Assoc. J.*, 131:1053–1057.
6. Subcommittee on Definition and Prevalence of the 1984 Joint National Committee (1985): Hypertension prevalence and the status of awareness, treatment, and control in the United States. *Hypertension*, 7:457–468.
7. Working Group on Risk and High Blood Pressure (1985): An epidemiological approach to describing risk associated with blood pressure levels. *Hypertension*, 7:641–651.
8. Moser, M. (1983): A decade of progress in the management of hypertension. *Hypertension*, 5:808–813.
9. Goldman, L., and Cook, E. F. (1984): The decline in ischemic heart disease mortality rates. *Ann. Intern. Med.*, 101:825–836.
10. Bulpitt, C. J., Beevers, D. G., Butler, A., et al. (1986): The survival of treated hypertensive patients and their causes of death: A report from the DHSS hypertensive care computing project (DHCCP). *J. Hypertension*, 4:93–99.
11. Forsyth, R. A. (1984): Coronary heart disease in treated hypertensive patients and risk-matched normotensive control subjects. *Am. Heart J.*, 108:305–310.
12. Yano, K., McGee, D., and Reed, D. M. (1983): The impact of elevated blood pressure upon 10-year mortality among Japanese men in Hawaii: The Honolulu heart program. *J. Chronic Dis.*, 36:569–579.
13. Management Committee (1980): The Australian therapeutic trial in mild hypertension. *Lancet*, 1:1261–1267.
14. Helgeland, A. (1980): Treatment of mild hypertension: A five year controlled drug trial. *Am. J. Med.*, 69:725–732.
15. Amery, A., Brixko, P., Clement, D., et al. (1985): Mortality and morbidity results from the European working party on high blood pressure in the elderly trial. *Lancet*, 1:1349–1354.
16. Medical Research Council Working Party (1985): MRC trial of treatment of mild hypertension: Principal results. *Br. Med. J.*, 291:97–104.
17. Hypertension Detection and Follow-Up Cooperative Group (1979): Five-year findings of the hypertension detection and follow-up program: I. Reduction in mortality of persons with high blood pressure, including mild hypertension. *JAMA*, 242:2562–2571.
18. Multiple Risk Factor Intervention Trial Research Group (1982): Multiple risk factor intervention trial: Risk factor changes and mortality results. *JAMA*, 248:1465–1477.
19. Management Committee of the Australian Therapeutic Trial in Mild Hypertension (1982): Untreated mild hypertension. *Lancet*, 1:185–191.
20. Horan, M. J., Kennedy, H. L., and Padgett, N. E. (1981): Do borderline hypertensive patients have labile blood pressure? *Ann. Intern. Med.*, 94:466–468.
21. Perloff, D., Soklow, M., and Cowan, R. (1983): The prognostic value of ambulatory blood pressure. *JAMA*, 249:2792–2798.
22. Castelli, W. P. (1984): Epidemiology of coronary heart disease: The Framingham study. *Am. J. Med.*, 76:4–12.
23. Garland, C., Barrett-Connor, E., Suarez, L., and Criqui, M. H. (1983): Isolated systolic hypertension and mortality after age 60 years: A prospective population-based study. *Am. J. Epidemiol.*, 118:365–376.
24. Hulley, S. B., Furberg, C. D., Gurland, B., et al. (1985): Systolic hypertension in the elderly program (SHEP): Antihypertensive efficacy of chlorthalidone. *Am. J. Cardiol.*, 56:913–920.
25. Parving, H. H., Anderson, A. R., Smidt, U. M., and Svendsen, P. A. (1983): Early aggressive antihypertensive treatment reduced rate of decline in kidney function in diabetic nephropathy. *Lancet*, 1:1175–1178.
26. Kaplan, N. M. (1986): *Clinical Hypertension*, 4th ed. Williams and Wilkins, Baltimore.
27. Kaplan, N. M. (1985): Non-drug treatment of hypertension. *Ann. Intern. Med.*, 102:359–373.
28. Modan, M., Halkin, H., Almog, S., et al. (1985): Hyperinsulinemia: A link between hypertension obesity and glucose intolerance. *J. Clin. Invest.*, 75:809–817.
29. Weinsier, R. L., Norris, D. J., Birch, R., et al. (1985): The relative contribution of body fat and fat pattern to blood pressure level. *Hypertension*, 7:578–585.
30. Barrett-Connor, E., and Khaw, K.-T. (1985): Is hypertension more benign when associated with obesity? *Circulation*, 72:53–60.
31. Bloom, E., Reed, D., Yano, K., and MacLean, C. (1986): Does obesity protect hypertensives against cardiovascular disease? *JAMA*, 256:2972–2975.
32. MacMahon, S. W., Macdonald, G. J., Bernstein, L., Andrews, G., and Blacket, R. B. (1985): Comparison of weight reduction with metoprolol in treatment of hypertension in young overweight patients. *Lancet*, 1:1233–1236.
33. MacMahon, S. W., Wilcken, D. E. L., and Macdonald, G. J. (1986): The effect of weight reduction on left ventricular mass: A randomized controlled trial in young, overweight hypertensive patients. *N. Engl. J. Med.*, 314:334–339.

34. Fagerberg, B., Andersson, O. K., Persson, B., and Hedner, T. (1985): Reactivity to norepinephrine and effect of sodium on blood pressure during weight loss. *Hypertension,* 7:586–592.
35. Brown, J. J., Lever, A. F., Robertson, J. I. S., et al. (1984): Salt and hypertension. *Lancet,* 2:456.
36. MacGregor, G. A. (1985): Sodium is more important than calcium in essential hypertension. *Hypertension,* 7:628–637.
37. Bittle, C. C., Jr., Molina, D. J., and Bartter, F. C. (1985): Salt sensitivity in essential hypertension as determined by the Cosinor method. *Hypertension,* 7:989–994.
38. Ram, C. V. S., Garrett, B. N., and Kaplan, N. M. (1981): Moderate sodium restriction and various diuretics in the treatment of hypertension: Effects on potassium wastage and blood pressure control. *Arch. Intern. Med.,* 141:1015–1019.
39. Landmann-Suter, R., and Struyvenberg, A. (1978): Initial potassium loss and hypokalaemia during chlorthalidone administration in patients with essential hypertension: The influence of dietary sodium restriction. *Eur. J. Clin. Invest.,* 8:155–164.
40. Meneely, G. R., and Battarbee, H. D. (1976): High sodium-low potassium environment and hypertension. *Am. J. Cardiol.,* 38:768–785.
41. Kaplan, N. M., Carnegie, A., Raskin, P., Heller, J. A., and Simmons, M. (1985): Potassium supplementation in hypertensive patients with diuretic-induced hypokalemia. *N. Engl. J. Med.,* 312:746–749.
42. Cappuccio, F. P., Markandu, N. D., Beynon, G. W., Shore, A. C., Sampson, B., and MacGregor, G. A. (1985): Lack of effect of oral magnesium on high blood pressure: A double blind study. *Br. Med. J.,* 291:235–238.
43. Rasmussen, H. S., Norregard, P., Lindeneg, O., McNair, P., Backer, V., and Balslev, S. (1986): Intravenous magnesium in acute myocardial infarction. *Lancet,* 1:234–235.
44. McCarron, D. A. (1985): Is calcium more important than sodium in the pathogenesis of essential hypertension? *Hypertension,* 7:607–627.
45. Meese, R. B., Gonzalez, D. G., Casparian, J. M., Ram, C. V. S., Pak, C. Y. C., and Kaplan, N. M. (1986): Failure of calcium supplements to relieve hypertension (Abstr.). *Clin. Res.,* 34:218A.
46. McCarron, D. A., and Morris, C. D. (1985): Blood pressure response to oral calcium in persons with mild to moderate hypertension: A randomized, double-blind, placebo-controlled, crossover trial. *Ann. Intern. Med.,* 103:825–831.
47. Resnick, L. M., Nicholson, J. P., and Laragh, J. H. (1984): Outpatient therapy of essential hypertension with dietary calcium supplementation (Abstr.). *J. Am. Coll. Cardiol.,* 3:616.
48. Puddey, I. B., Vandongen, R., Beilin, L. J., and Rouse, I. L. (1985): Alcohol stimulation of renin release in man: Its relation to the hemodynamic, electrolyte, and sympatho-adrenal responses to drinking. *J. Clin. Endocrinol. Metab.,* 61:37–42.
49. Jackson, R., Stewart, A., Beaglehole, R., and Scragg, R. (1985): Alcohol consumption and blood pressure. *Am. J. Epidemiol.,* 122:1037–1044.
50. Coldizt, G. A., Branch, L. G., Lipnick, R. J., et al. (1985): Moderate alcohol and decreased cardiovascular mortality in an elderly cohort. *Am. Heart J.,* 109:886–889.
51. Cade, R., Mars, D., Wagemaker, H., et al. (1984): Effect of aerobic exercise training on patients with systemic arterial hypertension. *Am. J. Med.,* 77:785–790.
52. Duncan, J. J., Farr, J. E., Upton, S. J., Hagan, R. D., Oglesby, M. E., and Blair, S. N. (1985): The effects of aerobic exercise on plasma catecholamines and blood pressure in patients with mild essential hypertension. *JAMA,* 254:2609–2613.
53. Jennings, G., Nelson, L., Nestel, P., et al. (1986): The effects of changes in physical activity on major cardiovascular risk factors, hemodynamics, sympathetic function, and glucose utilization in man: A controlled study of four levels of activity. *Circulation,* 73:30–40.
54. Stamler, R., Stamler, J., Grimm, R., et al. (1985): Nonpharmacological control of hypertension. *Prevent. Med.,* 14:336–345.
55. Langford, H. G., Blaufox, M. D., Oberman, A., et al. (1985): Dietary therapy slows the return of hypertension after stopping prolonged medication. *JAMA,* 253:657–664.
56. Andersen, B., Snorrason, S. P., Ragnarsson, J., and Hardarson, T. (1985): Hydrochlorothiazide and potassium chloride in comparison with hydrochlorothiazide and amiloride in the treatment of mild hypertension. *Acta Med. Scand.,* 218:449–454.
57. Kaplan, N. M. (1984): Our appropriate concern about hypokalemia. *Am. J. Med.,* 77:1–4.
58. Kannel, W. B., and Abbott, R. D. (1985): A prognostic comparison of asymptomatic left ventricular hypertrophy and unrecognized myocardial infarction: The Framingham study. *Am. Heart J.,* 111:391–397.
59. Struthers, A. D., Whitesmith, R., and Reid, J. L. (1983): Prior thiazide diuretic treatment increases adrenaline-induced hypokalaemia. *Lancet,* 1:1358–1360.
60. Dornhorst, A., Powell, S. H., and Pensky, J. (1985): Aggravation by propranolol of hyperglycaemic effect of hydrochlorothiazide in type II diabetics without alteration of insulin secretion. *Lancet,* 1:123–126.
61. Weidmann, P., Uehlinger, D. E., and Gerber, A. (1985): Antihypertensive treatment and serum lipoproteins. *J. Hypertension,* 3:297–306.
62. MacMahon, S. W., and Macdonald, G. J. (1986): Antihypertensive treatment and plasma lipoprotein levels: The associations in data from a population study. *Am. J. Med.,* 80(*Suppl.* 2A):40–47.
63. Participating Veterans Administration Medical Centers (1982): Low doses v standard dose of reserpine: A randomized, double-blind, multiclinic trial in patients taking chlorthalidone. *JAMA,* 248:2471–2477.
64. Kelton, J. G. (1985): Impaired reticuloendothelial function in patients treated with methyldopa. *N. Engl. J. Med.,* 313:596–600.
65. Kaplan, N. M. (1984): Effects of guanabenz on plasma lipid levels in hypertensive patients. *J. Cardiovasc. Pharmacol.,* 6:S841–S846.

66. Weber, M. A., Drayer, J. I. M., McMahon, F. G., Hamburger, R., Shah, A. R., and Kirk, L. N. (1984): Transdermal administration of clonidine for treatment of high BP. *Arch. Intern. Med.*, 144:1211–1213.
67. Sacks, F. M., and Dzau, V. J. (1986): Adrenergic effects on plasma lipoprotein metabolism. *Am. J. Med.*, 80(*Suppl.* 2A):71–81.
68. Graham, R. M. (1984): Selective alpha$_1$-adrenergic antagonists: Therapeutically relevant antihypertensive agents. *Am. J. Cardiol.*, 53:16A–20A.
69. Joint National Committee on Detection, Evaluation, and Treatment of High Blood Pressure (1984): The 1984 report of the Joint National Committee on Detection, Evaluation, and Treatment of High Blood Pressure. *Arch. Intern. Med.*, 144:1045–1057.
70. Hill, J. F., Bulpitt, C. J., and Fletcher, A. E. (1985): Angiotensin converting enzyme inhibitors and quality of life: The European trial. *J. Hypertension*, 3(*Suppl.* 2):S91–S94.
71. Smith, W. M., Kulaga, S. F., Moncloa, F., Pingeon, R., and Walker, J. F. (1984): Overall tolerance and safety of enalapril. *J. Hypertension*, 2(*Suppl.* 2): 113–117.
72. Williams, G. H., and Hollenberg, N. K. (1985): Are non-modulating patients with essential hypertension a distinct subgroup? *Am. J. Med.*, 79(*Suppl.* 3C):3–9.
73. Halperin, A. K., and Cubeddu, L. X. (1986): The role of calcium channel blockers in the treatment of hypertension. *Am. Heart J.*, 111:363–382.
74. Buhler, F. R., Bolli, P., Kiowski, W., Erne, P., Hulthen, U. L., and Block, L. H. (1984): Renin profiling to select antihypertensive baseline drugs: Renin inhibitors for high-renin and calcium entry blockers for low-renin patients. *Am. J. Med.*, 7:36–42.
75. Weinberger, M. H. (1985): Blood pressure and metabolic responses to hydrochlorothiazide, captopril, and the combination in black and white mild-to-moderate hypertensive patients. *J. Cardiovasc. Pharmacol.*, 7:S52–55.
76. Hulley, S. B., Furberg, C. D., Gurland, B., et al. (1985): Systolic hypertension in the elderly program (SHEP): Antihypertensive efficacy of chlorthalidone. *Am. J. Cardiol.*, 56:913–920.
77. M'Buyamba-Kabangu, J. R., Lepira, B., Fagard, R., et al. (1986): Relative potency of a beta-blocking and a calcium entry blocking agent as antihypertensive drugs in black patients. *Eur. J. Clin. Pharmacol.*, 29:523–527.
78. Laragh, J. H. (1984): Modification of stepped care approach to antihypertensive therapy. *Am. J. Med.*, 77:78–86.
79. Schlant, R. C. (1985): Reversal of left ventricular hypertrophy by drug treatment of hypertension. *Chest*, 88(*Suppl.*):194S–198S.
80. McAreavey, D., Ramsey, L. E., Latham, L., et al. (1984): "Third drug" trial: comparative study of antihypertensive agents added to treatment when blood pressure remains uncontrolled by a beta blocker plus thiazide diuretic. *Br. Med. J.*, 288:106–111.
81. White, W. B., Viadero, J. J., Lane, T. J., and Podesla, S. (1986): Effects of combination therapy with captopril and nifedipine in severe or resistant hypertension. *Clin. Pharmacol. Ther.*, 39:43–48.
82. Ahmed, M. E. K., Walker, J. M., Beevers, D. G., and Beevers, M. (1986): Lack of difference between malignant and accelerated hypertension. *Br. Med. J.*, 292:235–237.
83. Bakir, A. A., Bazilinski, N., and Dunea, G. (1986): Transient and sustained recovery from renal shutdown in accelerated hypertension. *Am. J. Med.*, 80:172–176.

The Kidney in Hypertension, edited by Norman M. Kaplan, Barry M. Brenner, and John H. Laragh. Raven Press, New York © 1987.

Vasodilators and Beta-Adrenergic Antagonists

Stephen C. Textor

Consultative Medicine/Nephrology, Renal Physiology Laboratory, City of Hope National Medical Center, Duarte, California 91010

BETA-ADRENERGIC ANTAGONISTS

Since the introduction of propranolol in the late 1960s for use in the treatment of cardiac arrhythmias and the observations that arterial pressure fell in many patients receiving beta-blockers, this class of drug has enjoyed rapid acceptance as a mainstay of antihypertensive therapy. Development of beta-adrenergic receptor blockers has expanded rapidly and constitutes one of the first departures from the "stepped-care" approach to hypertension therapy instituted in the 1950s utilizing sequential combinations of diuretics and sympatholytic agents.

A large part of this acceptance relates to the relative freedom from major side effects typical of previous agents, such as postural hypotension, sedation, and impotence. There has been a growing trend to utilize beta-blocking drugs as initial, and often sole therapy for essential hypertension, thereby avoiding some of the problems associated with diuretic administration.

There are currently seven beta-adrenergic antagonists and one combined alpha-beta antagonist available commercially in the United States and many more worldwide.

This chapter reviews the basic mechanisms and pharmacology of beta-adrenergic blocking agents, particularly as they relate to renal function. It became apparent soon after their introduction that the beta-blockers possessed cardiovascular features that effectively counter the less agreeable characteristics of potent direct vasodilators, e.g., reflex tachycardia. Hence, the combination of beta-blockers and vasodilators has proven to be an excellent choice for resistant or severe hypertension.

As understanding of circulatory regulation and pharmacotherapeutics has progressed, it has become evident that regional vascular beds may be selectively affected in different ways. Hence, consideration of the systemic and regional hemodynamic properties of beta-blockers is essential. The fact that alteration of cardiac output and blood pressure may have direct effects on renal function under some circumstances poses a concern to clinicians and will be expanded below.

Beta-Receptors and Mechanisms of Antihypertensive Activity

Neural control of the circulation derives primarily by peripheral sympathetic adrenergic outflow. The neurotransmitter emanating from nerve terminals in this limb is norepinephrine, which activates two major types of adrenergic receptors, designated alpha and beta. It has long been recognized that vascular smooth muscle may possess both alpha- and beta-receptors. The balance of alpha- and beta-adrenergic influences with individual vascular beds may vary widely, and typically they exert opposing actions, i.e., vasoconstriction induced by alpha-mediated neurons and vasodilation induced by beta-mediated neurons. Several subsets of receptors have been defined, including postsynaptic alpha receptors (alpha-1), which modulate vasoconstriction, and presynaptic alpha receptors (alpha-2),

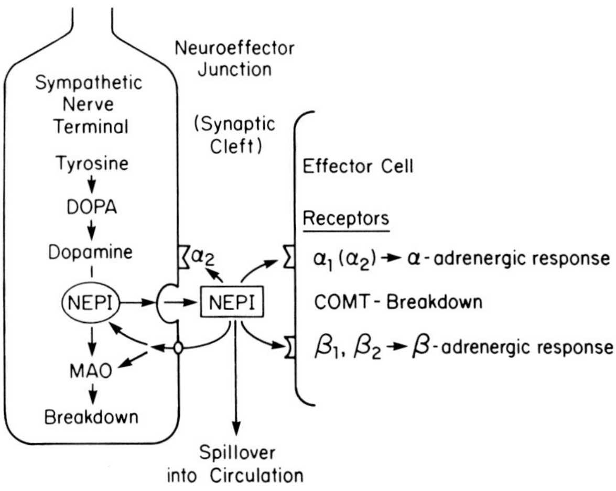

FIG. 1. Schematic representation of peripheral adrenergic neuroeffector junction. Axonal nerve transmission signals the release of prepackaged norepinephrine into the synaptic cleft. Alpha- and beta-receptors are thereby activated, depending on the relative density of each. Alpha-1 receptors are located at postsynaptic sites and usually mediate vasoconstriction, whereas alpha-2 receptors are primarily presynaptic as shown. Beta-receptors are postsynaptic and mediate a variety of functions, including peripheral vasodilation. (MAO) monoamine; (NEPI) norepinephrine; (COMT) catecholamine-0-methyl-transferase. (Modified from ref. 59.)

which feedback on nerve traffic (Fig. 1) (6,13,48,59).

Currently two major categories of peripheral beta-adrenoceptors, beta-1 and beta-2, have been identified. Both classes are widely represented, but various tissues are more heavily served with one or the other. In general, cardiac sympathetic tone is mediated by beta-1 receptors, and agents preferentially acting on beta-1 receptors have been termed "cardioselective," whereas peripheral vascular effects are predominantly beta-2. These receptors are identified by the characteristics of being selectively activated or inhibited by synthetic or endogenous catecholamines. Table 1 identifies some of the major localizing features of beta-1 and beta-2 receptors. It should be emphasized that these represent functional and pharmacologic classifications and may undergo modifications as further information accrues.

Table 1. *Functional classification of beta-adrenergic receptors*[a]

Beta-1	Beta-2
Heart	Smooth muscle cell contractility
Increase heart rate	Bronchioles
Increase contractility (inotropic)	Peripheral vessels
Increase conduction velocity	
Increase automatically	
Juxtaglomerular cell: renin release	Glycogenolysis
	Lipolysis
	Insulin release
	Potassium uptake—transcellular

[a]All classifications indicate relative activity; even "selective agents" possess some degree of activity in all receptors.

Beta-blocking agents owe their activity to structural resemblance to endogenous catecholamines and their receptor-blocking properties within neuroeffector beds. Hence, different compounds may be more or less specific for different receptor types, and in some instances activate the receptor to some degree, i.e., possess intrinsic sympathomimetic activity (ISA).

The precise mechanisms by which beta-adrenergic blockade cause a reduction in blood pressure have been controversial and are still unresolved (Fig. 2). Hemodynamic measurements indicate that a reduction in cardiac output, due primarily to the fall in heart rate, occurs promptly both in subjects developing a subsequent fall in blood pressure and in those who do not respond (40,50). The fact that arterial pressure falls some time after this reduction has been taken to indicate that the change in cardiac output *per se* is at best an initiator of circulatory adjustments and not a requirement for pressure reduction. This is consistent with the observation that agents with ISA may reduce pressure without a fall in resting heart rate or cardiac output (21). It has been proposed that a complex series of adjustments develops during which the

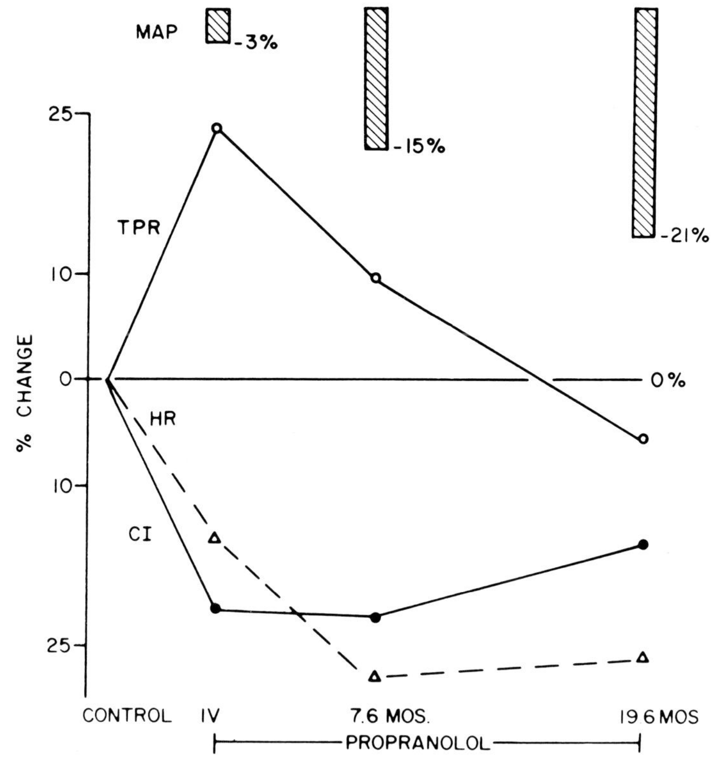

FIG. 2. Summary of hemodynamic changes observed after initiating beta-blockade. Acute alterations in cardiac output and resistance tend to be associated with pressure reduction only after a period of time has elapsed. The mechanism for the fall in resistance observed after an initial rise is still unresolved. (MAP) mean arterial pressure; (TPR) total peripheral resistance; (HR) heart rate; (CI) cardiac index. (From ref. 50.)

balance between beta- and alpha-adrenergic tone mediating vasoconstriction becomes reset, allowing reduction in both arterial pressure and peripheral resistance despite reduction in cardiac output and inotropic state (23,50).

Plasma renin activity falls during administration of many beta-blockers. However, the fall in plasma renin activity tends to be dissociated in time from pressure responses (9,24,49). Moreover, some investigators have noted additive effects of beta-blockade to treatment with angiotensin converting enzyme inhibitors, making it unlikely that renin suppression is a central mechanism.

CNS antihypertensive actions were proposed during early studies using high dose administration of propranolol (13,48). Certainly, some side effects, e.g., hallucinations, nightmares, etc., must represent central drug accumulation. However, many agents with demonstrably minimal CNS penetration are effective antihypertensive agents, making a primary CNS effect likely to be a secondary factor.

Despite the pharmacologically unique features of each beta-blocking agent, including variable degrees of receptor selectivity, ISA, CNS penetration, and other actions that may not be directly related to adrenergic blockade whatsoever, the relative homogeneity and predictability of blood pressure response from one agent to another has been remarkable. No clear characteristic related to beta-blockade has emerged to favor selection of one agent over another for purely antihypertensive efficacy.

Pharmacology of Beta-Blocking Agents

Table 2 contains a summary of the beta-adrenergic blocking agents currently available in the United States. Major pharmacologic features applicable to their use include the following:

Route of Excretion

Several of these are primarily excreted by hepatic metabolism and renal excretion of conjugates. These tend to be agents of short or intermediate duration. Nadolol and atenolol are excreted unchanged by renal routes primarily and therefore accumulate in patients with renal insufficiency. Active half-lives are considerably longer with these agents, making once-daily or even less frequent dosing possible.

Lipophilicity

The relative lipid solubility of these agents has been associated with greater or lesser penetration of the CNS (59). At usual doses, it is questionable whether this is commonly of clinical significance. Nonetheless, some individuals are particularly prone to CNS effects, such as vivid dreams or hallucinations. These may not occur in some patients with administration of an alternative compound not having CNS penetration.

Receptor Selectivity

Several agents, including atenolol, acebutolol, and metoprolol, have been developed with relative selectivity for beta-1 receptor. Others are considered "nonselective" and inhibit both beta-1 and beta-2 receptors. This selectivity is lost as doses are increased. Cardioselectivity offers the theoretical, and perhaps real, advantage of inducing less bronchospasm, less inhibition of glucose release, and less peripheral vasoconstriction in susceptible individuals (21,39). It must be emphasized that despite selectivity, problematic bronchospasm may occur with any of these compounds.

Intrinsic Sympathomimetic Activity

Some agents, notably pindolol and acebutolol in the United States, have a minor degree of beta-agonist activity. Hence, little or no diminution of resting heart rate or cardiac output is observed with these drugs, although responses to sympathetic stimulation during stress are blocked.

Combined Alpha- and Beta-Blockade

Labetatol possesses both alpha-1 and nonselective beta-adrenergic blocking properties in a ratio of 1:3 after oral administration. As a result, peripheral resistance is reduced and its anti-

Table 2. *Beta-blocking agents available in the United States*

Name	Brand name	Beta-receptors	Excretion	$t\frac{1}{2}$	ISA[a]	Usual dose
Acebutolol	Sectral	Beta-1	Renal	3	+	200 mg b.i.d.
Atenolol	Tenormin	Beta-1	Renal	6–8	—	50–100 mg q.d.
Metoprolol	Lopressor	Beta-1	Hepatic	3–4	—	50 mg b.i.d.
Nadolol	Corgard	Nonselective	Renal	14–18	—	40–120 mg q.d.
Pindolol	Visken	Nonselective	Hepatic	3–4	+ +	5–20 mg b.i.d. or t.i.d.
Propranolol	Inderal	Nonselective	Hepatic	3–5	—	40–120 mg b.i.d.
Timolol	Blocadren	Nonselective	Hepatic	4	—	10–20 mg b.i.d.
Combined alpha-beta						
Labetalol	Normodyne Trandate	Nonselective hepatic		4–6	—[b]	200 mg b.i.d.

[a](ISA) Intrinsic sympathomimetic activity.
[b]Small degree of beta-2-mediated vasodilation reported.

hypertensive potency achieves a level similar to combined blockade, e.g., the addition of prazosin and a beta-blocker. Postural hypotension secondary to alpha-blockade has been observed.

Beta-Adrenergic Blockade and the Kidney

Beta-blocking agents have profound effects on both the systemic and regional circulations (Table 3). Generally, they diminish the cardiovascular response to maximal effort, as peak heart rate and cardiac output are diminished. Each regional vascular bed may thereby experience some degree of circulatory reduction under certain conditions. This has been evident clinically as the frequent complaint of "cool hands" or, in more severe instances, exacerbation of underlying Raynaud's phenomenon or claudication (13). Under circumstances of marginal cardiac performance, congestive heart failure may ensue (20).

As a major recipient of cardiac output, the renal vasculature also may be affected during beta-blockade (Fig. 3). Although the renal circulation usually is well protected against perturbations in flow, several studies in patients receiving propranolol indicate that sustained falls in renal plasma flow and glomerular filtration rate (GFR) may occur. This phenomenon has been observed in both hypertensive patients and normotensive volunteers (4,5,14,19,42,60,61). Of greatest concern is the contention that a fall

Table 3. *Renal effects of beta-blocking agents*

Renal blood flow
Diminished: ?Secondary to cardiac output
?Unopposed alpha-vasoconstriction
Unchanged: Nadolol, pindolol, atenolol
Occasional severe fall in presence of underlying vascular disease
Glomerular filtration rate
Diminished: Usually transient
Unchanged:
Plasma renin activity: Often suppressed
Diuretic-stimulated renin release remains
Sodium excretion
Delayed/impaired excretion of sodium load
Overt sodium retention in compromised cardiac function
Potassium homeostasis
Adrenergic mediation of cellular shifts impaired

in glomerular filtration rate appeared that did not recover, despite withdrawal of the drug (5). The precise mechanism of this fall in blood flow and GFR is not well established, although one study indicated a general relationship between fall in renal plasma flow and unopposed alpha-adrenergic vascular constriction, as reflected by norepinephrine levels (14). The various beta-blockers appear to differ in this regard. Although numerous agents have been shown to reduce renal blood flow, nadolol appears to produce short-term increases in renal perfusion and is regularly associated with redistribution of cardiac output to the kidneys during chronic administration (51). Less extensive data indicate that atenolol and pindolol may spare the renal circulation also (8,61). The mechanisms behind nadolol-induced changes are not fully understood, although a structural resemblance to dopamine has been observed.

Regardless of the mechanism, these observations underscore the sensitivity of individual vascular beds to alterations in systemic hemodynamics during antihypertensive therapy. The widespread use of these agents without major decrements in renal function is reassuring and suggests that under normal circumstances, minor decrements in renal blood flow pose no clinical problem. However, when other factors, such as underlying vascular disease, render the renal circulation particularly susceptible, a fall in cardiac output and perfusion pressure may induce significant renal failure, which may be reversible on discontinuing the agent (52,57). Other instances of acute renal failure have been reported occasionally during therapy with beta-blockers but without detailed information about the underlying circulatory status of the patients. Although such cases are uncommon, they represent important instances of reversible acute renal failure that should be recognized when they occur.

Beta-adrenergic blockade may impair sodium excretion, although this may be subtle. These drugs are often used as monotherapy without a diuretic. However, if challenged with a sodium load, subjects taking propranolol have a delayed and incomplete natriuresis despite normal renal

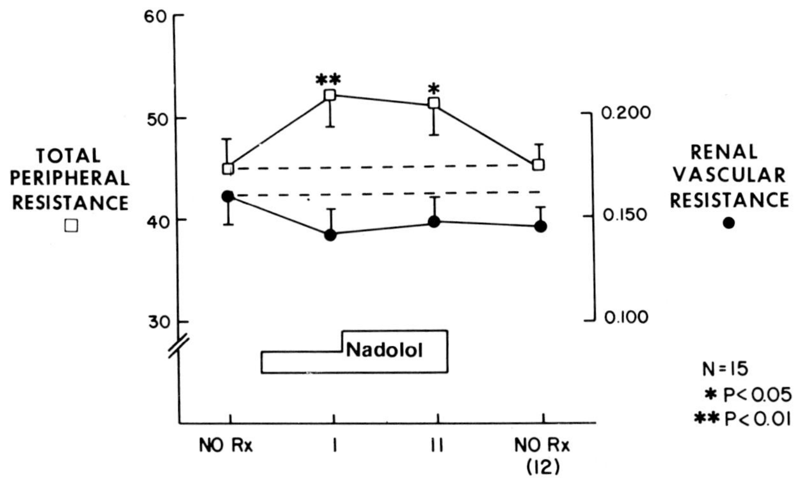

FIG. 3. Changes in peripheral vascular resistance as compared to renal vascular resistance before and during therapy with oral nadolol. The renal vascular bed did not share in the generalized increase in vasomotor tone; these data underscore the independent nature of regulation in individual vascular beds. (From ref. 51.)

function (33). Early observations in patients with borderline cardiovascular status showed progressive volume retention and edema formation also (20). These effects may be particularly evident in subjects with renal failure. In such instances, addition of diuretics or discontinuation of beta-blockade may be required.

Recent studies have indicated that adrenergic activity may modulate transmembrane shifts in potassium. Hence there has been concern that plasma levels of potassium may rise in patients receiving beta-blocking drugs during exercise or muscle breakdown (31,62). Although small increments in plasma levels of potassium have in fact occurred in hypertensive patients monitored closely, this has not posed a clinical problem. In patients receiving diuretics, a small but consistent reduction in hypokalemia has been observed (55).

VASODILATORS

Studies of cardiac output, arterial pressure, and circulatory volume in hypertensive patients have repeatedly indicated that elevated total peripheral resistance is the most common hemodynamic feature of most clinical hypertension (22,35). Mechanisms underlying the rise in vascular resistance are multifactorial. Under most clinical conditions, elevated sympathetic neural tone to the vasculature may be demonstrated. Circulating vasoconstrictor substances, such as angiotensin and perhaps vasopressin, may participate under specific pathophysiologic conditions (25). All of these ultimately act by augmenting smooth muscle contractile state, which appears to be modulated by the influx of sodium and calcium into smooth muscle cells. Hence, it follows that vasodilating agents should likely play a prominent role in antihypertensive therapy. Despite the apparent logic of this strategy, therapy with direct vasodilating agents alone is rarely effective or tolerated. This is due to the complex range of responses induced by vasodilation, including stimulation of renin secretion, adrenergic outflow, reflex tachycardia, flushing, and headaches. They are currently most commonly used as third-line agents after diuretics and sympatholytic or beta-blocking drugs. Nonetheless, direct vasodilators are an important part of the armamentarium in treating patients with renal disease, particularly as renal failure develops. Progressive renal disease of many etiologies, particularly glomerulonephritis and nephrosclerosis, is often accompanied by moderate to severe hypertension that requires complex drug regimens (7). Often it is desirable to avoid excessive diuretic use and volume depletion, which may diminish glomerular filtration. Hence, it may be preferable to allow mild volume excess and accept the need for potent antihypertensives, including the direct vasodilators (2,32).

Taken in the context of this discussion, "vasodilator" refers to an agent producing direct relaxation of smooth muscle leading to reduction of peripheral resistance. This definition limits the group to agents listed in Table 4. In a broader context, most antihypertensive agents, including diuretics, sympatholytic agents, or angiotensin converting enzyme inhibitors, indirectly lead to reductions in resistance and thus could be construed as being "vasodilators." These agents are discussed elsewhere.

Pharmacology of Direct Vasodilators

Usual dosages and basic characteristics of these compounds are listed in Table 4.

Intravenous Agents

Nitroprusside. This agent is a prototype of compounds producing direct smooth muscle relaxation (Figs. 4 and 5). It is limited to use in hypertensive emergencies or cardiac afterload reduction (see Chapter 13). It has the advantage of being extremely short acting and allowing precise titration, but requires careful monitoring. Thiocyanate accumulation after several days

Table 4. *Vasodilators used in antihypertensive therapy*

	Forms available	Usual dose	Comments
Intravenous only			
Sodium nitroprusside	(50 mg/500 ml D5W)		
Nipride		0.5–10 μg/kg/min	Titrate to effect
Nipress			Thiocyanate accumulation over days. Rapid disappearance (minutes)
Diazoxide	(300 mg/ampule)		
Hyperstat		50–150 mg/bolus	May repeat bolus dose q.10 min. Fluid retention regularly
Oral agents			
Hydralazine	(10,25,50,100 mg)		
Apresoline		25–100 mg b.i.d.	Reflex adrenergic stimulation. Occasional lupus-like syndrome. (Rare at daily dose < 200 mg/day)
Minoxidil	(2.5,10 mg)	2.5–20 mg b.i.d.	Hirsutism regularly. Fluid retention universal
Loniten			
Prazosin	(1,2,5 mg)	2–10 mg b.i.d.	Post-synaptic alpha-1 blocking agent
Minipress			First dose occurrence of hypotension. Less effective than direct vasodilators. Fewer reflex adrenergic effects
Calcium channel blockers			
Nifedipine	(10 mg)	10–20 mg t.i.d.	Direct arterial effects reflex adrenergic stimulation
Procardia			
Diltiazem	(30,60 mg)	30–60 mg t.i.d. or q.i.d.	Intermediate effects to nifedipine/verapamil
Cardizem			
Verapamil	(80,120 mg)	80 mg t.i.d.	Negative inotropic effects: should not be used with beta-blockers. Modest vasodilating properties
Isoptin			
Calan			

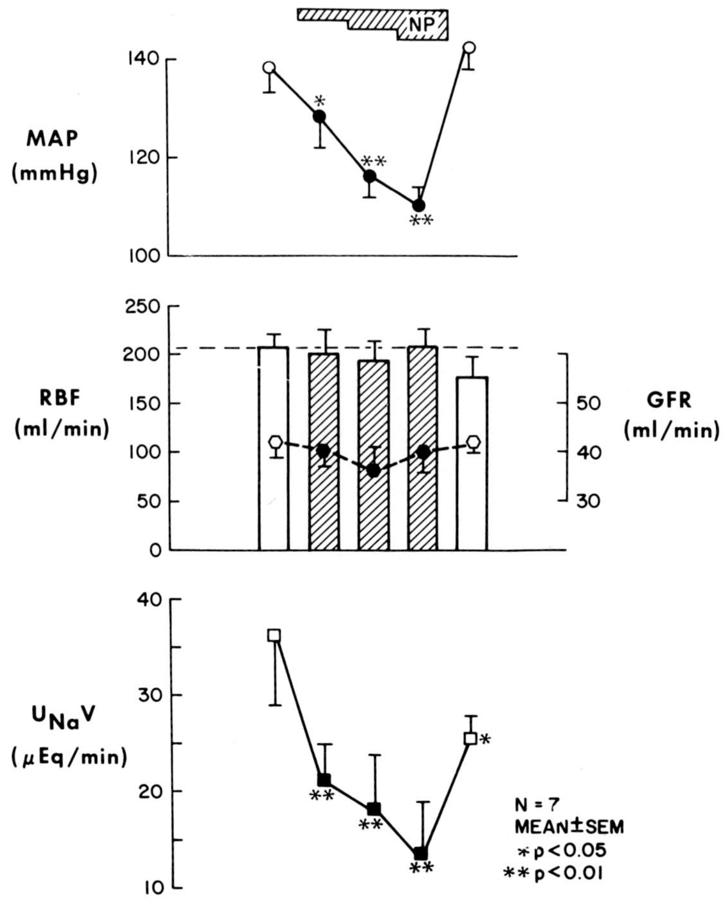

FIG. 4. Mean arterial pressure (MAP), renal hemodynamics, and sodium excretion during infusion of sodium nitroprusside in the dog. Over the range studied, vasodilator therapy had no discernible effect on renal blood flow (RBF) and glomerular filtration rate (GFR). Sodium excretion fell in parallel with renal perfusion pressure. ($U_{Na}V$) sodium excretion.

may limit its sustained use, particularly in patients with impaired glomerular filtration.

Diazoxide. Structurally related to thiazide diuretics, diazoxide is reserved for use in hypertensive emergencies. Given either in bolus or sequential "miniboluses," it may be effective for several hours. However, it induces reflex tachycardia, volume retention, and occasionally hyperglycemia, particularly when administered repeatedly. Its chief limitation is the difficulty in titrating blood pressure response in a specific case. Undesirable hypotension and worsening myocardial ischemia have been reported during its use (30).

Orally Active Vasodilators

Prazosin. Initially considered to be a direct vasodilator, prazosin (minipress) was subsequently characterized as a peripheral alpha-1-receptor antagonist. It is moderately effective as an antihypertensive agent but less potent than hydralazine or minoxidil. Rapid pressure reduction after the first dose is occasionally en-

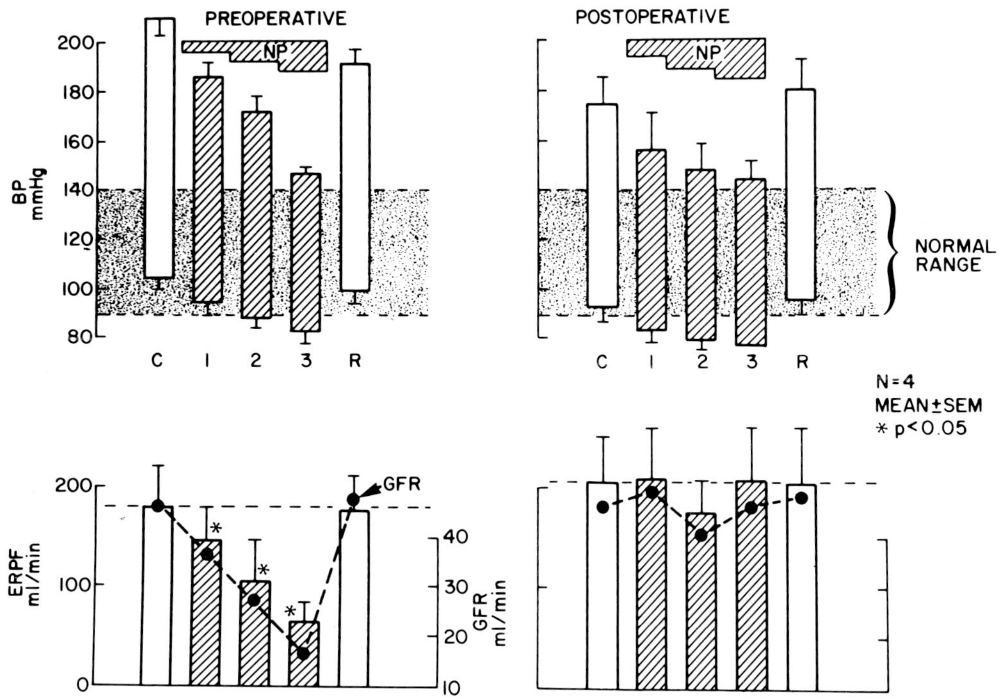

FIG. 5. Arterial pressure (BP) and renal hemodynamics in patients with underlying renal vascular disease during infusion of sodium nitroprusside. Reduction in pressure to normotensive levels produced marked impairment of renal function under conditions of near-critical vascular stenosis. After revascularization of one kidney, a similar pressure reduction, shown in the right panel, produced no such impairment. These data illustrate the sensitivity of the kidney to blood pressure reduction by vasodilators in the presence of renovascular compromise. (NP) nitroprusside; (ERPF) effective renal plasma flow; (GFR) glomerular filtration rate. (From ref. 53.)

countered, leading to the recommendation to start therapy in the evening.

Hydralazine. This agent acts as a direct arteriolar smooth muscle dilator and is active when administered orally. Previous use as a single agent met with generally unacceptable prevalence of palpitations, flushing, headache, etc., due to reflex adrenergic stimulation. Part of its vasodilation is achieved via activation of cyclic AMP. When used with adrenergic blocking agents, its effectiveness as an antihypertensive drug is enhanced and these problems are reduced (63). Renal excretion is achieved after hepatic acetylation. Occasional lupus-like reactions with positive serologies, arthralgias, and serous effusions have occurred during hydralazine administration. In general these have occurred in patients receiving high doses (400 mg/day) or having impaired acetylation (3).

Minoxidil. Acting as a direct arteriolar dilator, this compound is more potent than hydralazine (Fig. 6). Its use is regularly accompanied by hirsutism, which may be distressing, particularly for females. Reflex sympathetic activation must be countered as with other vasodilators and fluid retention may be substantial. Experimental data indicate that intrarenal minoxidil increases renal blood flow but diminishes sodium excretion, perhaps by modifying proximal peritubular capillary hemodynamic forces (38,64). Plasma renin activity and aldosterone stimulation regularly occur. It seems likely that

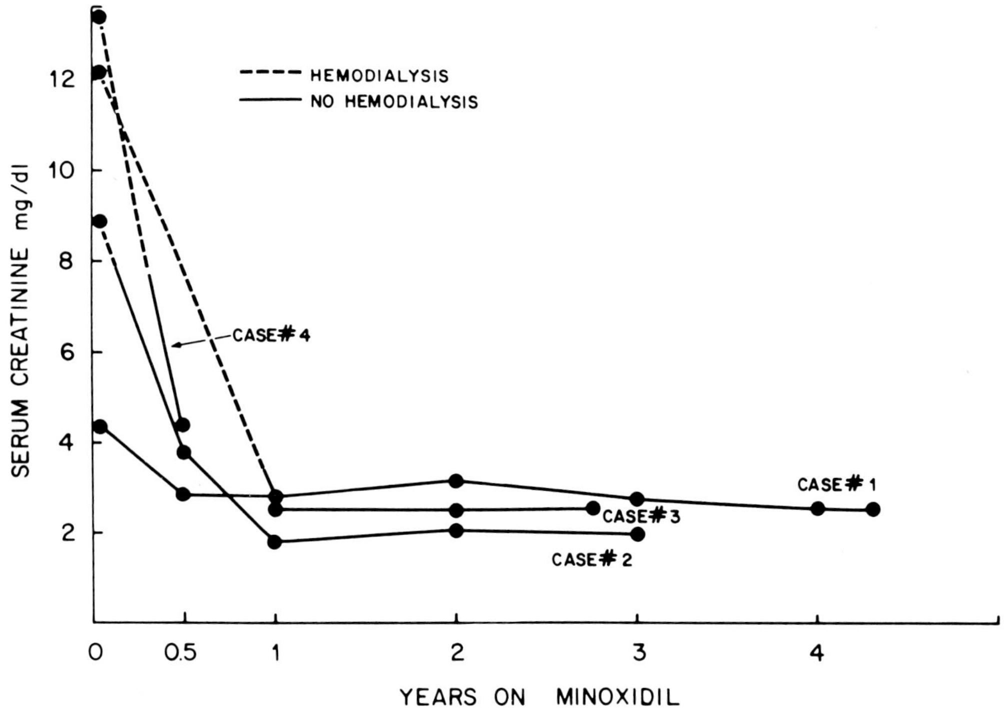

FIG. 6. Serum creatinine levels before and after long-term therapy with antihypertensive regimens containing minoxidil. In these patients, substantial improvements in renal function were observed after initial therapy for malignant hypertension, indicating the potential for recovery from renal damage during effective blood pressure control. (From ref. 40.)

systemic precapillary sphinchter dilation adds local hydrostatic pressure forces to favor nonrenal edema formation also. Because of unexplained occurrence of pericardial effusion in some patients and rare instances of myocardial fibrosis, its use has been reserved generally for refractory and severe hypertension. It is nearly universally effective, however, and has been a major factor in successfully reversing hypertensive crises associated with malignant nephrosclerosis and scleroderma (26,45,58).

Calcium Channel Blockers

These agents are a heterogeneous collection of compounds characterized by their ability to retard "slow-channel"-mediated calcium entry into cells *in vitro*. Some of these agents are effective antihypertensive drugs, primarily by vasodilator actions. A special interest in the cardiovascular effects of these agents derives from the information they may provide regarding the pathogenetic role of smooth muscle calcium fluxes in the causation of hypertensive disorders. Experimental data indicate that vascular tone relates directly to calcium entry and intracellular compartmental distribution. These may be regulated by numerous factors, including alpha-adrenergic stimulation and vasoconstrictors (28,29). However, it should be emphasized that calcium channel blocking drugs are remarkably heterogeneous in their actions, unlike the beta-blockers. It is not clear that clinical and cardiovascular effects are limited to or even primarily determined by their properties of calcium entry blockade.

Nifedipine. This agent is the most widely utilized for antihypertensive therapy. It has been well tolerated for treatment of hypertensive emergencies, particularly when administered sublingually (1,44). Limitations have been most directly related to side effects of vasodilation, including flushing, palpitation, headache, etc., similar to other such compounds. Localized fluid retention, usually around the ankles, is common. Initial studies have suggested that nifedipine, and related compounds such as nitrendipine, were most effective in elderly patients and those whose plasma renin activity is low (44). It produces coronary vasodilation but has relatively little effect upon cardiac performance.

Verapamil. This compound is at the other end of a spectrum from nifedipine: It has the least vascular activity and the most cardiac effects. Cardiac conduction is slowed and negative inotropic effect is regularly observed. Occasional cardiac decompensation has been encountered when verapamil was combined with beta-blockers. Some studies have indicated modest activity in mild to moderate hypertension (29).

Diltiazem. This agent has actions intermediate between those of nifedipine and verapamil. Early trials have indicated a modest response when used as monotherapy in mild-to-moderate hypertension (47).

Systemic and Renal Effects of Vasodilation

Administration of vasodilating agents may profoundly alter systemic and regional hemodynamics. In general, cardiac output increases due to a rise in heart rate mediated by reflex adrenergic stimulation. The rise may be sufficient to effectively counter the expected fall in blood pressure (43) and may provoke symptoms of cardiac discomfort, palpitations, and overt angina. As a practical matter, direct vasodilators must be administered either with an adrenergic sympatholytic agent, such as clonidine or methyldopa, or with a beta-blocking drug to be tolerable to most patients. Blunting the change in cardiac output enhances antihypertensive efficacy (26,63).

Local vasodilation may be prominent. Cerebral vascular changes may produce headaches and a "pounding" sensation. Cutaneous changes are described as "burning" and may be locally circumscribed resembling a rash. Often these effects are temporally related to administration of the drugs. Depending on the particular structural features of the individual and underlying vascular lesions, regional "steal" phenomena may occur, leading to shunting of blood away from particular beds as other beds dilate.

In some instances, particularly during use of minoxidil and nifedipine, local arteriolar vasodilation has been suggested to explain localized edema formation despite intravascular volume contraction (36).

Considering the widespread actions of these drugs and the complexity of the renal blood supply, it is no surprise that the kidney may register a variety of responses (Table 5). As with many agents that lower arterial pressure, diminish stretch receptor tone in the kidney, and provoke widespread sympathetic discharge, stimulation of renin release is widely observed. Pretreatment with a vasodilator has been commonly used to stimulate renin release during renal vein sampling for the diagnosis of renovascular hypertension (36,44,54). In some con-

Table 5. *Renal effects of vasodilators*

Renal blood flow
Increased in acute studies
Increased in low flow states, e.g., congestive heart failure
Unchanged in long-term studies
Glomerular filtration rate
Usually unchanged
May fall in parallel with renal blood flow
Plasma renin activity
Stimulated: adrenergic reflex stimulation
Fall in arterial pressure: Stretch receptors
?Direct stimulation: CA^{2+} channel blockers
Sodium excretion
Intrarenal administration: Variable, occasional increase
Minoxidil decreases sodium excretion
Net effect during systemic administration: Sodium retention
Reduction of renal perfusion pressure
Alteration of peritubular capillary forces
Stimulation of renin-angiotensin-aldosterone axis
Venous pooling in capacitance bed
Direct renal effects?

ditions, it is clear that the associated generation of angiotensin counters arterial pressure reduction as a result.

Regional blood flow to the kidney may temporarily increase. Studies during initial administration often reveal vasodilation, increases in flow, and occasionally increases in sodium excretion (16,27,37,38). Such changes are usually variable and short-lived. Multiple counterregulatory mechanisms in the kidney buffer the circulation and tend to prevent sustained changes in perfusion. Depending on the localization of intrarenal effects, peritubular hydrostatic pressures may change in a variety of ways, leading to net reabsorption of excretion of sodium (44,64). Hence it has been difficult to predict the sum total effect of renal hemodynamic changes, particularly when coupled with overall changes in systemic perfusion pressure.

As a rule, however, clinical administration of vasodilators produces net sodium retention. Diazoxide, nitroprusside, minoxidil, and hydralazine all have limited effectiveness unless diuretics are administered concomitantly. The same is probably true with calcium channel blocking drugs, although some were effective as monotherapy in short-term studies (1,44, 47,56).

There are important exceptions to these observations, which underscore the importance of considering the underlying circulatory conditions as they relate to renal function. In states of low cardiac output, such as congestive heart failure, generalized vasoconstriction in the periphery, including the kidney, may lead to reduced renal blood flow, glomerular filtration, and sodium excretion. Effective vasodilation under these conditions has been observed to lower vascular impedance and improve perfusion in many organs. These changes may occasionally be enough to produce measurable improvements in renal hemodynamics and lead to improved sodium homeostasis (10,11,17,37).

A second exception relates to patients with fixed anatomic vascular disease affecting the kidney. Administration of vasodilators may lead to pressure reduction beyond the limits of perfusion needed for continued glomerular filtration. This has been documented during nitroprusside infusion in patients with tight bilateral renal arterial stenosis or stenosis affecting a solitary kidney (52,53). Although recent emphasis has been focused on selective loss of filtration due to efferent arteriolar vasodilation associated with inhibition of angiotensin converting enzyme, it is likely that this represents a subset of patients at risk of losing renal function due to critical levels of perfusion. A similar form of functional acute renal failure has occurred during administration of minoxidil and calcium channel blockers (12,15,46).

In this regard, several series of patients with impaired renal function and accelerated or malignant hypertension treated with vasodilators have been reported. The general results have been encouraging as regards improved short-term survival and control of blood pressure, when compared to previous high morbidity and mortality from untreated disease. However, close review of the kidney function data from these series indicates that loss of renal function, requiring subsequent chronic dialysis, occurs commonly (34,40,41,46,58). Whether this partly reflects hemodynamic impairment of the renal circulation beyond diseased small vessels deserves further investigation.

From a clinical standpoint, recognition of the potential for pharmacologic manipulation of blood pressure to affect renal hemodynamics is paramount. Unexplained deterioration of glomerular filtration or intractable sodium retention should raise the possibility of underlying vascular disease to the kidney.

Combination of Beta-Blocking Drugs and Vasodilators

As implied in the above sections, many of the hemodynamic effects of beta-blocking compounds effectively inhibit undesirable reflex responses to vasodilators. Conversely, vasodilators augment the efficacy of beta-blockers by offsetting unopposed alpha-mediated vasoconstriction remaining during beta-blocker therapy.

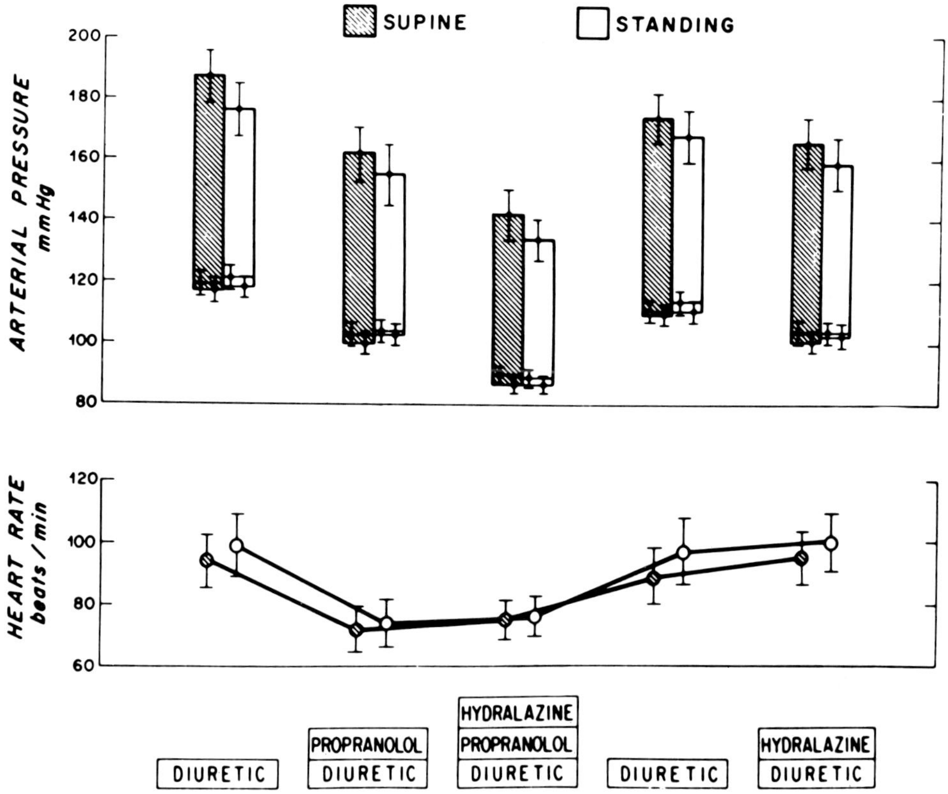

FIG. 7. Blood pressure and heart rates determined during therapy with combinations of propranolol or hydralazine in essential hypertensive patients. The antihypertensive actions were additive between these agents, and unacceptable results of vasodilators, e.g., tachycardia, were markedly blunted by using the combination.

Hence, combination of vasodilator and beta-blockade has proven to be well tolerated and to be a mainstay in the management of resistant hypertension requiring three drugs or more (Fig. 7).

There are few quantitative data regarding the effects of combination therapy on renal function and hemodynamics. In general, it may be rationally inferred that the effects within the kidney represent some combined expression of the individual agents (8,18,26,27).

SUMMARY

Beta-adrenergic blocking drugs have widespread cardiovascular effects and alter regional hemodynamics in many vascular beds, including that of the kidney. Under normal circumstances, the bulk of clinical data would indicate that diminished renal blood flow and glomerular filtration associated with propranolol administration has little clinical significance, although impaired sodium excretion may be observed. However, under particular circumstances, losses of renal function during cardiac output reduction may be observed and should raise the possibility of underlying intrinsic vascular disease. Some of the other beta-blockers, in particular nadolol, atenolol, and pindolol, appear to allow more efficient redistribution of cardiac output as regards the kidney.

In evaluating clinical reports in this area, the difference between acute, first-dose studies and those results obtained during chronic therapy must be emphasized. Although many short-term effects have been described, the overall stability of the renal blood supply despite pharmacologic manipulation is remarkable. It is likely that improved understanding in this area will depend on better definition of the microcirculation, e.g., glomerular transcapillary pressure changes, and the interaction between systemic hemodynamic alterations and the kidney.

Despite concerns about the renal effects of these agents, several points merit reemphasis. The clear benefits of vigorous control of arterial pressure in terms of reduced mortality from cerebrovascular and cardiac events have been well established. Despite progressive and occasionally advanced renal dysfunction associated with malignant hypertension, it is clear that azotemia may improve during long-term antihypertensive therapy following malignant hypertension. Reversal of scleroderma renal crisis presents a case in point (58). It is in these settings that combinations of beta-blockers and vasodilators are most commonly employed.

Nonetheless, the observation that progressive renal failure may ensue, despite good pressure control and improved survival, ought to be sobering. Whether the fate of the injured kidney depends partly on intrarenal hemodynamic effects of the pharmacologic agents employed must remain an open question.

REFERENCES

1. Ambroso, G. C., Como, G., Scalamogna, A., Citterio, A., Casati, S., and Ponticelli, C. (1985): Treatment of arterial hypertension with nifedipine in patients with chronic renal insufficiency. *Clin. Nephrol.*, 23:41–45.
2. Baldwin, D. S., and Neugarten, J. (1985): Treatment of hypertension in renal disease. *Am. J. Kid. Dis.*, 5(4):A57–A70.
3. Batchelor, J. R., Welsh, K. I., Tinoco, R. M., Dollery, C. T., Hughes, G. V. R., Bernstein, R., Ryan, P., Naish, P. F., Aber, G. M., Bing, R. F., and Russell, G. I. (1980): Hydralazine induced systemic lupus erythematosus: Influence of HLA-DR and sex on susceptibility. *Lancet*, 1:1107–1109.
4. Bauer, J. H. (1983): Effects of propranolol therapy on renal function and body fluid composition. *Arch. Int. Med.*, 143:927–931.
5. Bauer, J. H., and Brooks, C. S. (1979): The long-term effect of propranolol therapy on renal function. *Am. J. Med.*, 66:405–410.
6. Birkenhager, W. H., and De Leeuw, P. W. (1983): Adrenergic vasoconstriction as a cause of inadequate hypotensive response to beta-adrenergic blockade. *Hypertension*, 5:III31–35.
7. Blythe, W. B. (1985): Natural history of hypertension in renal parenchymal disease. *Am. J. Kid. Dis.*, 5(4):A50–A56.
8. Bolt, G. R., and Saxena, P. R. (1984): Interaction of atenolol with the systemic and regional hemodynamic effects of hydralazine in conscious renal hypertensive rabbits. *J. Pharmacol. Exp. Ther.*, 230:205–213.
9. Buhler, F. R., Laragh, J. H., Baer, L., Vaughn, D. E., and Brunner, H. R. (1972): Propranolol inhibition of renin secretion. *N. Engl. J. Med.*, 287:1209–1214.
10. Cogan, J. J., Humphreys, M. H., Carlson, C. J., Benowitz, N. I., and Rapaport, E. (1981): Acute vasodilator therapy increases renal clearance of digoxin in patients with congestive heart failure. *Circulation*, 64:973–976.
11. Cohn, J. N., and Franciosa, J. A. (1977): Vasodilator therapy of cardiac failure. *N. Engl. J. Med.*, 297:27–31.
12. Collste, P., Haglund, K., Lundgren, G., et al. (1979): Reversible renal failure during treatment with captopril. *Br. Med. J.*, 2:612–613.
13. Conolly, M. E., Kersting, F., and Dollery, C. T. (1976): The clinical pharmacology of beta-adrenoceptor blocking drugs. *Prog. Cardiovasc. Dis.*, 19:203–234.
14. De Leeuw, P. W., and Birkenhager, W. H. (1982): Renal response to propranolol treatment in hypertensive humans. *Hypertension*, 4:125–131.
15. Diamond, J. R., Cheuns, J. Y., and Fans, L. S. (1984): Nifedipine-induced renal dysfunction. Alterations in renal hemodynamics. *Am. J. Med.*, 77:905–909.
16. Dietz, J. R., Davis, J. O., Freeman, R. H., Villarreal, D., and Echtenkamp, S. F. (1983): Effects of intrarenal infusion of calcium entry blockers in anesthetized dogs. *Hypertension*, 5:482–488.
17. Elkayam, U., Weber, L., Campese, V. M., Massry, S. G., and Rahimtoola, S. H. (1984): Renal hemodynamic effects of vasodilation with nifedipine and hydralazine in patients with heart failure. *J. Am. Coll. Cardiol.*, 4:1261–1267.
18. Elliott, H. L., McLean, K., Sumner, D. J., Meredith, P. A., and Reid, J. L. (1981): Immediate cardiovascular responses to oral prazosin. Effects of concurrent β-blockers. *Clin. Pharmacol. Ther.*, 29:303–309.
19. Epstein, M., and Oster, J. R. (1982): Beta-blockers and the kidney. *Mineral and Electrolyte Metabolism.*, 8:237–254.
20. Epstein, S. E., and Braunwald, E. (1966): The effect of beta-adrenergic blockade on patterns of urinary sodium excretion: Studies in normal subjects and in patients with heart disease. *Ann. Intern. Med.*, 65:20–27.
21. Frishman, W. H. (1981): Beta-adrenoceptor antagonists: New drugs and new indications. *N. Engl. J. Med.*, 305:500–506.
22. Frohlich, E. D. (1977): Hemodynamics of hypertension. In: *Hypertension: Pathophysiology and Treatment*, edited by J. Genest, E. Kiow, and O. Kuchel, pp. 15–48. McGraw-Hill, New York.

23. Frohlich, E. D., Tarazi, R. C., Dustan, H. P., and Page, I. H. (1968): The paradox of beta-adrenergic blockade in hypertension. *Circulation,* 37:417–423.
24. Garrett, B. N., and Kaplan, N. M. (1980): Plasma renin activity suppression: Duration after withdrawal from β-adrenergic blockade. *Arch. Intern. Med.,* 140:1316–1318.
25. Gavras, H., Hatzinikolaou, P., North, W. G., et al. (1982): Interaction of the sympathetic nervous system with vasopressin and renin in the maintenance of blood pressure. *Hypertension,* 4:400–405.
26. Gottlieb, T. B., Katz, F. H., and Chidsey, C. A. (1972): Combined therapy with vasodilator drugs and beta adrenergic blockade in hypertension. A comparative study of minoxidil and hydralazine. *Circulation,* 45:571–582.
27. Green, T. P. (1984): Systemic vasodilation and renal sodium excretion: Effects of hydralazine and diazoxide. *Life Sci.,* 34:2169–2176.
28. Huelseman, J. L., Sterzel, R. B., McKenzie, D. F., and Wilcox, C. S. (1985): Effects of a calcium entry blocker on blood pressure and renal function during angiotensin-induced hypertension. *Hypertension,* 7:374–379.
29. Hulthen, U. L., Bolli, P., Amann, F. W., Kiowski, W., and Buhler, F. R. (1982): Enhanced vasodilation in essential hypertension by calcium channel blockade with verapamil. *Hypertension,* 4:26–31.
30. Kanada, S. A., Kanada, D. J., Hutchinson, R. A., and Wu, D. (1976): Angina-like syndrome with diazoxide therapy for hypertensive crisis. *Ann. Intern. Med.,* 84:696–699.
31. Katz, L. D., D'Avella, J., and De Fronzo, R. A. (1984): Effect of epinephrine on renal potassium excretion in the isolated perfused rat kidney. *Am. J. Physiol.,* 247:F331–F338.
32. Kaufman, A. M., and Levitt, M. F. (1985): The effect of diuretics on systemic and renal hemodynamics in patients with renal insufficiency. *Am. J. Kid. Dis.,* 5(4):A71–A78.
33. Krauss, X. H., Schalekamp, M. A. D. H., Kolsters, G., Zaal, G. A., and Birkenhager, W. H. (1972): Effects of chronic beta-adrenergic blockade on systemic and renal haemodynamic responses to hyperosmotic saline in hypertensive patients. *Clin. Sci.,* 43:385–391.
34. Ledingham, J. G. G., and Beutow, G. (1979): Cerebral complications in the treatment of accelerated hypertension. *Q. J. Med.,* 189:25–41.
35. London, G. M., Safar, M. E., Sassard, J. E., Levenson, J. A., and Simon, A. C. (1984): Renal and systemic hemodynamics in sustained essential hypertension. *Hypertension,* 6:743–754.
36. Loutzenhiser, R., Epstein, M., Horton, C., and Hamburser, R. (1985): Nitrendipine-induced stimulation of renin release by the isolated perfused rat kidney. *Proc. Congr. Exp. Biol. Med.,* 180:133–136.
37. Mantle, J. A., Russell, R. O., Tauxe, W. N., Dustan, H. P., and Rogers, W. J. (1980): Effects of vasodilators on renal function in severe heart failure. *Nouv. Presse Med.,* 9:2399–2403.
38. Mertz, J. I., Haas, J. A., Berndt, T. J., Burnett, J. C., and Know, F. G. (1983): Effects of secretion on peritubular capillary Starling forces and proximal fluid reabsorption in the rat. *J. Clin. Invest.,* 72:622–625.
39. Minneman, K. P., Hegstrand, L. R., and Molinoff, P. B. (1979): The pharmacological specificity of beta-1 and beta-2 adrenergic receptors in rat heart and lung *in vitro. Mol. Pharmacol.,* 15:21–33.
40. Mitchell, J. C., Graham, R. M., and Pettinger, W. A. (1981): Renal function during long-term treatment of hypertension with Minoxidil. Comparison of benign and malignant hypertension. *Ann. Intern. Med.,* 93:676–681.
41. Mroczek, W. J., Davidov, M., Gavrilovich, L., and Finnerty, F. A. (1969): The value of aggressive therapy in the hypertensive patient with azotemia. *Circulation,* 40:893–904.
42. Nayler, W. G., McInnes, I., Swann, J. B., Carson, V., and Lowe, T. E. (1967): Effect of propranolol, a beta-adrenergic antagonist, on blood flow in the coronary and other vascular beds. *Am. Heart J.,* 73:207–216.
43. Pagani, M., Vatner, S. F., and Braunwald, E. (1978): Hemodynamic effects of intravenous sodium nitroprusside in the conscious dog. *Circulation,* 57:144–151.
44. Pedrinelli, R., Fouad, F. M., Tarazi, R. C., Bravo, E. L., and Textor, S. C. (1986): Nitrendipine, a calcium-entry blocker: Renal and humoral effects in human arterial hypertension. *Arch. Intern. Med.,* 146:62–65.
45. Pettinger, W. A., and Mitchell, H. C. (1973): Minoxidil—An alternative to nephrectomy for refractory hypertension. *N. Engl. J. Med.,* 289:167–171.
46. Pohl, J. E. F., Thurston, H., and Swales, J. D. (1974): Hypertension with renal impairment: Influence of intensive therapy. *Q. J. Med.,* 43:561–589.
47. Pool, P. E., Massie, B. M., Venkataraman, K., Hirsch, A. T., Samant, D. R., Seagren, S., Gaw, J., Salel, A. F., and Tabau, J. F. (1986): Diltiazem monotherapy for systemic hypertension: A multicenter, randomized placebo-controlled trial. *Am. J. Cardiol.,* 57:212–217.
48. Pritchard, B. N. C. (1978): Beta-adrenergic receptor blockade in hypertension: Past, present and future. *Br. J. Pharmacol.,* 5:379–399.
49. Stokes, G. S., Weber, M. A., and Thornell, I. R. (1974): Beta-blockers and plasma renin activity in hypertension. *Br. Med. J.,* 1:60–62.
50. Tarazi, R. C., and Dustan, H. P. (1972): Beta-adrenergic blockade in hypertension: Practical and theoretical implications of long-term hemodynamic variations. *Am. J. Cardiol.,* 29:633–640.
51. Textor, S. C., Fouad, F. M., Bravo, E. L., Tarazi, R. C., Vidt, D. G., and Gifford, R. W. (1982): Redistribution of cardiac output to the kidneys during oral nadolol administration. *N. Engl. J. Med.,* 307:601–605.
52. Textor, S. C., Novick, A. D., Steinmuller, D. R., and Streem, S. B. (1983): Renal failure limiting antihypertensive therapy as an indication for renal revascularization: A case report. *Arch. Intern. Med.,* 143:2208–2211.
53. Textor, S. C., Novick, A. D., Tarazi, R. C., Klimas, V., Vidt, D. G., and Pohl, M. (1985): Critical per-

fusion pressure for renal function in patients with bilateral atherosclerotic renal vascular disease. *Ann. Intern. Med.*, 102:308–314.

54. Thind, G. S., Montojo, P. M., Johnson, A., and Amin, F. (1983): Enhancement of renal venous renin ratios by intravenous hydralazine in renovascular hypertension. *Am. J. Cardiol.*, 53:109–115.
55. Vincent, H. H., Veld, A. H., Boomsma, F., and Schalekamp, M. A. (1985): Prevention of epinephrine-induced hypokalemia by nonselective beta blockers. *Am. J. Cardiol.*, 56:10D–14D.
56. Waeber, B., Nussberger, J., and Brunner, H. R. (1985): Does renin determine the blood pressure response to calcium entry blockers? *Hypertension*, 7:223–227.
57. Warren, D. J., Swainson, C. P., and Wright, N. (1974): Deterioration in renal function after beta-blockade in patients with chronic renal failure and hypertension. *Br. Med. J.*, 2:193–194.
58. Wasner, C., Coode, C. R., and Fries, J. F. (1978): Successful medical treatment of scleroderma renal crisis. *N. Engl. J. Med.*, 299:873–875.
59. Weiner, N., and Taylor, P. (1985): Neurohumoral transmission: The autonomic and somatic motor nervous systems. In: *The Pharmacologic Basis of Therapeutics*, edited by A. G. Goodman and L. S. Gilman, pp. 66 –100. Macmillan, New York.
60. Wilkinson, R. (1982): Beta-blockers and renal function. *Drugs*, 23:195–206.
61. Wilkinson, R., Stevens, I. M., Pickering, M., Robson, V., Hawkins, T., Kerr, D. N., and Harry, J. D. (1980): A study of the effects of atenolol and propranolol on renal function in patients with essential hypertension. *Br. J. Clin. Pharmacol.*, 10:51–59.
62. Williams, M. E., Gervino, E. V., Rosa, R. M., Landsberg, L., Young, J. B., Silva, P., and Epstein, F. H. (1985): Catecholamine modulation of rapid potassium shifts during exercise. *N. Engl. J. Med.*, 312:823–827.
63. Zacest, R., Gilmore, E., and Koch-Weser, J. (1972): Treatment of essential hypertension with combined vasodilation and beta-adrenergic blockade. *N. Engl. J. Med.*, 286:617–622.
64. Zins, G. R. (1974): Alterations in renal function during vasodilator therapy. In: *Recent Advances in Renal Physiology and Pharmacology*, edited by L. G. Wesson and G. M. Fanelli. pp. 165–186.

The Kidney in Hypertension, edited by
Norman M. Kaplan, Barry M. Brenner,
and John H. Laragh. Raven Press,
New York © 1987.

Angiotensin Converting Enzyme Inhibitors: Evidence for Renin-Dependent and Renin-Independent Mechanisms of Action

Randall M. Zusman

Hypertension Division, Cardiac Unit, Massachusetts General Hospital and Harvard Medical School, Boston, Massachusetts 02114

The circulating renin-angiotensin system, along with the adrenergic nervous system, the kallikrein-kinin system, and the vasopressin system, plays an important role in the regulation of systemic vascular resistance, blood pressure, and fluid-electrolyte metabolism. The contribution of the renin-angiotensin system under various physiologic conditions has been elucidated through the use of inhibitors of the renin-angiotensin cascade. In attempting to determine the role of the renin-angiotensin system in the physiology and pathophysiology of blood pressure regulation and disorders of cardiovascular function, such as congestive heart failure, specific antagonists of renin activity, including antibodies directed against the active site of the renin enzymatic protein, angiotensin converting enzyme inhibitors, and angiotensin receptor antagonists, have been utilized. In each of these attempts, specific inhibitors of an important step in the renin-angiotensin cascade were designed as unique agents to be used for the dissection of the role of renin in blood pressure regulation. However, invariably, these agents have been found to produce surprising changes in blood pressure under conditions where the activity would otherwise be thought to be minimal. The purpose of this chapter is to outline the use of these inhibitors as tools to elucidate the role of the renin-angiotensin system in the regulation of blood pressure, with particular attention to the effects of angiotensin converting enzyme inhibitors not explicable on the basis of the inhibition of the "plasma" renin-angiotensin system.

THE RENIN-ANGIOTENSIN CASCADE

Angiotensin II stimulates vascular smooth muscle and the adrenal gland and causes vasoconstriction, aldosterone production, and sodium retention. Because both vasoconstriction and sodium retention increase blood pressure, considerable attention has been directed toward the development of a clinically useful inhibitor of the renin-angiotensin cascade. Three steps in the generation of angiotensin II or its cellular action can be attacked (1). Renin, a proteolytic enzyme produced by the juxtaglomerular apparatus, cleaves angiotensinogen to produce angiotensin I, which has no vasopressor activity. Angiotensin converting enzyme, located within the pulmonary circulation (2), then cleaves two amino acids from angiotensin I, yielding the octapeptide angiotensin II; the latter compound, through interaction with its receptor, constricts vascular smooth muscle and stimulates aldosterone biosynthesis. Inhibition of the renin-angiotensinogen reaction, blockade of the angiotensin II receptor, or inhibition of converting enzyme diminishes the physiologic effect of angiotensin II *in vivo* and theoretically should decrease blood pressure in experimental models of hypertension and in patients with renin-dependent hypertension.

Renin Antibodies

Renin has been purified from many sources (3–6). Using purified renin as an antigen, Haber and co-workers raised antibodies against the catalytic site of the enzyme; these antibodies serve as a probe for the investigation of the role of renin in normal cardiovascular homeostasis and in experimental models of hypertension (7). These antibodies prevent an increase in blood pressure in response to injections of purified canine renin but do not prevent the increase in blood pressure induced by angiotensin I or angiotensin II (8). Similarly, the injection of renin-specific antibodies reduces the blood pressure in sodium-depleted dogs, thus demonstrating that maintenance of blood pressure in this physiologic state is renin dependent (7,8). Because the antibody is specific for renin, no significant hemodynamic response to antibody injection occurs in animals given a high-salt diet; under these conditions, the role of renin in maintaining blood pressure is minimal. The administration of renin-specific antibody to dogs with acute renovascular hypertension promptly eliminates renin from the peripheral circulation and restores normal blood pressure. The redevelopment of hypertension 24 to 36 hr following antibody injection coincides with the gradual metabolism of the renin-specific antibody and the reappearance of renin activity in the peripheral circulation (7,8). Monoclonal, antihuman, renin-specific antibodies have been isolated using cell fusion techniques (9). These antibodies do not bind nonrenin proteolytic enzymes and are species specific. Because they are directed toward the catalytic site, these highly potent antibodies are specific tools for physiologic studies in subhuman primates and in humans.

Competitive Renin Inhibitors

Since Skeggs and colleagues reported that an octapeptide was the shortest peptide capable both of serving as a substrate for renin and of functioning as a competitive inhibitor of the renin-angiotensinogen reaction (10,11), a number of analogs have been synthesized that exhibit stronger inhibitory properties than those of this original octapeptide. Renin normally cleaves a leucine-leucine bond in angiotensinogen. Burton and co-workers reported that the substitution of phenylalanine for these leucine residues yielded a molecule that served as a poor substrate for renin's proteolytic activity, and that prevented its reaction with angiotensinogen by competitive inhibition (12).

The intravenous injection of this peptide caused a reduction in blood pressure in sodium-depleted *Macaca fascicularis* monkeys that was not observed following injection of the peptide into normotensive, sodium-replete animals (12). Because peptide infusion blocked the pressor response to purified human renin but not to angiotensin I or angiotensin II in these animals, the investigators concluded that this renin inhibitory peptide had no effect on the converting enzyme, but that its effect was specific for inhibition of the renin-angiotensinogen reaction. In a separate study, administration of this renin inhibitory peptide in a monkey model of acute renovascular hypertension promptly lowered blood pressure, presumably because of inhibition of the renin-angiotensinogen reaction (13).

Clinical investigation of the renin inhibitory peptide extended these experimental findings. When administered to sodium-depleted humans, the peptide produced a more complex hemodynamic response (14). While the subjects were in the supine position, intravenous administration of the inhibitor reduced blood pressure only moderately; when in the upright position, however, the blood pressure of these same subjects fell precipitously. In addition, in contrast to the tachycardia that usually accompanies vasodilation in sodium-depleted subjects, the nadir of the blood pressure response was associated with sinus bradycardia.

In a preliminary study, the effect on blood pressure of giving the renin inhibitory peptide to one subject after administration of a high-salt diet (200 mEq/day) was determined. Because plasma renin activity is known to be suppressed under these conditions, a minimal hypotensive response to inhibition of the renin-angiotensin cascade was expected. Strikingly, the subject's blood pressure fell markedly in both supine and upright positions, and the decrease again was associated with bradycardia. During renin inhibitory peptide infusion, the plasma renin activity of this one subject increased. This finding suggests that effective blockade of the generation of angiotensin II occurred with release of the negative feedback pathways that normally suppress renin release. In contrast to the fall in plasma aldosterone concentration that frequently accompanies the inhibition of the renin-angiotensin system with other substances, however, plasma aldosterone concentration increased during renin inhibitory peptide infusion.

These data suggest that, although designed as a specific inhibitor of the renin-angiotensinogen reaction, the renin inhibitory peptide has multiple mechanisms of action. In addition to inhibiting peripheral renin activity, the peptide might inhibit renin within the blood vessel wall, brain, or other sites. If so, a previously unrecognized role for these tissue renins in the regulation of cardiovascular homeostasis will be unmasked. The peptide might produce parasympathetic stimulation that results in sinus bradycardia, venous dilation, and a fall in cardiac output. Alternatively, it might interact with another system and release vasodilating substances. Finally, the peptide might activate cardiac reflexes such as the Bezold-Jarisch reflex, which results in peripheral vasodilation, bradycardia, and hypotension. Recently experimental evidence for negative inotropic activity of this peptide has been obtained; thus the development of left ventricular dysfunction and a fall in cardiac output is a contributing factor to the production of hypotension in response to this substance (15).

Other investigators also have explored the hemodynamic effects of renin-specific inhibitors. Boger and colleagues have developed a highly potent renin inhibitor through substitution of statine into the angiotensinogen peptide sequence (16). Administration of this material to sodium-depleted dogs also decreased blood pressure and reduced heart rate instead of producing tachycardia (17). These studies lend credence to the suggestion that although renin inhibitory peptides were synthesized as specific inhibitors of the renin-angiotensinogen reaction, they might have multiple mechanisms of action, either dependent or independent of the renin-angiotensin cascade.

ANGIOTENSIN II RECEPTOR ANTAGONISTS

A similar multiplicity of activity characterizes the action of angiotensin analogs, competitive antagonists of the angiotensin-receptor interaction. The substitution of sarcosine and alanine for the naturally occurring amino acids at positions one and eight in the angiotensin II molecule yields the highly competitive receptor antagonist, saralasin (18). Administration of this peptide to experimental animals with acute renovascular hypertension and to patients with high-renin hypertension significantly reduces blood pressure. In low-renin states, however, saralasin exhibits agonistic activity and increases blood pressure (19). The clinical utility of this compound thus is limited to the identification of renin-dependent states, and even here its lack of specificity has prevented its widespread adoption as a diagnostic tool.

CONVERTING ENZYME INHIBITION

The importance of the angiotensin converting enzyme was first recognized by Skeggs and colleagues, who found that the product of the reaction of crudely purified porcine renin with equine angiotensinogen was a mixture of two peptide hormones (20). Subsequent study revealed that production of the second hormone, later shown to be angiotensin II, was due to contamination of the angiotensinogen substrate by an enzyme that released a dipeptide from the carboxy terminus of angiotensin I (21,22). Both angiotensins had vasopressor properties following intravenous infusion. But Helmer, using a superfusion assay system measuring rabbit aortic strip contraction, later identified angiotensin II as the biologically active moiety (22). The vasopressor response to angiotensin I infusion therefore was attributable to its conversion to angiotensin II. Ng and Vane demonstrated that angiotensin I was converted to angiotensin II during passage through the pulmonary circulation (23,24). Their work suggested that a pulmonary enzyme in intimate contact with the blood as it passed through the pulmonary circulation accounted for the rapid metabolism of the precursor peptide to angiotensin II. Subsequent studies have demonstrated that the converting enzyme is a component of the vascular endothelium of many tissues and that its localization on the luminal surface of the plasma membrane is ideally suited for its function (2). Because of the parallelism of proteolytic deactivation and activation of bradykinin and angiotensin I, respectively, during transit through the pulmonary circulation, it was suggested that the same protein, the angiotensin converting enzyme, might be responsible for the catalysis of both reactions (25). In 1968 Bakhle reported that bradykinin potentiating factor, a mixture of polypeptides isolated from venom of the snake *Bothrops jararaca,* inhibited the conversion of angiotensin I to angiotensin II by canine pulmonary tissue (26). Ferreira previously had demonstrated that this peptide mixture potentiated the action of bradykinin on smooth muscle by inhibiting kininase activity and kinin degradation (27). After purifying individual peptides from the snake venom, Ferreira and colleagues confirmed that the substances could inhibit both angiotensin converting activity and bradykininase activity of a pulmonary homogenate (28,29).

The first angiotensin converting enzyme inhibitor studied in humans was teprotide, a synthetic nonapeptide. Teprotide blocks the vasopressor response to intravenous infusions of angiotensin I, and effectively reduces blood pressure in patients with elevated plasma renin activity (30).

Studies with synthetic substrates and inhibitors of angiotensin converting enzyme led to the conclusion that the angiotensin converting enzyme was a carboxypeptidase similar to pancreatic carboxypeptidase A (31). Additional studies revealed that the angiotensin converting enzyme is a zinc-containing metalloprotein, also similar to carboxypeptidase A (32). It therefore was assumed that the site and mechanism of action of the angiotensin converting enzyme would be similar to those of the pancreatic enzyme (33). In 1973 Byers and Wofenden reported that *d*-2-benzylsuccinic acid was a potent competitive inhibitor of carboxypeptidase A. This competitive activity was thought to be secondary to the simultaneous and stereospecific interaction of the inhibitor with three substrate binding sites at the active site of the carboxypeptidase enzyme (34). Reasoning that similar stereospecificity might characterize the active site of angiotensin converting enzyme, Cushman and colleagues sequentially analyzed compounds that might serve as orally active converting enzyme inhibitors. These investigators demonstrated that an analogue of proline, D-3-mercapto-2-methyl-propanoyl-1-proline, was a highly specific inhibitor of the converting enzyme *in vitro* (35). The alpha-methyl group and the carboxyl groups of proline later were shown to interact with hydrophobic sites of the angiotensin converting enzyme. The mercapto substitution on the beta carbon resulted in specific interaction with the zinc atom, which is a crucial portion of the catalytic site of the enzyme, and accounts for the marked inhibitory properties of the molecule (36). This compound, captopril, was later found to be a potent competitive inhibitor of converting enzyme activity.

Based on the foregoing discussion of the synthesis of the converting enzyme inhibitor captopril and the properties of the converting enzyme as both the activator of angiotensin II and deactivator of bradykinin, it was assumed that the response of animals and humans to captopril could be explained by changes in the levels of angiotensin II and bradykinin in the plasma. However, this assumption cannot explain many of the responses to captopril in normal and hypertensive animals and humans. In renin-independent models of hypertension, the efficacy of captopril can only be explained by a non-renin-mediated antihypertensive activity. The non-renin-mediated activity of captopril may be accounted for in part by captopril's stimulation of arachidonic acid release and a consequent increase in the synthesis of vasodilatory prostaglandins.

The theoretical mechanism of action of a converting enzyme inhibitor involves changes in both the renin-angiotensin and the kallikrein-kinin systems (37). Inhibition of the converting enzyme by captopril decreases generation of angiotensin II from angiotensin I. The decrease in angiotensin II diminishes vasoconstrictor activity and decreases adrenal aldosterone biosynthesis. The consequent decrease in vasoconstrictor activity (and in theory, a sodium diuresis) thus lowers blood pressure. Because angiotensin II participates in a negative feedback loop that inhibits renin release by the juxtaglomerular apparatus, the fall in angiotensin II concentration produces a reflex increase in renin activity and an increased concentration of angiotensin I. Because of the inhibition of the converting enzyme, however, this increase in angiotensin I concentration cannot elevate plasma angiotensin II concentration. In addition, because the converting enzyme is responsible for the destruction of bradykinin, the accumulation of increased concentrations of the vasodilator bradykinin reduces peripheral vascular resistance and lowers systemic blood pressure. Many clinical and laboratory studies have confirmed that the administration of teprotide or captopril significantly decreases plasma angiotensin II concentration, plasma aldosterone concentration, and blood pressure. Systemic vascular resistance falls and cardiac output is maintained or increased, consistent with a reduction in the vasoconstrictor effects of angiotensin II (38). The acute response to converting enzyme inhibition appears to correlate closely with the pretreatment plasma renin activity, and the response thus is consistent with the theoretical mechanism of action of these compounds (39).

Although theoretically expected to increase plasma kinin levels, converting enzyme inhibition has not been consistently proved to alter circulating kinin concentration. Occasional studies have reported an elevation in plasma kinin concentration (40–45), but most investigators have failed to demonstrate any significant increase (46–56). Kinins are local mediators rather than circulating substances, and many enzymes other than the angiotensin converting enzyme can inactivate them through kininase activity. Therefore, a failure to demonstrate an increase in circulating kinin concentration is not totally unexpected. Carretero and colleagues examined the role of kinins in the acute and chronic hypotensive effect of converting enzyme inhibitors, using specific antikinin antibodies that block the depressor effect of exogenously administered bradykinin. Because the administration of antikinin antibodies had no effect on the hypotensive response to captopril in sodium-depleted rats, the authors concluded that the antihypertensive activity of captopril in this model could be attributed solely to its inhibition of the renin-angiotensin cascade. Administration of the antikinin antibodies in the spontaneously hypertensive rat or in two-kidney, one-clip hypertensive rats significantly attenuated the decrease in blood pressure following captopril administration, however (57). Although a consistent change in plasma kinin levels has not been found, the possibility that tissue kinins not accessible to the antikinin antibodies played a role in the antihypertensive activity of captopril cannot be excluded by such studies.

In addition to the possible role of kinins in the antihypertensive activity of captopril, additional evidence for a non-renin-mediated antihypertensive activity of captopril has been obtained in studies involving experimental animals and normotensive and antihypertensive humans. Marks and co-workers reported that captopril decreased blood pressure by 15% in normal rats. Following nephrectomy, the blood pressure of the animals fell by 30%; however, the administration of captopril produced a further 10% drop in blood pressure despite the absence of renin in the peripheral circulation. In animals with early Goldblatt two-kidney, one-clip hypertension (a model known to be renin dependent), captopril produced a 50% decrease in blood pressure that was associated with marked elevations in plasma renin activity. On the other hand, in rats with late two-kidney, one-clip hypertension (a model of hypertension thought not to depend on the plasma renin-angiotensin system), captopril also produced a substantial drop in blood pressure. In addition, in animals made hypertensive by the chronic administration of deoxycorticosterone and a high-salt diet, captopril reduced blood pressure by 20 mm Hg. These rats have markedly suppressed plasma renin activity and represent an experimental model of volume-expansion, low-renin hypertension (58). Moreover in salt-depleted rats in which the endogenous renin-angiotensin system has been blocked by infusion of the competitive angiotensin II antagonist saralasin, captopril further reduces blood pressure (59).

Muirhead and colleagues reported that the administration of captopril to rats receiving exogenous angiotensin II and high-salt diets significantly decreased blood pressure (60). The reduction of blood pressure in this experimental model could not be explained on the basis of a reduction in plasma angiotensin II concentration, as the exogenous administration of angiotensin II maintained a high level of this vasoconstrictor polypeptide in the peripheral circulation, raised the blood pressure to hypertensive levels, and suppressed endogenous renin release. In contrast, Textor and co-workers reported that chronic angiotensin II infusion to conscious rats prevented any hemodynamic response to converting enzyme inhibition. These investigators concluded that neither bradykinin nor vasodilator hormones contributed to the long-term antihypertensive activity of captopril (61).

Additional studies by Muirhead and associates revealed that administration of captopril significantly decreases blood pressure in spontaneously hypertensive rats, an experimental model in which the hypertension is thought to be independent of the renin-angiotensin system (62). The decrease in peripheral vascular resistance in these studies also suggests a non-renin-mediated antihypertensive activity of captopril.

If captopril's antihypertensive activity were solely due to the antagonism of the generation of angiotensin II by renin in the peripheral circulation, bilateral nephrectomy would be expected to totally eliminate any hemodynamic response to the administration of this converting enzyme inhibitor. Leslie and co-workers reported that captopril failed to reduce the blood pressure of anephric patients. These authors concluded that if captopril had an angiotensin-independent antihypertensive activity, this action would depend on the presence of functional renal tissue (63). Man In't Veld, however, reported that the volume status of anephric patients dramatically affected the hemodynamic response to captopril. Salt- and water-repleted patients showed no response to captopril prior to hemodialysis. Following hemodialysis and relative salt and water depletion, however, captopril significantly reduced blood pressure (64,65).

The relative activities of saralasin and captopril in early and late Goldblatt two-kidney, one-clip hypertension were studied by Thurston and colleagues. They found that in the early phase of hypertension, both saralasin and captopril reduced blood pressure significantly. In the chronic phase of hypertension, however, only captopril evoked a statistically significant decrease in blood pressure, again suggesting that captopril has an antihypertensive effect independent of the renin-angiotensin system. They further found that in salt-loaded or salt-restricted animals, or those with chronic two-kidney Goldblatt hypertension, converting enzyme inhibition resulted in reduction in blood pressure beyond that observed following angiotensin receptor blockade with saralasin (66).

An additional approach to the study of a possible non-renin-mediated antihypertensive activity of captopril was reported by Tree and Morton. Investigating the blood pressure of sodium-loaded dogs as a function of the plasma angiotensin II concentration before and after captopril administration, they found that a higher concentration of angiotensin II was required to produce the same blood pressure in dogs that had received captopril than in those animals that had not (67). In a similar study, Swartz and co-workers found that following infusion of teprotide, the plasma angiotensin II level had to be raised by a mean value of 45 pg/ml above the control plasma angiotensin II concentration to maintain the same blood pressure. Because an increase in plasma bradykinin levels following converting enzyme inhibition was found in this study, the authors suggested that one or more other factors, perhaps bradykinin, was responsible for the greater-than-expected hypotensive response to converting enzyme inhibition based on the fall in angiotensin II concentration (45). Crantz and colleagues reported that captopril elicited a greater drop in blood pressure than did teprotide in a group of patients with normal-renin essential hypertension. Unlike the response to teprotide, captopril administration was not associated with an increase in plasma kinin concentration (46). Finally, in a study of 26 hypertensive patients, Fagard and co-workers reported that captopril had a greater antihypertensive effect than did saralasin (68). Their findings again suggested a non-renin-mediated antihypertensive activity for this orally active converting enzyme inhibitor.

Prostaglandin Synthesis and the Non-Renin-Mediated Antihypertensive Effect of Converting Enzyme Inhibitors

Vinci and co-workers published the first study suggesting that the non-renin-mediated antihypertensive activity of converting enzyme inhibitors was due to prostaglandin release. They infused teprotide at a rate sufficient to lower blood pressure by 10 mm Hg in subjects with mild essential hypertension. The concentration of prostaglandin E in arterial blood, as measured by radioimmunoassay, increased threefold during teprotide infusion (69). Plasma arterial bradykinin concentration remained unchanged during teprotide infusion. Swartz and co-workers subsequently reported the effect of captopril on the prostaglandin system in normal subjects on both high- and low-sodium diets. Captopril induced a significant increase in the excretion of the 13,14-dihydro-15-keto metabolite of prostaglandin E_2. The depressor response to captopril correlated closely with the change in urinary prostaglandin E_2 metabolite excretion, but did not correlate with changes in plasma angiotensin II and kinin levels (70).

Abe and co-workers reported an increase in urinary prostaglandin E excretion following captopril administration in patients with essential hypertension. Administration of a prostaglandin synthesis inhibitor to these same patients abolished the antihypertensive activity of captopril (71). Moore and colleagues reported an increase in the urinary excretion of the prostaglandin E_2 metabolite following captopril administration in sodium-restricted patients with essential hypertension. In these patients, the administration of indomethacin or aspirin was associated with decreased prostaglandin E_2 excretion and a significant blunting of the depressor response to captopril (72). Similarly, Silberbauer et al. (73), Ogihara et al. (74), Witzgall et al. (75), and Goldstone et al. (76) have demonstrated that the administration of a prostaglandin synthesis inhibitor blunts the hemodynamic response to captopril in hypertensive and normal subjects. Finally, Provoost reported that aspirin and indomethacin diminished the hemodynamic response to captopril administration in rats (77).

This series of studies led to the conclusion that the antihypertensive activity of captopril is not solely related to its inhibition of the renin-angiotensin cascade. Nor is there consistent evidence to suggest that an increase in plasma kinin concentration plays an important role in the reduction in blood pressure following captopril administration. The accumulated studies of captopril's effect in models of low-renin hypertension, as well as the evidence for an increase in plasma and urinary prostaglandins, and the inhibitory effect of prostaglandin synthesis inhibitors on captopril's hemodynamic response, suggest that captopril has major prostaglandin-mediated antihypertensive activity.

The prostaglandin-mediated vasodilation is particularly important in the hypotensive response to captopril in experimental animals or in humans with a low plasma renin activity. What is the cellular mechanism by which captopril stimulates prostaglandin biosynthesis? The chemical pathways leading to prostaglandin biosynthesis have been exquisitely elucidated in numerous laboratories (78). Prostaglandins are derived from arachidonic acid, a polyunsaturated fatty acid stored within the phospholipid storage pool of every cell in the body. Activation of a phospholipase—predominantly phospholipase A_2, but phospholipase C in some tissues—results in the release of arachidonic acid, which subsequently is converted to the precursor prostaglandin G_2 by the cyclooxygenase enzyme. Prostaglandin G_2 is converted to prostaglandin E_2, or prostaglandin $F_{2\alpha}$ by peroxidation and isomerization, to thromboxane A_2 by thromboxane synthetase, or to prostacyclin by prostacyclin synthetase. The production of prostaglandin E_2 and prostaglandin $F_{2\alpha}$ locally might have a significant effect on individual vascular beds (79). Thromboxane A_2, a strikingly potent vasoconstrictor (80) predominantly synthesized in the platelet, is a potent stimulant of platelet aggregation (81). Although thromboxane A_2 can be synthesized by other tissues, it probably is not a vasoconstricting hormone. Prostacyclin, a potent vasodilating substance produced predominantly by the vascular endothelium (82), causes vasodilation and inhibition of platelet aggregation. Because prostacyclin is stable in aqueous solution and has a half-life in biologic systems of up to 5 min, it might be an important circulating vasodilator or antiaggregating substance (83).

The development of a technique for the isolation of renomedullary interstitial cells in tissue culture provided an opportunity for the study of the regulation of cellular prostaglandin biosynthesis (84). The addition of vasoactive peptides such as angiotensin II, vasopressin, and importantly, bradykinin, to these cells causes an increase in prostaglandin synthesis (85). Subsequent stimulation by vasoactive peptides activates the phospholipase and releases arachidonic acid from the phospholipid fraction; the arachidonic acid subsequently is converted to prostaglandins (86). This prostaglandin synthetic response to angiotensin II stimulation has been studied in detail, and the interaction of angiotensin II with its receptor, the binding characteristics of this receptor, the stimulation of phospholipase activity, and the release of arachidonic acid and subsequent conversion to prostaglandin E_2 demonstrate parallel dose-response curves and receptor binding kinetics (87).

When added to the tissue culture medium of these cells, captopril produced up to a 30-fold stimulation of prostaglandin biosynthesis. Half-maximal stimulation of prostaglandin biosynthesis occurred at a captopril concentration of approximately 8 μM. Like the vasoactive peptides, captopril stimulates prostaglandin biosynthesis through activation of the phospholipase and through an increase in the rate of release of the precursor fatty acid leading to prostaglandin E_2 biosynthesis. In similar studies, captopril increased prostacyclin biosynthesis from aortic vascular endothelium (L. Levine, *personal communication*) and increased prostacyclin and prostaglandin E_2 biosynthesis by isolated renal glomeruli (88).

Using the *in vitro* renomedullary interstitial cell system, it has been possible to elucidate the mechanism by which converting enzyme inhibition, prostaglandins, and bradykinin interact in a way that might explain the captopril-related antihypertensive response. Previous studies have demonstrated that potentiation of bradykinin following captopril administration was secondary to the stimulation of prostaglandin biosynthesis, particularly in the kidney (89). Mullane and Moncada reported increased prostacyclin release following bradykinin administration in beagles (90). The administration of a prostaglandin synthesis inhibitor markedly attenuated the potentiation of bradykinin following captopril administration. Both captopril and bradykinin independently stimulated arachidonic acid release and prostaglandin biosynthesis by renomedullary interstitial cells in tissue culture (37). However, incubation of cells in the simultaneous presence of captopril and bradykinin increased prostaglandin biosynthesis and arachidonic acid release; these alterations exceeded the additive effects of the two agents' independent effects.

The augmented prostaglandin synthesis in response to captopril and bradykinin is particularly noteworthy in view of the data of Vinci et al. (69). In addition to the increase in prostaglandin biosynthesis observed following converting enzyme inhibition with teprotide, Vinci and co-workers found that the reduction in blood pressure correlated with the increase in arterial blood prostaglandin concentration of their patients; these same patients were found to have significantly increased urinary kinin excretion. A small number of hemodynamic nonresponders failed to demonstrate the increase in prostaglandins and urinary kinin. An increase in urinary kinin excretion was observed by Olsen and Arrigoni-Martelli following captopril administration and blood pressure reduction in normal conscious dogs (91).

An important consideration in the study of captopril-stimulated prostaglandin biosynthesis is, What structural characteristics of the molecule result in its ability to promote phospholipase activation, arachidonic acid release, and the subsequent formation of vasodilating prostaglandins? To address this question, the effects of captopril and three of its chemical analogs as well as the effects of enalapril and its biologically active metabolite, enalaprilic acid, on prostaglandin biosynthesis were studied (Fig. 1). Although a simple chemical molecule and an analog of proline, captopril has an optically active center at the beta carbon that allows for chemical modification. The formation of the optical enantiomer of captopril (SQ 14534) produces a molecule with less converting enzyme inhibitory activity but does not diminish its ability to stimulate prostaglandin biosynthesis. As Fig. 1 illustrates, the increase in prostaglandin concentration evoked by this captopril analog at a concentration of 7.5 μM was approximately eightfold. In addition, a doubling of prostaglandin biosynthesis was achieved at a concentration of approximately 2 μM; these values are identical to those of captopril. Indeed, even removal of the methyl group at the optically active center, which produces an optically inactive molecule (SQ 13863) and affects its ability to serve as converting enzyme inhibitor, has absolutely no effect on prostaglandin biosynthesis *in vitro*. However, the substitution of the sulfhydryl group by a carboxyl group (SQ 13297) totally eliminates the ability of the compound to stimulate prostaglandin biosynthesis even at levels 1,000-fold greater than those at which an effect is observed for the parent molecule.

Enalapril and enalaprilic acid are converting enzyme inhibitors recently demonstrated to have significant antihypertensive activity in the treatment of patients. These two compounds do not have sulfhydryl group substitutions as part of the chemical structure (57). After oral administration, enalapril (MK 421), an ethylester of its active metabolite enalaprilic acid (MK 422), is converted via bioactivation in the liver to a very potent angiotensin-converting inhibitor. Addition of either enalapril or enalaprilic acid to the incubation medium of renomedullary interstitial cells in tissue culture has no effect on prostaglandin biosynthesis (92).

This sequence of studies on the relationship between chemical structure and prostaglandin stimulation indicates that the stimulation of prostaglandin biosynthesis is not a general property of the converting enzyme inhibitors but rather depends on specific chemical characteristics of the molecule involved. The sulfhydryl component of captopril is the critical chemical characteristic of this molecule. This group confers on the molecule the ability to stimulate prostaglandin production. L. Levine (*personal communication*) and Galler et al. (93) have confirmed the ability of captopril to stimulate

COMPOUND	STRUCTURE	INHIBITION OF ANGIOTENSIN CONVERTING ENZYME (IC_{50}), μm	STIMULATION OF PROSTAGLANDIN E_2 BIOSYNTHESIS	
			AT 7.5 μm	ED_{2X} (μm)
SQ 14225 (Captopril)	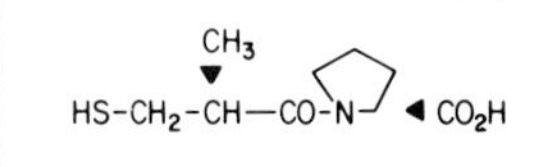	0.023	8X	2.1
SQ 14534	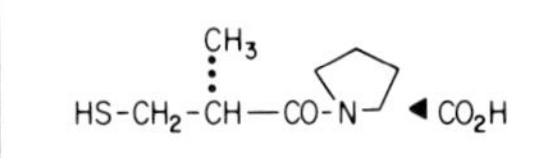	2.4	7.8X	2.4
SQ 13863	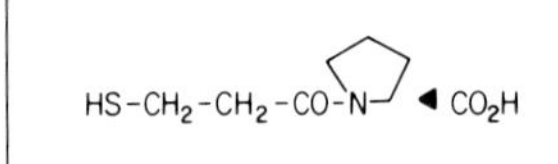	0.20	7.6X	2.2
SQ 13297	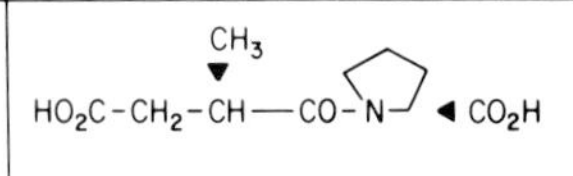	22.0	0	>1000
MK-421 (Enalapril)	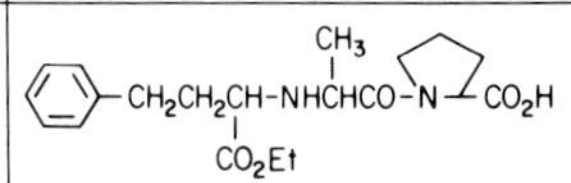	1.2	0	>1000
MK-422	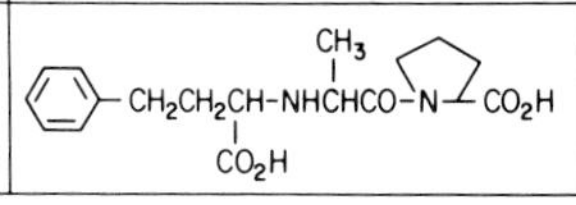	0.0012	0	>1000

FIG. 1. Effects of converting enzyme inhibitors on prostaglandin biosynthesis *in vitro*. (From ref. 92.)

prostaglandin biosynthesis by aortic endothelial cells in tissue culture and in isolated renal glomeruli, respectively. In the latter study it is of interest to note that although glomeruli synthesize PGE_2, $PGF_{2\alpha}$, thromboxane A_2, and prostaglandin, only PGE_2 and prostacyclin synthesis was increased. This observation suggests the presence of compartmentalization of the enzymes leading to the synthesis of these vasodilating substances.

A second important effect of captopril on the prostaglandin system is the synergistic activity of bradykinin and captopril in stimulating prostaglandin biosynthesis by renomedullary interstitial cells in tissue culture. Although captopril has no significant effect on plasma bradykinin concentrations, Vinci and co-workers noted a significant increase in urinary kinin excretion in those patients experiencing a drop in blood pressure (43). Thus, although bradykinin concentrations were unaffected in plasma, the authors did observe an increase in bradykinin in tissue, where kinins can potentially stimulate endogenous prostaglandin biosynthesis. Bradykinin is a potent stimulant of prostaglandin biosynthesis by the renomedullary interstitial cells in tissue culture. The combination of captopril and bradykinin, however, increases the rate of arachidonic acid release and prostaglandin synthesis above and beyond that to be expected by the simple additive effects of the two compounds. This observation points to the possibility of a synergistic prostaglandin-stimulating activity of captopril and bradykinin, leading to enhanced prostaglandin synthesis *in vivo*. This synergism is similar to the effects of bradykinin and high-density lipoproteins on prostacyclin synthesis in vascular endothelial and smooth muscle cells *in vitro*.

The significance of captopril-stimulated prostaglandin biosynthesis as an important aspect of its mechanism of antihypertensive activity is indicated by a number of clinical and experimental studies. Captopril administration to experimental animals made hypertensive by the administration of deoxycorticosterone and sodium chloride resulted in a 23 mm Hg drop in blood pressure (94). Pretreatment of these animals with indomethacin, a nonsteroidal antiinflammatory drug and a potent inhibitor of prostaglandin biosynthesis, resulted in complete attenuation of the antihypertensive response to captopril. Thus, in this model of low-renin hypertension, the sole mechanism of the antihypertensive activity of captopril was increased prostaglandin biosynthesis; this finding explains the antihypertensive response to converting enzyme inhibition in a model thought to be independent of the renin-angiotensin cascade. Goldstone and co-workers assessed the effect of the prostaglandin system and the renin angiotensin system on captopril's antihypertensive activity in normal volunteers on low- and high-salt diets (95). Plasma renin activity was elevated in patients placed on a sodium-restricted diet. The administration of captopril to these subjects resulted in an approximately 12 mm Hg drop in blood pressure. In these individuals the administration of a prostaglandin synthesis inhibitor prior to captopril administration did not attenuate the antihypertensive response. In contrast, in the individuals on a high-salt diet with low plasma renin activity, captopril produced a similar 12 mm Hg drop in blood pressure. Prior administration of a prostaglandin synthesis inhibitor totally attenuated the antihypertensive response, however (95). These studies point to the importance of a prostaglandin-mediated antihypertensive activity in individuals with low plasma renin activity.

The contrasting effects of captopril and enalapril on prostaglandin stimulation also explain the difference in the response to these molecules in experimental models of hypertension. Whereas captopril administration reduces the blood pressure of animals made hypertensive by the administration of deoxycorticosterone and sodium chloride through its ability to stimulate prostaglandin formation and produce peripheral vasodilation, enalapril has no significant antihypertensive activity in this model of hypertension (96). In addition, whereas captopril reduces the blood pressure of animals made hypertensive by the chronic infusion of angiotensin II, enalapril has no antihypertensive activity when employed in this experimental model (97). In contrast, both captopril and enalapril are effective antihypertensive agents when administered to experimental models of hypertension known to be dependent on the renin-angiotensin cascade (98). Finally, the contrast between these two converting enzyme inhibitors has been demonstrated by Shoback and co-workers, who administered both captopril and enalapril to human subjects and measured the plasma concentration of prostaglandin E metabolites. Whereas captopril is a potent stimulant of prostaglandin E_2 synthesis, enalapril did not affect plasma prostaglandin E_2 metabolite concentrations (99).

A proposed summary of captopril's mechanism of action is shown in Fig. 2. Inhibition of the angiotensin converting enzyme in the pulmonary circulation reduces the rate of conversion of angiotensin I to angiotensin II. The falling angiotensin II concentration and the concomitant decrease in plasma aldosterone concentration cause a decrease in peripheral vascular resistance and a decrease in sodium retention that lead to a drop in blood pressure. This effect is the predominant mechanism of action of captopril in patients with high plasma renin activity, such as those in sodium-depleted state and in patients with high-renin hypertension. Although the angiotensin converting enzyme can metabolize bradykinin to inactive metabolites, no consistent and significant change in plasma bradykinin concentrations has been documented, probably because of the multiple other enzymes capable of metabolizing bradykinin that are not affected by captopril. Despite the absence of a significant change in plasma kinin concentrations, however, an increase in tissue levels of this potent polypeptide—in particular, augmented kinin formation by the kidney—may result in increased vasodilation within those tissues and heightened stimulation of prostaglandin biosynthesis. Finally, captopril directly stimulates prostaglandin biosynthesis and thus raises the arterial concentration of prostaglandin

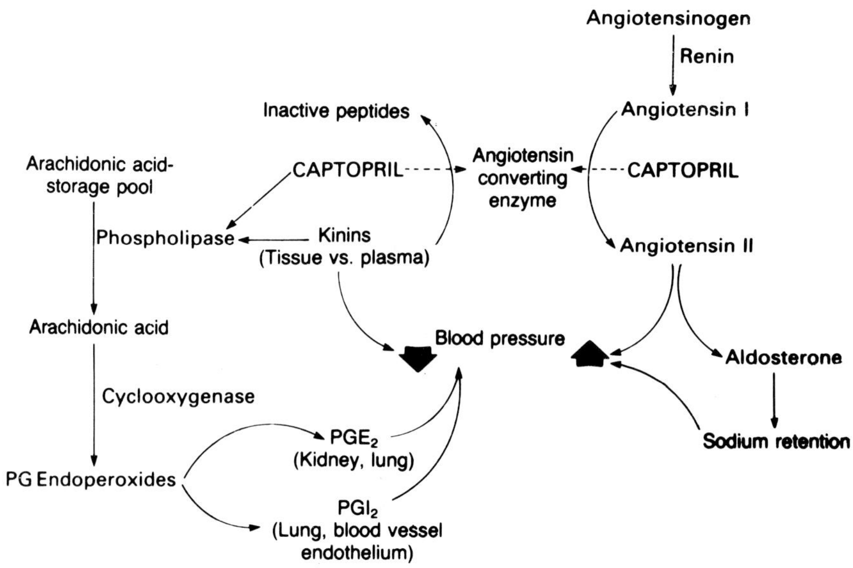

FIG. 2. Biochemical effects of angiotensin converting enzyme inhibition following captopril administration. (From ref. 107.)

E_2, produced predominantly by the kidney and the lung, and prostacyclin (PGI_2), produced by the lung, the kidney, and the blood vessel endothelium. Increases in prostaglandin biosynthesis might result from the direct effects of captopril on cellular arachidonic acid release or from the accentuation and possible acceleration of the stimulation of prostaglandin biosynthesis by bradykinin both within the peripheral circulation and at the tissue level. The vasodilation that occurs because of increased arterial prostaglandin concentrations is the major mechanism for the antihypertensive activity of captopril in the sodium-replete state and in patients with low renin hypertension. Enalapril's mechanism of action is limited to its effect on the renin-angiotensin-aldosterone cascade.

The mechanism of the synergistic effect of captopril and bradykinin on cellular prostaglandin biosynthesis remains unknown. Indeed, the mechanism of captopril-stimulated arachidonic acid release has yet to be elucidated. Although peptide hormone-stimulated prostaglandin biosynthesis depends on increased calcium influx following receptor activation, captopril-stimulated prostaglandin biosynthesis does not appear to be a calcium-dependent process. Additional evidence for an important role of captopril-stimulated prostaglandin/prostacyclin biosynthesis *in vivo* is provided by studies of platelet function in patients receiving captopril for the treatment of hypertension. Platelet aggregation is diminished in patients following captopril therapy compared to pretreatment values. *Ex vivo* incubation of platelets with captopril does not affect aggregation parameters and thus the decrease in aggregability must result from an *in vivo* response to drug therapy. This effect may be secondary to the decreased angiotensin II levels in these patients or to the antiplatelet effects of captopril-stimulated prostacyclin biosynthesis and release. Indeed it might be speculated that the decreased mortality observed in experimental models of myocardial infarction after captopril therapy or of patients receiving captopril for the treatment of congestive heart failure might reflect the beneficial effects of an increase in the synthesis of PGE_2 and prostacyclin by vascular endothelium, myocardial, and other arachidonic acid-metabolizing tissues. If in fact this hypothesis is true, a difference in platelet function should be observed in patients during captopril vs enalapril treatment, since the former, but not the latter, directly stimulates prostaglandin formation.

Whether renin-specific antibodies, renin inhibitory peptides, or converting enzyme inhibitors have been used, there has been a direct correlation between the acute response of the blood pressure with the initial plasma renin activity. But the chronic response to therapy with these agents, especially the response to converting enzyme inhibition, has been clearly dissociated from the pretreatment plasma renin and angiotensin concentrations. Recently, it has been suggested that the reason for the dissociation is related to differential importance of the plasma renin-angiotensin system and the renin-angiotensin cascade within tissues, specifically the vascular endothelium and vascular smooth musculature (100).

The vascular renin system may be more important as a mediator of chronic converting enzyme inhibition than is the sympathetic nervous system, through reduction in catecholamine release at noradrenergic nerve endings by converting enzyme inhibitors, or possible alterations in baroreceptor reflex activity (101,102). Recent studies by Okamura and colleagues have shown a dissociation between vascular and circulating renin-angiotensin activities such that a reduction in blood pressure was observed in response to converting enzyme inhibition with enalapril or angiotensin II receptor antagonism with sarcosine-1, isoleucine-8, angiotensin II in rats with chronic two-kidney, one-clip hypertension, despite insignificant abnormalities of the plasma angiotensin concentration (103). Additional studies have shown that the long-term response to converting enzyme inhibition correlates better with inhibition of converting enzyme activity within the vasculature and the kidney than with changes in the plasma renin-angiotensin cascade (104).

The possibility of an importance of the vascular renin-angiotensin system also suggests potential differences among the converting enzyme inhibitors due to differential effects in the individual tissues secondary to the rate of transport into the cellular site of converting enzyme activity as well as different rates of metabolism and duration of intracellular converting enzyme inhibition. The vascular renin-angiotensin system thus accounts for a possible "non-renin-mediated" antihypertensive activity, which is not prostaglandin dependent, for converting enzyme inhibitors such as enalapril, which do not stimulate cellular prostaglandin release. The potential for abnormalities of the tissue renin-angiotensin system accounting for abnormalities of blood pressure regulation should not be discounted as a potential mechanism for the induction of increased vascular tone and thus, an increase in systemic blood pressure despite a normal plasma renin activity (100).

Recent evidence that certain hypertensive patients fail to appropriately modify renal blood flow and their adrenal responsivity to changes in sodium diet as would normal subjects has led to the term renal nonmodulation. These abnormalities can be corrected by the administration of captopril and suggest that at least in a minority of patients with essential hypertension, the physiologic responses to saline administration and exogenous angiotensin II infusion might be explained on the basis of abnormalities of tissue renin-angiotensin generation (104). Thus, abnormalities of the vascular renin-angiotensin pathway must be considered as potential pathogenetic mediators in the development of the hypertensive process (105).

There are at present innumerable converting enzyme inhibitors under investigation (106). Although each converting enzyme inhibitor is a proline analog, they differ dramatically in their chemical structures. In addition to sulfhydryl- and nonsulfhydryl-containing converting enzyme inhibitors, prodrugs, or drugs that are active as administered, there are phosphoric acid derivatives as well as chemical compounds having unique side-chain substitutions. In comparing currently available and soon to become available agents, it will be important to assess both "renin-dependent" and "renin-independent" activities of these agents. In addition to effects on the plasma renin-angiotensin cascade, on the vascular and tissue renin-angiotensin cascade, and on the metabolism of vasodilators such as bradykinin and prostaglandins, the effects of these agents on other modifiers of vascular smooth muscle tone and blood pressure should not be ignored. Despite attempts to specifically design drugs having unique chemical activities, these agents appear to have effects on blood pressure regulation that could not have been predicted at the time of their discovery and initial investigation.

REFERENCES

1. Haber, E. (1979): Nephrology Forum: The renin-angiotensin system and hypertension. *Kidney Int.*, 15:427–444.
2. Soffer, R. L. (1976): Angiotensin-converting enzyme and the regulation of vasoactive peptides. *Annu. Rev. Biochem.*, 45:73–94.
3. Dzau, V. J., Slater, E. E., and Haber, E. (1978): Complete purification of dog renal renin. *Biochemistry,* 18:5224–5228.
4. Corvol, P., Devaux, C., Ito, T., Sicard, P., Duclox, J., and Menard, J. (1977): Large scale purification of hog renin: Physiologic characterization. *Circ. Res.*, 41:616–620.
5. Inagami, T., Murakami, K., (1977): Pure renin. Isolation for hog kidney and characterization. *J. Biol. Chem.*, 252:2978–2983.
6. Slater, E. E., Cohn, R. C., Dzau, V., and Haber, E. (1978): Purification of human renin. *Clin. Sci. Mol. Med.* 55:117S–121S.
7. Haber, E., Dzau, V., Kopelman, R., Slater, E. E., and Barger, A. C. (1980): Renin-specific antibody as a physiologic tool. In *Enzymatic Release of Vasoactive Peptides,* edited by F. Gross and G. Vogel, pp. 73–88. Raven Press, New York.
8. Dzau, V. J., Kopelman, R. I., Barger, A. C., Slater, E. E., and Haber, E. (1980): Renin-specific antibody for study of cardiovascular homeostasis. *Science,* 207:1091–1093.
9. Dzau, V. J., Devine, D., Mudgett-Hunter, M., Kopelman, R. I., Barger, A. C., and Haber, E. (1983): Antibodies as specific renin inhibitors: Studies with polyclonal and monoclonal antibodies and Fab fragments. In *Proceedings of a Symposium on the Renin-Angiotensin System. Biochemistry, Pharmacology, and Clinical Aspects* (*Suppl*), Heidelberg. *Clin. Exp. Hypertens.*, 85 (7 and 8):1207–1220.
10. Skeggs, L. T., Jr., Kahn, J. R., Lentz, K., and Shurnway, N. P. (1957): The preparation, purification and amino acid sequence of polypeptide renin substrate. *J. Exp. Med.*, 106:439–453.
11. Skeggs, L. T., Jr., Lentz, K. E., Hahn, J. R., and Hochstrasse, H. (1968): Kinetics of the renin reaction with nine synthetic peptide substrates. *J. Exp. Med.*, 128:13–34.
12. Burton, J., Cody, R. J., Herd, J. A., and Haber, E. (1980): Specific inhibition of renin by an angiotensinogen analog: Studies in sodium depletion and renin-dependent hypertension. *Proc. Natl. Acad. Sci. USA,* 77:5476–5479.
13. Cody, R. J., Burton, J., Evin, G., Poulsen, K., Herd, J. A., and Haber, E. (1980): A substrate analog inhibitor of renin that is effective *in vivo*. *Biochem. Biophys. Res. Comm.* 97:230–235.
14. Zusman, R. M., Christensen, D., Burton, J., Nussberger, J., Dodds, A., and Haber, R. (1983): Hemodynamic effects of a competitive renin inhibitory peptide in humans: Evidence for multiple mechanisms of action. *Trans. Assoc. Am. Physicians.,* 96:365–374.
15. Zusman, R. M., Hartley, L. H., Burton, J., and Haber, E. (1987): Evidence for a non-renin dependent cardiovascular effect of a renin inhibitory peptide: Negative inotropic activity and suppressed cardiac output. *Hypertension* (*in press*).
16. Boger, J., Lohr, N. S., Ulm, E. H., Poe, M., Blaine, E. H., Fanelli, G. M., Lin, T. -Y., Payne, L. S., Schorn, T. W., LaMont, B. I., Vassil, T. C., Stabilito, I. I., Verger, D. F., Rich, D. G., and Bopari, A. S. (1983): Novel renin inhibitors containing the amino acid statine. *Nature,* 303:81–84.
17. Blaine, E. H., Schorn, T. W., and Boger, J. S. (1984): Statine-containing renin inhibitor: Dissociation of blood pressure lowering and renin inhibition in Na-deficient dogs. *Hypertension,* 6(*Suppl. I*): 1111–1118.
18. Khosla, M. O., Smeby, R. R., and Bumpers, F. M. (1974): Structure-activity relationships in angiotensin II analogs. In *Angiotensin,* edited by I. Page and F. M. Bumpers, p. 126. Springer-Verlag, Berlin.
19. Pals, D. T., Masucci, F. D., Sipos, F., and Denning, G. S., Jr. (1971): A specific competitive antagonist of the vascular action of angiotensin II. *Circ. Res.*, 29:664–672.
20. Skeggs, L. T., Marsh, W. M., and Kahn, J. R. (1954): Existence of two forms of hypertension. *J. Exp. Med.*, 99:275–282.
21. Lentz, K. E., Skeggs, L. T., and Wood, K. R. (1956): The amino acid composition of hypertensin II and its biochemical relationship to hypertensin I. *J. Exp. Med.*, 104:183–191.
22. Helmer, O. (1957): Differentiation between two forms of angiotinin by means of spirally cut strips of rabbit aorta. *Am. J. Physiol.*, 188:571–577.
23. Ng, K. K. F., and Vane, J. R. (1967): Conversion of angiotensin I to angiotensin II. *Nature,* 215: 762–766.
24. Ng, K. K. F., and Vane, J. R. (1968): Fate of angiotensin I in the circulation. *Nature,* 218:144–150.
25. Ferreira, S. H., and Vane, J. R. (1967): The disappearance of bradykinin and eledosin from the circulation and vascular beds of the cat. *Br. J. Pharmacol. Chemother.*, 30:417–424.
26. Bakhle, Y. S. (1968): Conversion of angiotensin I to angiotensin II by cell free extracts of dog lung. *Nature,* 220:919–921.
27. Ferreira, S. H. (1965): A bradykinin-potentiating factor (BPF) present in venom of *Bothrops jararaca*. *Br. J. Pharmacol.*, 24:163–169.
28. Ferreira, S. H., Greene, L. J., Alabaster, V. A., Bakhle, Y. S., and Vane, J. R. (1970): Activity of

various fractions of bradykinin potentiating factor against angiotensin I converting enzyme. *Nature,* 225:379–380.

29. Ferreira, S. H., Bartelt, D. C., and Greene, L. J. (1970): Isolation of bradykinin-potentiating peptides from *Bothrops jararaca* venom. *Biochemistry,* 9:2583–2593.
30. Antonaccio, M. J. (1982): Angiotensin converting (ACE) inhibitors. *Am. Rev. Pharmacol. Toxicol.,* 22:57–87.
31. Hartsuck, J. A., and Lipscomb, W. N. (1971): Carboxy peptidase A. In: *The Enzyme, Vol. 3,* edited by P. D. Boyer, pp. 1–56. Academic Press, New York.
32. Das, M., and Soffer, R. L. (1975): Pulmonary angiotensin-converting enzyme: Structural and catalytic properties. *J. Biol. Chem.,* 250:6762–6768.
33. Cushman, D. W., Cheung, H. S., Sabo, E. F., and Ondetti, M. A. (1978): Design of new antihypertensive drugs: Potent and specific inhibitors of angiotensin-converting enzyme. *Prog. Card. Dis.,* 21:176–182.
34. Byers, L. D., and Wolfenden, P. (1973): Binding of the bi-product analog benzylsuccinic acid by carboxypeptidase A. *Biochemistry,* 12:2070–2072.
35. Cushman, D. W., Cheung, H. S., Sabo, E. F., and Ondetti, A. (1977): Design of potent competitive inhibitors of angiotensin-converting enzyme. *Biochemistry,* 16:5484–5491.
36. Cushman, D. W., and Ondetti, M. A. (1980): Inhibitors of angiotensin-converting enzyme. *Prog. Med. Chem.,* 174:41–104.
37. Zusman, R. M. (1983): Regulation of the prostaglandin biosynthesis in cultured renal medullary interstitial cells. In: *Prostaglandins and the Kidney,* edited by M. J. Dunn, C. Patrono, and G. A. Cinotti, pp. 17–25. Plenum, New York.
38. Horovitz, Z. P., ed. (1981): *Angiotensin Converting Enzyme Inhibitors: Mechanisms of Action and Clinical Implications. Urban and Schwarzenberg, Baltimore.*
39. Case, D. B., Atlas, S. A., Laragh, J. H., Sealey, J. E., Sullivan, P. A., and McKinstry, D. N. (1978): Clinical experience with blockade of the renin-angiotensin system by an oral converting-enzyme inhibitor (SQ 14225, captopril) in hypertensive patients. *Prog. Cardiovasc. Dis.,* 21:195–206.
40. McCaa, R. E., Hall, J. E., and McCaa, C. S. (1978): The effects of angiotensin I-converting enzyme inhibitors on arterial blood pressure and urinary sodium excretion: Role of the renal renin-angiotensin and kallikrein-kinin systems. *Circulation,* 43(*Suppl.* I):I32–I39.
41. Koffer, H., Vlasses, P. H., Ferguson, R. K., Weis, M., and Adler, A. G. (1980): Captopril in diuretic-treated hypertensive patients. *JAMA,* 244:2532–2535.
42. Kono, T., Ikeda, F., Oseko, F., Imura, H., and Endo, J. (1979): Effects of angiotensin I-converting enzyme inhibitor, SQ 14.225, in normal man. *Endocrinol. Jpn.,* 26:441–518.
43. Johnston, C. I., Yasujima, M., and Clappison, B. H. (1981): The kallikrein-kinin system and angiotensin converting enzyme inhibition in hypertension. In: *Angiotensin Converting Enzyme Inhibitors,* edited by Z. P. Horovitz, pp. 1257–1264. Urban and Schwarzenberg, Baltimore.
44. Swartz, S. L., Williams, G. H., Hollenberg, N. K., Levine, L., Dluhy, R. G., and Moore, T. J. (1980): Captopril-induced changes in prostaglandin production: Relationship to vascular responses in normal man. *J. Clin. Invest.,* 65:1257–1264.
45. Swartz, S. L., Williams, G. H., Hollenberg, N. K., Moore, T. J., and Dluhy, R. G. (1979): Converting enzyme inhibition in essential hypertension: The hypotensive response does not reflect only reduced angiotensin II formation. *Hypertension,* 1:106–111.
46. Crantz, F. R., Swartz, S. L., Hollenberg, N. K., Moore, T. J., Dluhy, R. G., Williams, G. H. (1980): Differences in response to the peptidyldipeptide hydrolase inhibitors SQ 20,881 and SQ 14,225 in normal-renin essential hypertension. *Hypertension,* 2:604–609.
47. Johnston, C. I., McGrath, B. P., and Matthews, P. G. (1979): Comparison of the hormonal effects of captopril (SQ 14225) and hydrochlorothiazide in the treatment of essential hypertension. *Med. J. Aust.* (*Suppl.* 2), 2:R15–R22.
48. Johnston, C. I., Millar, J. A., Casley, D. J., McGrath, B. P., and Matthews, P. G. (1980): Hormonal responses to angiotensin blockade. Comparison between receptor antagonism and converting enzyme inhibition. *Circ. Res.* (*Suppl* 1), 46:1128–1134.
49. Johnston, C. I., Millar, J. A., McGrath, B. P., and Matthews, P. G. (1979): Long-term effects of captopril (SQ 14,225) on blood pressure and hormone levels in essential hypertension. *Lancet,* 2:493–496.
50. McGrath, B. P., Matthews, P. G., and Johnston, C. I. (1980): Acute changes in blood pressure and vasoactive hormones after captopril in hypertensive patients. *Clin. Exp. Pharmacol. Physiol.,* 7:487–492.
51. Millar, J. A., and Johnston, C. I. (1979): Sequential changes in circulating levels of angiotensin I and II, renin, and bradykinin after captopril. *Med. J. Aust.,* 2(*Suppl.* 2):R15–R17.
52. Kondo, K., Okuno, T., Konishi, K., Saruta, T., and Kato, E. (1979): Central and peripheral effects of bradykinin and prostaglandin E_2 on blood pressure in conscious rats. *Arch. Pharmacol.,* 308:111–115.
53. Matthews, P. G., and Johnston, C. I. (1979): Responses of the renin-angiotensin system and kallikrein-kinin system to sodium and converting enzyme inhibitor (SQ 14,225). *Adv. Exp. Med. Biol.,* 120B:447–457.
54. Matthews, P. G., and Johnston, C. I. (1979): Changes in endogenous circulating angiotensin and bradykinin after inhibition of converting enzyme (kinanase II). *Med. J. Aust.* (*Suppl.* 2), 2:R12–R15.
55. Matthews, P. G., McGrath, B. P., and Johnston, C. I. (1979): Hormonal changes with long-term converting enzyme inhibition by captopril in essential hypertension. *Clin. Sci.* (*Suppl.* 5), 57:135s–138s.
56. Swartz, S. L., Williams, G. H., Hollenberg, N. K., Crantz, F. R., Moore, T. J., Levin, L., Sasahara, A. A., and Dluhy, R. G. (1980): Endocrine profile in the long-term phase of converting-enzyme inhibition. *Clin. Pharmacol. Ther.,* 28:499–508.

57. Carretero, O. A., Scicli, A. G., and Maitra, S. R. (1981): Role of kinins in the pharmacological effects of converting enzyme inhibitors. In: *Angiotensin Converting Enzyme Inhibitors: Mechanisms of Action and Clinical Implications,* edited by Z. P. Horovitz, pp. 105–122. Urban and Schwarzenberg, Baltimore.
58. Marks, E. S., Bing, R. F., Thurston, H., and Swales, J. D. (1980): Vasodepressor property of the converting enzyme inhibitor captopril (SQ 14,225): The role of factors other than renin-angiotensin blockade in the rat. *Clin. Sci.,* 58:1–6.
59. Thurston, H., and Swales, J. D. (1978): Converting enzyme inhibitor and saralasin infusion in rats: Evidence for an additional vasodepressor property of converting enzyme inhibitor. *Circ. Res.,* 42:588–592.
60. Muirhead, E. E., Brooks, B., and Brosius, W. L. (1980): Antihypertensive action of captopril in angiotensin-salt hypertension. *Arch. Pathol. Lab. Med.,* 104:631–634.
61. Textor, S. C., Brunner, H. R., and Gavras, H. (1981): Converting enzyme inhibition during chronic angiotensin II infusion in rats: Evidence against a nonangiotensin mechanism. *Hypertension,* 3:269–276.
62. Muirhead, E. E., Prewitt, R. L., Jr., Brooks, B., and Brosius, W. L., Jr. (1978): Antihypertensive action of the orally active converting enzyme inhibitor (SQ 14,225) in spontaneously hypertensive rats. *Circ. Res.,* (*Suppl.* 1)43:153–158.
63. Leslie, B. R., Case, D. B., Sullivan, J. F., and Vaughan, E. D., Jr. (1980): Absence of blood-pressure lowering effect of captopril in anephric patients.
64. Man In't Veld, A. J., Schicht, I. M., Derkx, F. H. M., de Bruyn, J. H. B., and Schalekamp, M. A. D. H. (1980): Effects of an angiotensin-converting enzyme inhibitor (captopril) on blood pressure in anephric subjects. *Br. Med. J.,* 1:288–290.
65. Man In't Veld, A. J., Schicht, I. M., Derkx, F. H. M., de Bruyn, J. H. B., and Schalekamp, M. A. D. H. (1980): Effects of an angiotensin-converting enzyme inhibitor (captopril) on blood pressure in anephric subjects. *Br. Med. J.,* 1:288–290.
66. Thurston, H., Bing, R. F., Russeli, G. I., and Swales, J. D. (1981): The vasodepressor mechanism of converting enzyme inhibitors. In: *Angiotensin Converting Enzyme Inhibitors: Mechanisms of Action and Clinical Implications,* edited by Z. P. Horovitz, pp. 105–122. Urban and Schwarzenberg, Baltimore.
67. Tree, M., and Morton, J. J. (1980): Evidence that the acute hypotensive effect of captopril in dogs is not wholly explained by a reduction of plasma angiotensin II and its direct vasoconstrictor effect. *Clin. Sci.,* 59:451–456.
68. Fagard, F., Amery, A., Lijnen, P., and Reybrouck, T. (1979): Haemodynamic effects of captopril in hypertensive patients: Comparison with saralasin. *Clin. Sci.,* 57:131s–134s.
69. Vinci, J. M., Horowitz, D., Zusman, R. M., Pisano, J. J., Catt, K. J., and Keiser, H. R. (1979): The effect of converting enzyme inhibition with SQ 20881 on plasma and urinary kinins, prostaglandin E and angiotensin II in hypertensive man. *Hypertension,* 1:416–426.
70. Swartz, S. L., Williams, G. H., Hollenberg, N. K., Crantz, F. R., Levine, L., Moore, T. J., and Dluhy, R. G. (1980): Increase in prostaglandins during converting enzyme inhibition. *Clin. Sci.,* 59:133s–135s.
71. Abe, K., Ito, T., Sato, M., Haruyama, T., Sato, K., Omata, K., Hiwatari, M., Sakurai, Y., Imai, Y., and Yoshinaga, K. (1980): Role of prostaglandin in the antihypertensive mechanism of captopril in low renin hypertension. *Clin. Sci.,* 59:141s–144s.
72. Moore, T. J., Crantz, F. R., Hollenberg, N. K., Koletsky, R. J., Leboff, M. S., Swartz, S. L., Levine, L., Podolsky, S., Dluhy, R. G., and Williams, G. H. (1981): Contribution of prostaglandins to the antihypertensive action of captopril in essential hypertension. *Hypertension,* 3:168–173.
73. Silberbauer, K., Stanek, B., and Templ, H. (1982): Acute hypotensive effect of captopril in man modified by prostaglandin synthesis inhibition. *Br. J. Clin. Pharmacol.,* 14:87S–93S.
74. Ogihara, T., Maruyama, A., Hata, T., Mikami, H., Nakamaru, M., Naka, T., Ohde, H., and Kumahara, Y. (1981): Hormonal responses to long-term converting enzyme inhibition in hypertensive patients. *Clin. Pharmacol. Ther.,* 30:328–335.
75. Witzgall, H., Hirsch, B., Scherer, B., and Weber, P. C. (1982): Acute haemodynamic and hormonal effects of captopril are diminished by indomethacin. *Clin. Sci.,* 62:611–615.
76. Goldstone, R. M., Martin, K., Zipser, R., and Horton, R. (1981): Evidence for a dual action of converting enzyme inhibitor on blood pressure in normal man. *Prostaglandins,* 22:587–598.
77. Provoost, A. (1980): The effect of prostaglandin synthesis inhibition of the acute blood pressure reduction by captopril in pentobarbitol-anaesthetized rats. *Eur. J. Pharmacol.,* 65:425–428.
78. Samuelsson, B., Ramwell, P., and Paoletti, R. eds. (1976–1983): *Advances in Prostaglandin, Thromboxane, and Prostacyclin Research, Vols. 1–11.* Raven Press. New York.
79. Vane, J. R. (1969): The release and fate of vasoactive hormones in circulation. *Br. J. Pharmacol.,* 35:209–213.
80. Samuelsson, B. (1977): The role of prostaglandin endoperoxides and thromboxanes in human platelet aggregation. In *Prostaglandins in Hematology,* edited by M. J. Silver, J. B. Smith, and J. J. Kocsis, pp. 1–10. Spectrum Publications, New York.
81. Needleman, P., Minkes, M., And Raz, A. (1976): Thromboxanes: Selective biosynthesis and distinct biological properties. *Science,* 193:163–165.
82. Vane, J. R., and Bergstrom, S., eds. (1980): *Prostacyclin.* Raven Press, New York.
83. Moncada, S., Korbut, R., Bunting, S., and Vane, J. R. (1978): Prostacyclin is a circulating hormone. *Nature,* 273:767–768.
84. Muirhead, E. E., Germain, G. S., Armstrong, F. B., Brooks, B., Leach, B. E., Byers, L. W., Pitcock, J. A., and Brown, P. B. (1975): Endocrine-type antihypertensive function of renomedullary interstitial cells. *Kidney Int.,* 8:S271–S282.
85. Zusman, R. M., and Keiser, H. R. (1977): Prostaglandin biosynthesis by rabbit renomedullary inter-

stitial cells in tissue culture: Stimulation by angiotensin II, bradykinin and arginine vasopressin. *J. Clin. Invest.*, 60:215–223.

86. Zusman, R. M., and Keiser, H. R. (1977): Prostaglandin E_2 biosynthesis by rabbit renomedullary interstitial cells in culture: Mechanisms of stimulation by angiotensin II, bradykinin and arginine vasopressin. *J. Biol. Chem.*, 252:2069–2071.
87. Brown, C. A. Zusman, R. M., and Haber, E. (1980): Identification of an angiotensin receptor in rabbit renomedullary interstitial cells in tissue culture: Correlation with prostaglandin biosynthesis. *Circ. Res.*, 48:802–807.
88. Galler, M., Folkert, V. W., and Schlondorff, D. (1981): Effect of converting enzyme inhibitor on prostaglandin synthesis by isolated rat glomeruli (*Abstr.*) *Clin. Res.*, 29:271A.
89. Murthy, V. S., Waldron, T. L., and Goldberg, M. E. (1978): The mechanism of bradykinin potentiation after inhibition of angiotensin-converting enzyme by SQ 14,225 in conscious rabbits. *Circ. Res.*, 43:140–145.
90. Mullane, K. M., and Moncada, S. (1980): Prostacyclin mediates the potentiated hypotensive effect of bradykinin following captopril treatment. *Eur. J. Pharmacol.*, 66:355–365.
91. Olsen, U. B., and Arrigoni-Martelli, E. (1979): The effects of kininase II inhibition by SQ 14,225 on kidney kallikrein-kinin and prostaglandin systems in conscious dogs. *Eur. J. Pharmacol.*, 54:229–234.
92. Zusman, R. M. (1987): Effects of converting enzyme inhibitors on the renin-angiotensin-aldosterone, bradykinin, and arachidonic-prostaglandin systems: Correlation of chemical structure and biologic activity. *Am. J. Kidney Dis.* (*in press*).
93. Galler, M., Folkert, V. W., and Schlondorff, D. (1981): Effect of converting enzyme inhibitor on prostaglandin synthesis by isolated rat glomeruli (*Abstr.*). *Clin. Res.*, 29:271A.
94. Dollery, C. T., and Miyamori, I. (1979): Indomethacin and the hypotensive action of captopril in DOCA salt hypertensive rats. *Br. J. Pharmacol.*, 68:117P–118P.
95. Goldstone, R. M., Martin, K., Zipser, R., and Horton, R. (1981): Evidence for a dual action of converting enzyme inhibitor on blood pressure in normal man. *Prostaglandins*, 22:587–598.
96. Sweet, C. S., Gaul, S. L., Reitz, P. M., Blaine, E. H., and Ribeiro, L. T. (1983): Mechanism of action of enalapril in experimental hypertension and acute left ventricular failure. *J. Hypertens.*, 1:53–63.
97. Sweet, C. S., Gross, D. M., Arbegast, P. T., Gaul, S. L., Britt, P. M., Ludden, C. T., Weitz, D., and Stone, C. A. (1981): Antihypertensive activity of *N*-[(*S*)-1-(ethoxycarboxyl)-3-phenylpropyll-L-Ala-L-Pro (MK 421) on orally active converting enzyme inhibitor. *J. Pharmacol. Exp. Ther.*, 216:548–556.
98. Sweet, C. S., and Ulm, E. H. (1984): Enalapril. *New Drugs Annual: Cardiovascular Drugs*, 2:1–17.
99. Shoback, D. M., Williams, G. H., Swartz, S. L., Davies, R. O., and Hollenberg, N. K. (1983): Time course and effect of sodium intake on vascular and hormonal responses to enalapril (MK 421) in normal subjects. *J. Cardiovasc. Pharmacol.*, 5:1010–1018.
100. Dzau, V. J. (1986): Significance of the vascular renin-angiotensin pathway. *Hypertension*, 8:553–559.
101. Malik, K. U., and Nasjletti, A. (1976): Facilitation of adrenergic transmission by locally generated angiotensin II in rat mesenteric arteries. *Circ. Res.*, 38:26–30.
102. Zimmerman, B. G. (1981): Adrenergic facilitation by angiotensin: Does it serve a physiological function? *Clin. Sci.*, 60:343–348.
103. Okamura, T., Miyazaki, M., Inagami, T., and Toda, N. (1986): Vascular renin-angiotensin system in two-kidney, one-clip hypertensive rats. *Hypertension*, 8:560–565.
104. Shoback, D. M., Williams, G. H., Moore, T. J., Dluhy, R. G., Podolsky, S., and Hollenberg, N. K. (1983): Defect in the sodium-modulated tissue responsiveness to angiotensin II in essential hypertension. *J. Clin. Invest.*, 72:2115–2124.
105. Dzau, V. J. (1984): Renin inhibitors and angiotensin converting enzyme inhibitors: Rationale and comparison of results. In: *Endocrinology*, edited by F. Labire and I. Proulx, Elsevier, New York. pp. 412–418.
106. Brunner, H. R., Nussberger, J., and Waeber, B. (1985): The present molecules of converting enzyme inhibitors. *J. Cardiovasc. Pharmacol.*, 7:S2–S11.
107. Zusman, R. M. (1984): Renin- and non-renin-mediated antihypertensive actions of converting enzyme inhibitors. *Kidney Int.*, 25:969–983.

The Kidney in Hypertension, edited by Norman M. Kaplan, Barry M. Brenner, and John H. Laragh. Raven Press, New York © 1987.

Diuretics

Burton D. Rose and Laurence A. Turka

The Brigham and Women's Hospital, Boston, Massachusetts 02115

Diuretics, particularly the thiazides, have been effectively used in the treatment of hypertension for more than 30 years. When given as monotherapy, these drugs are as effective as, or more effective than newer agents such as the β-adrenergic blockers or converting enzyme inhibitors (71,76,113–115). Despite this proven efficacy, however, many questions remain unanswered concerning the mechanisms responsible for their diuretic and antihypertensive actions, the metabolic complications that can occur, and the long-term safety of diuretic therapy, particularly in patients with underlying heart disease (57). There is, for example, suggestive evidence that diuretics may actually increase coronary mortality in some patients with mild hypertension. This review will deal primarily with these issues and will be limited to the use of diuretics as antihypertensive agents. The role of diuretic therapy in other conditions, such as edematous states and nephrolithiasis, will not be discussed.

MECHANISM OF DIURESIS

All diuretics act by inhibiting the tubular reabsorption of sodium, primarily by diminishing the movement of sodium from the tubular lumen into the cell (29). Their diuretic ability is a secondary effect, since water transport directly or indirectly follows that of sodium. Loop diuretics, for example, impair sodium chloride reabsorption in the medullary and cortical aspects of the thick ascending limb of the loop of Henle (45). Although these segments are relatively impermeable to water, a diuresis ensues because of a reduction in water reabsorption in the *descending* limb of the loop and in the medullary collecting tubule, segments in which passive water transport is dependent on the osmotic gradient normally created by sodium chloride reabsorption in the ascending limb (50).

Diuretics are usually classified by their primary site of action within the nephron: loop diuretics in the thick ascending limb, thiazide-type diuretics in the distal tubule, and potassium-sparing diuretics in the cortical collecting tubule[1] (29,82,89). The site of action is physiologically important because it determines both the diuretic potency and the concomitant effects on potassium and hydrogen excretion (89). For example, the proximal tubule is responsible for the reabsorption of approximately 65% of the filtered sodium. Nevertheless, proximally acting diuretics (such as the carbonic anhydrase inhibitor acetazolamide) are weak agents for two reasons: (a) most of the increase in sodium delivery out of the proximal tubule can be reabsorbed more distally, particularly in the loop of Henle; and (b) several mechanisms contribute to proximal sodium transport, so that inhibition of a single one has a relatively small total effect (22,29).

This section will cover only those diuretics that are used in the treatment of hypertension.

[1] These diuretics may also have less important effects in other nephron segments. The thiazides, for example, decrease sodium reabsorption in the proximal tubule (perhaps due to carbonic anhydrase inhibitory activity that is common to sulfonamide diuretics) (50,58), and the loop diuretic furosemide may have some activity in both the proximal tubule (again due to carbonic anhydrase inhibition) and the distal tubule (103,109).

Table 1. *Characteristic of commonly used diuretics in the treatment of hypertension*

Drug	Trade name	Usual daily dose in hypertension (mg)	Duration of action (hr)
Loop diuretics			
Furosemide	Lasix	20–80	6–8
Bumetanide	Bumex	0.5–2	4–6
Ethacrynic acid	Edecrin	25–100	6–8
Thiazide-type diuretics			
Hydrochlorothiazide	Hydrodiuril	25–100	6–12
	Esidrix		
	Oretic		
Chlorothiazide	Diuril	250–1,000	6–12
Chlorthalidone	Hygroton	25–100	24–72
Metolazone	Zaroxolyn	2.5–10	6–12
Potassium-sparing diuretics			
Amiloride	Midamor	5–10	18–24
	Moduretic[a]		
Triamterene	Dyrenium	50–100	7–9
	Dyazide[a]		
	Maxzide[a]		
Spironolactone	Aldactone	25–100	12–96
	Aldactazide[a]		

[a]A fixed dose combination with hydrochlorothiazide.

Table 1 lists the individual agents, their trade names, site of action, daily dose, and duration of diuresis.

Loop Diuretics

The loop diuretics furosemide, bumetanide, and ethacrynic acid are the most potent diuretics currently available, leading to the excretion of up to 25% of the filtered sodium load when used in high doses (82,125). The ability to produce such a large diuresis is related to two primary factors: The loop of Henle reabsorbs approximately 20 to 25% of the filtered sodium load; and the more distal segments have a limited capacity to reclaim the increased delivery out of the loop (14,82).

All active sodium transport in the loop of Henle takes place in the thick ascending limb. The energy required for this process is provided by the Na-K-ATPase pump in the basolateral membrane of the tubular cell (14,41). This pump actively transports sodium out of the cell, where it returns to the systemic circulation via the vasa recta capillaries. This transport system also maintains the cell sodium concentration at very low levels, thereby allowing sodium in the tubular lumen to enter the cells down a concentration gradient across the luminal membrane. Passive sodium entry is mediated by an electrically neutral Na:K:2Cl carrier that is most effective when all four sites on the carrier protein are occupied (41,45).

Furosemide and bumetanide (and possibly ethacrynic acid) act in the tubular lumen, apparently by competing for the Cl sites on the Na-K-2Cl carrier (29,41). All three drugs have equal efficacy, although bumetanide is approximately 40 to 50 times more potent than furosemide on a milligram per milligram basis. It also has a quicker onset and shorter duration of action (Table 1).[2] Ethacrynic acid has the least predictable dose-response curve. Furosemide and bumetanide are sulfonamide derivatives (as are the thiazides); ethacrynic acid, in comparison,

[2]The shorter duration of the diuresis with bumetanide is not necessarily beneficial. As will be discussed below, the diuretic-induced fluid loss activates compensatory sodium retaining mechanisms that markedly reduce sodium excretion once the diuretic effect has worn off (54). Once-a-day bumetanide results in more "diuretic-free" hours, an effect that can lead to a lesser total sodium loss.

is a phenoxyacetic acid derivative that may be preferable in patients who are allergic to sulfonamides.

Thiazide-Type Diuretics

Thiazide diuretics were initially synthesized as part of an effort to develop more potent inhibitors of carbonic anhydrase. It is now clear, however, that the primary site of action of these drugs is in the distal convoluted tubule (50,58,109), where they inhibit carrier-mediated sodium entry into the cell. The carrier protein in the distal tubule appears to be a simple Na:Cl carrier (99,109); this protein is different from the Na:K:2Cl carrier in the loop of Henle, which probably accounts for the different sites of action of the thiazides and loop diuretics.

When given in maximum dosage, the thiazides can inhibit the reabsorption of as much as 3 to 5% of the filtered sodium (82). The decrease in potency in relation to the loop diuretics is a simple result of the smaller amount of sodium that is normally reabsorbed in the distal tubule as compared to the loop of Henle. This is usually not a problem in the treatment of uncomplicated essential hypertension, however, since a large diuresis is neither required nor desirable. When used in conventional doses, thiazide diuretics tend to be relatively ineffective once the creatinine clearance falls below 20 to 25 ml/min (85). It is usually necessary to use a loop diuretic in this setting.

The various thiazide-type diuretics differ primarily in their duration of action (Table 1). Thus, the choice between these drugs should be based primarily on convenience of dosing and cost. The longer-acting agents, such as chlorthalidone, have a possible disadvantage in that they may induce more prominent potassium loss (4,83).

Potassium-Sparing Diuretics

The potassium-sparing diuretics, spironolactone, amiloride, and triamterene, act primarily in the cortical collecting tubule, the major site of action of aldosterone (29,50). In this portion of the nephron, sodium entry into the cell is again passive because the Na-K-ATPase pump maintains the cell sodium concentration at a relatively low level. Rather than being carrier mediated, however, sodium entry occurs through selective amiloride-sensitive sodium "channels" in the luminal membrane (55). The luminal membrane also has selective potassium channels, through which potassium is passively secreted into the lumen (55,100).

The ability of aldosterone to promote sodium reabsorption and potassium secretion in this segment is related in part to an increase in the number of open sodium and potassium channels in the luminal membrane (92,100). Potassium secretion is also indirectly related to sodium reabsorption: The movement of the cationic sodium from the lumen into the cell creates an electrical gradient that promotes potassium secretion (35,88). As a result, a diuretic that inhibits sodium reabsorption at this site also diminishes potassium secretion (and is therefore potassium-sparing) (35).

The three potassium-sparing diuretics have somewhat different modes of action. Spironolactone is an antagonist of aldosterone (16). It is unique among the diuretics in that it does not act at the luminal membrane and thus does not require access to the tubular fluid. Instead, it enters the cell by moving from the plasma across the basolateral membrane. Within the cell, it competes with aldosterone for binding to the cytosolic aldosterone receptor (16).

In comparison, amiloride specifically blocks the sodium channel in the luminal membrane, an effect that is independent of aldosterone (8). Amiloride can also inhibit Na-H exchange and the Na-K-ATPase pump, but these effects are not seen at the usual pharmacologic doses (8). The mechanism by which triamterene acts is not well understood, but may be similar to that of amiloride (50).

The potassium-sparing diuretics have relatively weak natriuretic activity, since the cortical collecting tubule normally reabsorbs only 1 to 2% of the filtered sodium (82). As a result, they are most often used in conjunction with the thiazide diuretics to treat or prevent potassium depletion (50,68,69,86). In this setting, they may also induce additional fluid loss and a further reduction in blood pressure (128).

MECHANISM OF ANTIHYPERTENSIVE EFFECT

The mechanism by which diuretics lower the blood pressure in essential hypertension is incompletely understood. Although fluid loss is important initially, other factors appear to play an important role in the maintenance phase of the hypotensive response.

Initial Diuresis

When a thiazide is given to a patient with essential hypertension, the systemic blood pressure typically falls (in responders) within the first week, but a slow decline can continue for up to 12 weeks (107). This hemodynamic response appears to be mediated by hypovolemia-induced reductions in plasma volume[3] (of 10–15%) and cardiac output (15,94,107). In some patients, however, volume depletion does not occur because the patient is relatively insensitive to the dose used or more commonly because the net diuresis is limited by a high sodium intake (20,83). In this setting, the hypotensive effect is minimized or prevented (20,83).

The initial reduction in blood pressure can also be limited by the neurohumoral responses that frequently are activated by volume depletion. For example, some patients with an adequate diuresis also have a marked increase in the production of angiotensin II; this vasoconstrictor can raise the systemic vascular resistance, thereby counteracting the direct effect of the diuretic (107,108).

Late Response

The mechanisms underlying the continued hypotensive response to diuretic therapy are incompletely understood. Most studies have shown that the plasma volume remains reduced, although there may be a partial return to pretreatment levels (15,94,127). Furthermore, this hypovolemia appears to be physiologically important, since volume expansion with intravenous saline or dextran raises the blood pressure toward the pretreatment level (32,127). A similar response (volume expansion and an elevation in blood pressure) can be achieved by discontinuation of the diuretic (106,127).

Maintenance of the antihypertensive effect of diuretics also may involve a decrease in systemic vascular resistance, which counteracts the frequent increase in plasma volume and cardiac output toward normal[4] (Fig. 1) (15,94,107). The factors responsible for this vasodilation are not well defined, since the thiazide diuretics do not appear to have a direct vascular effect (7). One possibility is related to the role of a putative endogenous, digitalis-like natriuretic hormone (which is clearly distinct from the atrial natriuretic peptides) in the genesis of salt-sensitive hypertension (10,21). There is both experimental and human evidence that an inherited defect in renal sodium excretion may be the primary abnormality in some forms of "essential" hypertension (91). Such a defect would lead initially to sodium retention and volume expansion, changes that promote the release of the natriuretic hormone, which, like digitalis, inhibits the cellular Na-K-ATPase pump (most importantly in renal tubular and vascular smooth muscle cells). The net effect is that euvolemia

[3]The baseline plasma volume in patients with essential hypertension tends to be somewhat below normal and to be inversely related to the severity of the hypertension (24). This apparently paradoxical effect is thought to reflect an increase in capillary hydrostatic pressure, which would favor the movement of fluid from the vascular space into the interstitium. This rise in intracapillary pressure could result from venous constriction (perhaps induced by enhanced sympathetic tone) or from incomplete autoregulation by the precapillary sphincters, which would allow some of the elevation in systemic blood pressure to be transmitted to the capillary.

[4]Although the plasma volume may be near normal after chronic diuretic therapy for essential hypertension, the decrease in vascular resistance means that vascular capacity has risen. Thus, the plasma volume may actually be diminished in relation to the enhanced vascular capacity. This would explain the initial fluid retention associated with discontinuation of the diuretic.

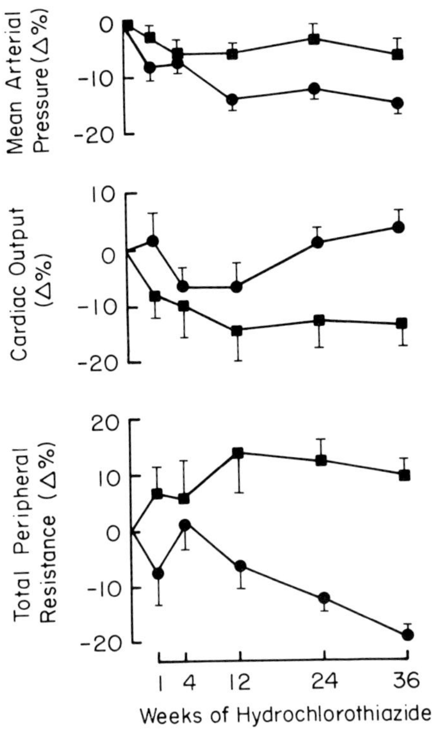

FIG. 1. Percentage changes in mean arterial pressure, cardiac output, and systemic vascular resistance in seven responders (●) and six nonresponders (■) to antihypertensive treatment with a thiazide diuretic. The fall in blood pressure in responders was mediated initially by a reduction in cardiac output; with time, the cardiac output returned to baseline and the hypotensive response was maintained by a decrease in systemic vascular resistance. The nonresponders had a persistent reduction in cardiac output that was counteracted by a rise in vascular resistance. (Adapted from ref. 107.)

is restored at the expense of a reduction in Na-K-ATPase activity, which impairs sodium extrusion from cells. The ensuing elevation in cell sodium concentration leads secondarily to decreased calcium efflux from the cell and a rise in the cell calcium concentration. This change in calcium regulation in vascular smooth muscle cells can produce vasoconstriction. Thus, the new steady state is characterized by hypertension, a normal cardiac output, and increased vascular resistance, findings typical of established essential hypertension (91).

This as yet unproven sequence would be reversible with diuretic therapy. The associated volume depletion inhibits secretion of the natriuretic hormone, thereby allowing the cell calcium concentration and vascular tone to return toward normal. One manifestation of this diuretic-induced fall in vascular resistance is diminished responsiveness to vasoconstrictors such as norepinephrine and angiotensin II (32,120), hormones which have a vascular action that is in part mediated by an increase in free cytosolic calcium.

MAJOR METABOLIC COMPLICATIONS

Diuretic therapy may be associated with a variety of fluid, electrolyte, and metabolic disturbances (Table 2). Although generally mild, these problems can be life-threatening, and may account for the possible increase in cardiac mortality that may occur in some treated patients with mild hypertension (see below). As a result, it is important to be aware of when these complications usually occur, their general relation to diuretic dosage, and which diuretics are most likely to produce a given side effect. This section will review those side effects that can lead to serious symptoms or that can increase coronary risk. Space limitations prevent a discussion of all of the side effects that may occur.

Time Course of Diuretic Effects

Diuretic-induced changes in urinary solute and water excretion are generally *self-limited* as long

Table 2. *Major metabolic complications of diuretic therapy*

Volume depletion
Azotemia
Hyponatremia
Hypokalemia (often with metabolic alkalosis)
Hyperkalemia (with potassium-sparing diuretics)
Hyperuricemia
Hypomagnesemia
Hyperlipidemia
Hyperglycemia

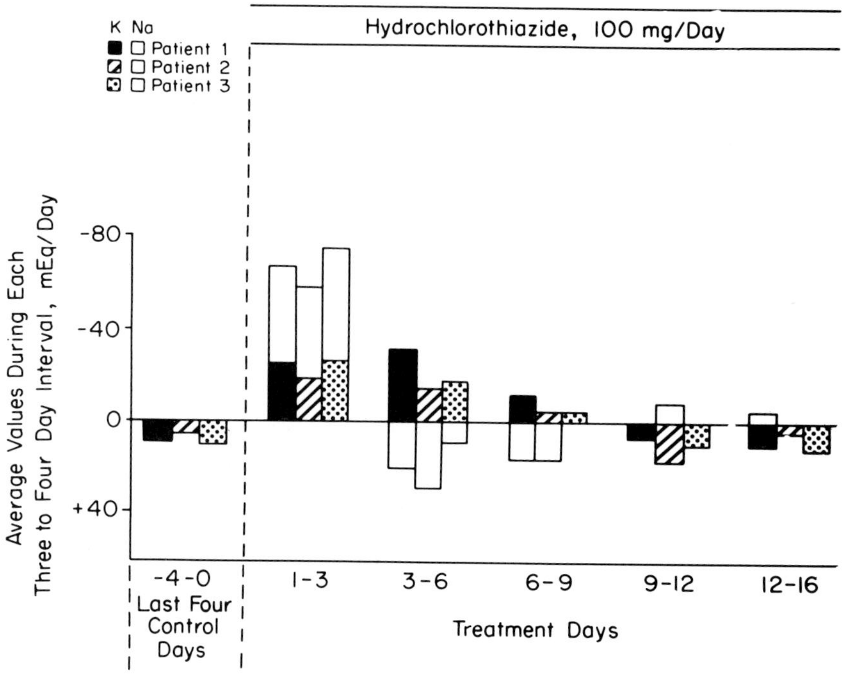

FIG. 2. Sodium and potassium balance in three nonedematous patients receiving 100 mg of hydrochlorothiazide per day. Data are presented for each patient as the average balance during each 3- or 4-day period. A net negative balance occurred for 3 days for sodium (open bars) and for 6 to 9 days for potassium (shaded bars) before a new steady state was established. (Adapted from ref. 69.)

as the diuretic dose and dietary intake are relatively constant. This principle can be appreciated from Fig. 2, which depicts the response of three normal subjects to the administration of 100 mg of hydrochlorothiazide per day (69). As can be seen, sodium loss occurs for only 3 days and potassium loss for only 6 to 9 days. After this period of negative sodium and potassium balance, intake and output again become equal, even though the diuretic is continued.

This *reestablishment of the steady state* is largely related to adaptive changes in renal and neurohumoral function. In terms of sodium balance, the initial volume depletion progressively enhances sodium reabsorption in the proximal and collecting tubules in an appropriate attempt to minimize further volume loss (22,54). This response is mediated by a variety of factors, including increased activity of the renin-angiotensin-aldosterone and sympathetic nervous systems and alterations in intrarenal hemodynamics (54). In comparison, the return of potassium balance is associated with a reduction in the initially high rate of distal potassium secretion. Two factors contribute to this phenomenon (88): a direct inhibitory effect of hypokalemia on potassium secretion (63), and a decrease in flow to the distal nephron induced by volume depletion (39).

The new steady state does not mean that the diuretic has ceased being effective. What has happened is a marked change in the pattern of solute and water excretion during the day: relatively high when the diuretic is acting, and very low once the diuretic effect has worn off due to the secondary adaptive responses (54).

These observations have important clinical implications. If one assumes that the diuretic dose and dietary intake are relatively constant (assumptions that are generally true in the otherwise healthy patient with essential hypertension), then all of the fluid and electrolyte disturbances listed in Table 2 are *most likely to occur in the first few weeks of therapy* (6,69,75,86,114,126). Thereafter, the patient is in a new steady state and the laboratory values tend to remain stable with prolonged therapy (75,86,114,126). For example, the administration of a potassium-sparing diuretic to correct thiazide-induced hypokalemia raises the plasma potassium concentration during the first 2 to 3 weeks of therapy, with no further change with time (Fig. 3).

As a result, it is most important to monitor volume status and the plasma sodium and potassium concentrations soon after the initiation of diuretic therapy. If these parameters are normal at 3 weeks, then late abnormalities are unlikely as long as the diuretic dose remains constant. The late development of hypokalemia or hyponatremia is usually related to some superimposed problem, such as a decrease in dietary intake or enhanced losses due to vomiting or diarrhea.

Hyponatremia

Diuretic-induced hyponatremia is not a common problem, but a marked reduction in the plasma sodium concentration leading to potentially irreversible neurologic damage or death can rarely occur (6). Elderly patients who have a large initial diuresis appear to be at greatest risk (5,6).

The fall in the plasma sodium concentration is primarily related to effective volume depletion. In this setting, two factors interact to diminish the excretion of ingested water: The release of antidiuretic hormone (ADH) is enhanced; and, due in part to increased proximal reabsorption, fluid delivery to the diluting segments in the loop of Henle and distal nephron is re-

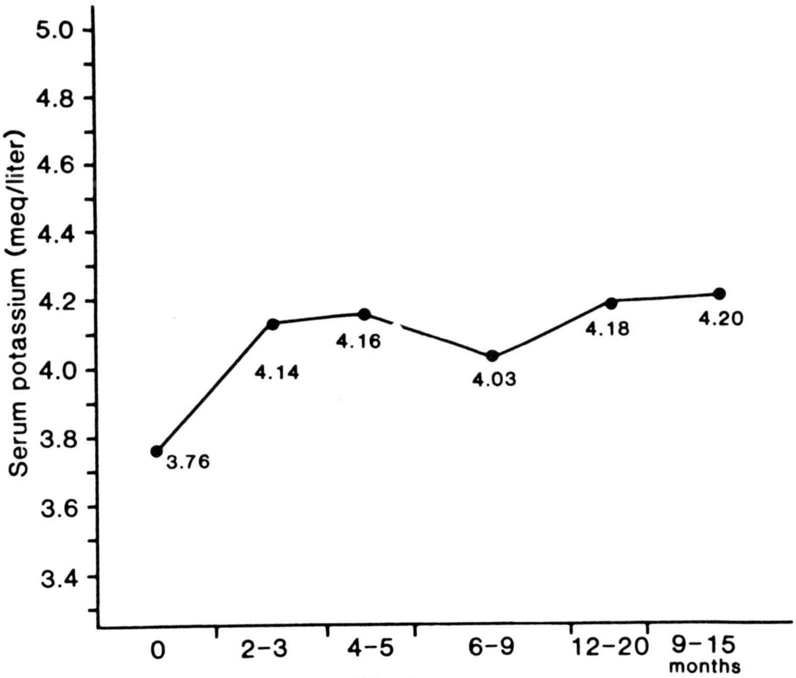

FIG. 3. Mean serum potassium levels after 5 mg of amiloride was added to the therapy of 32 patients who were being treated with 50 mg of hydrochlorothiazide. The serum potassium concentration rose in the first 2 to 3 weeks and was then stable for 9 to 15 months. (From ref. 86.)

duced. The net effect is water retention and the development of hyponatremia. The level of water intake and concurrent potassium depletion (which represents the loss of intracellular solute) also may contribute to the fall in the plasma sodium concentration (90).

Within this framework, it might be expected that the more potent loop diuretics would be more likely to produce hyponatremia. However, *almost all reported cases of marked diuretic-induced hyponatremia have resulted from the use of thiazide-type diuretics* (5,6,28). This unique susceptibility is related to the different sites of action of the loop and thiazide diuretics and their consequent effects on urinary concentrating ability. A concentrated urine is normally produced by equilibration of fluid in the medullary collecting tubule (in the presence of ADH) with the hyperosmotic medullary interstitium. The primary step in the generation of the medullary osmotic gradient is sodium chloride reabsorption without water in the ascending limb of the loop of Henle. This step, however, is specifically inhibited by the loop diuretics. As a result, the ability of ADH to promote water reabsorption is impaired, thereby lessening the risk of developing hyponatremia.

In comparison, the thiazides act in the cortex in the distal tubule, *do not interfere* with urinary concentration or the efficacy of ADH (105), and therefore are more likely to produce hyponatremia. Furthermore, the use of a thiazide also represents the major clinical setting in which effective *solute may be lost in excess of water,* directly leading to hyponatremia even in the absence of water intake. The combination of diuretic-induced sodium and potassium loss plus ADH-mediated water reabsorption can result in the excretion of a concentrated urine in which the sum of the sodium and potassium concentrations is greater than that in the plasma (6).

Hypokalemia

Potassium loss with a thiazide or loop diuretic results from the interplay of several factors, including increased flow to the distal potassium secretory site, hypovolemia-induced hyperaldosteronism, and, with a loop diuretic, direct inhibition of loop potassium reabsorption by interference with the Na:K:2Cl carrier in the luminal membrane (see above) (50). The incidence of hypokalemia (plasma potassium concentration below 3.5 mEq/liter) in patients treated with 50 to 100 mg of hydrochlorothiazide or chlorthalidone per day for essential hypertension has been reported to be between 30 and 50% (75,86,114).

The degree of urinary potassium loss is affected by three primary factors: diuretic dose, which diuretic is used, and the level of sodium intake.

1. The fall in the plasma potassium concentration is in part dose-related, increasing as the dose of hydrochlorothiazide or chlorthalidone is raised from 25 to 200 mg per day (49,75). This is an important consideration, because the antihypertensive effect does not increase as directly with dose, as many patients respond to 25 to 50 mg per day with little further effect from a higher dose (see below) (49,67,70,113). It is likely that, in many patients, increasing the degree of volume depletion by raising the dose is counterbalanced by enhanced renin secretion and increased production of the vasoconstrictor angiotensin II (107,108).
2. Loop diuretics, although more potent natriuretic agents if given in high doses, may induce less potassium loss than a thiazide when used in the treatment of hypertension (4,83). This seeming paradox may be related to the relatively short duration of action of these drugs (about 6 hr with oral furosemide, for example). As a result, more "diuretic-free" time is available each day to conserve potassium. Conversely, there is some evidence that a long-acting agent such as chlorthalidone may produce more potassium loss than an equal dose of the shorter-acting hydrochlorothiazide (83).
3. Moderately limiting sodium intake to approximately 70 to 80 mEq per day can reduce potassium loss by approximately 50% when compared to a nonrestricted diet containing almost 200 mEq of sodium

(83). This effect is probably related at least in part to decreased flow to the distal secretory site with sodium restriction.

The necessity to treat mild diuretic-induced hypokalemia is controversial. It has been argued that a reduction in the plasma potassium concentration to between 3.0 and 3.4 mEq/liter is too small to substantially increase cardiac risk (43). However, several observations suggest a possible link between diuretic use in essential hypertension, hypokalemia, and potentially serious cardiac arrhythmias.

First, the administration of a diuretic to normal subjects or patients with uncomplicated hypertension has been reported to induce hypokalemia as well as ventricular arrhythmias in some (48,49,73) but not all (66) studies. In some of these patients, however, potassium supplementation raised the plasma potassium concentration but did not decrease the frequency of premature beats, suggesting that some non-potassium-related mechanism may be involved (73). One possibility is diuretic-induced magnesium depletion, which can both cause arrhythmias and prevent repletion of the cellular potassium deficit (25,104).

Second, mild hypokalemia can become severe hypokalemia during a stress response. This effect appears to be mediated by epinephrine, which, acting via the β_2-adrenergic receptors, drives potassium from the extracellular fluid into the cells (13,102). The potential importance of this effect in patients treated with a diuretic is illustrated in Fig. 4. Epinephrine was infused into normal subjects to achieve a plasma concentration similar to that occurring in patients with a myocardial infarction. In the basal state, epinephrine lowered the plasma potassium concentration from 3.8 to 3.2 mEq/liter. However, when these subjects were pretreated with a thiazide, the baseline plasma potassium concentration fell to approximately 3.3 mEq/liter and, after epinephrine, to below 2.5 mEq/liter in some patients.

It is possible that, during an episode of coronary ischemia, this hypokalemic effect of epinephrine could predispose to ventricular arrhythmias. There is some evidence in support of this hypothesis, as an increased incidence of

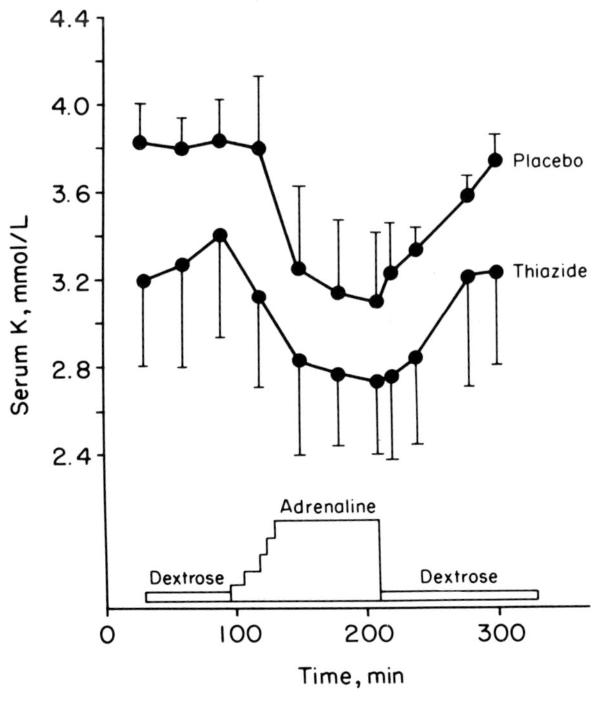

FIG. 4. Serum potassium concentration during infusion of adrenaline (epinephrine) in six patients who had pretreatment with a placebo or a thiazide for seven days. (From ref. 102.)

both ventricular fibrillation and ventricular tachycardia has been described in patients with an acute myocardial infarction who were initially hypokalemic, particularly if the plasma potassium concentration was below 3.0 mEq/liter (a measurement that includes a possible epinephrine effect) (79,80).

Taken together, these observations provide circumstantial evidence in favor of treating mild hypokalemia in hypertension. How and when this should be done will be discussed below after consideration of the possible adverse effects of therapy in patients with mild hypertension.

Hyperkalemia

The potassium-sparing diuretics tend to raise the plasma potassium concentration by impairing distal potassium secretion (50). This change is generally mild (34), with the risk of hyperkalemia being particularly small when these drugs are given to reverse thiazide-induced potassium depletion (69,86). However, a clinically significant elevation in the plasma potassium concentration can occur when one of these drugs is given to a patient who has renal insufficiency or who is concurrently taking potassium supplements or a converting enzyme inhibitor (which, by diminishing the production of angiotensin II. can decrease the release of aldosterone) (40).

There are currently three potassium-sparing diuretics available: amiloride, triamterene, and spironolactone. Although each is effective, amiloride has the advantages of once a day dosage and of probably having the fewest side effects. Spironolactone can lead to a variety of endocrine (impotence, gynecomastia, menstrual irregularities) and gastrointestinal problems, whereas triamterene has been associated with renal abnormalities including crystals and casts in the urine (97), kidney stones (96), an unusual form of acute renal failure in patients also taking indomethacin (27,122), and possibly acute interstitial nephritis (97).

Lipid and Carbohydrate Metabolism

The effect of diuretics on lipid metabolism is somewhat unclear. Short-term studies (generally 3 months or less) have revealed a 5 to 15% increase in the plasma concentration of cholesterol carried by low-density lipoproteins (2,42, 121,124). This effect is demonstrable in men and postmenopausal women but not in premenopausal women (11). It can be produced by thiazide-type and loop diuretics (121), but does not appear to occur with a potassium-sparing diuretic such as spironolactone (3).

In contrast to these findings, long-term follow-up of 1 to 6 years has not generally shown any increase in the plasma cholesterol level when compared to the pretreatment level (9,72,114). One possible explanation for this time dependence is that the reduction in cholesterol with time is related to concurrent dietary modification and not to waning of the diuretic effect. In the only one of the long-term studies that included a placebo group, the plasma cholesterol concentration fell during prolonged observation to *below* the baseline level in untreated patients, presumably due to a change in diet (72). As a result, the mean plasma cholesterol level remained approximately 7 mg/dl higher in the diuretic-treated group.

This numerically small change (2–3%) might be clinically important. Studies in hypercholesterolemic men given hypolipidemic therapy have suggested that there is approximately a 2% decrease in coronary risk for every 1% reduction in the plasma cholesterol concentration (64). If these results can be extrapolated to patients receiving diuretics, then the small elevation in the plasma cholesterol concentration might enhance coronary risk by 4 to 6%.

Diuretics can also increase coronary risk by their effects on carbohydrate metabolism (2). Chronic thiazide therapy has been shown to raise the plasma glucose concentration by a mean of 5 mg/dl in the fasting state and by 18 mg/dl 2 hr after a carbohydrate meal (117), although more marked hyperglycemia can occur in some patients. Both decreased insulin release and peripheral insulin resistance may contribute to the glycemic effect of diuretic therapy (101). Potassium depletion appears to be of primary importance in this setting, but a direct drug effect may also play a role (46,101).

ADVERSE EFFECTS OF THE TREATMENT OF MILD HYPERTENSION

The metabolic complications of thiazide therapy may be particularly important because of recent studies that suggest that the treatment of mild hypertension might be associated with *increased cardiac mortality* in some patients (57). This possibility was first suggested by the Multiple Risk Factor Intervention Trial (MRFIT). Treated men with mild hypertension who began with a normal electrocardiogram had almost a 25% reduction in coronary mortality at 7 years when compared to men who received less or no treatment. In contrast, men with an abnormal resting electrocardiogram had more than a *65% increase in cardiac mortality* with antihypertensive therapy (Table 3) (77,78).

The findings of this study have been criticized because it was designed to assess the efficacy of reversing a variety of cardiac risk factors (including hypercholesterolemia and smoking), not specifically the treatment of hypertension. As a result, the data above represent subgroup analysis that may lack statistical power. However, data from the Hypertension Detection and Follow-Up Program (HDFP) and the Oslo Hypertension Study also suggest that antihypertensive therapy can increase coronary risk in at least some patients (51,61). In the HDFP, for example, patients in the stepped (intensive) care group who began with a normal electrocardiogram had reduced mortality from both coronary heart disease and stroke when compared to the referred care group that received less or no therapy (Table 3). In contrast, those patients in the stepped care group who began with an *abnormal* electrocardiogram still had fewer cerebrovascular events but, as in the MRFIT, had a higher, although not statistically significant, coronary mortality (Table 3). The persistent benefit in terms of cerebrovascular disease may be explained by the observation that hypertension is the *primary risk factor* for stroke but only one of several important risk factors (including smoking and hypercholesterolemia) for cardiac disease (19,44). Thus, the potentially adverse metabolic effects of treatment would not substantially counteract the positive cerebrovascular effect of lowering the blood pressure.

Table 3. *Coronary heart disease deaths (per 1,000 patient-years) in patients with mild hypertension according to the resting electrocardiogram*[a]

	Normal EKG		Abnormal EKG	
MRFIT[b]	SI[c]	UC[d]	SI	UC
	2.3	3.0	4.2	2.5
HDFP[e]	SC[f]	RC[g]	SC	RC
	2.0	3.1	4.3	3.5

*Data from Refs. 51 and 78. Abbreviations: SI = Special intervention, UC = Usual care. SC = Stepped care, RC = Referred care.

[a]Data from refs. 51 and 78.

[b]Multiple Risk Factor Intervention Trial; [c]special intervention; [d]usual care; [e]Hypertension Detection and Follow-up Program; [f]stepped care; [g]referred care.

The MRFIT also found that the increase in coronary deaths was entirely due to sudden death (consistent with an arrhythmic event) and that the *enhanced risk was limited to those patients receiving a diuretic* (78). A similar adverse effect of diuretic therapy was suggested in the Medical Research Council trial: In nonsmokers, coronary events were reduced by one-third in patients treated with propranolol (versus placebo); this beneficial response was lost in those receiving a thiazide diuretic, even though there was a fall in blood pressure (averaging 13/6 mm Hg) that was equivalent to or slightly greater than that obtained with propranolol (71).

This seemingly deleterious effect of diuretics may be dose-related. In men with an abnormal electrocardiogram in the MRFIT, the percentage receiving more than 50 mg of hydrochlorothiazide or chlorthalidone per day was 51% in the special intervention group (which had a higher coronary mortality) but only 15% in the usual care group (78).

However, the mechanism by which diuretics may be harmful is unclear; as described above, hypokalemia (particularly when exacerbated during a stress response), hypomagnesemia, hyperlipidemia, and hyperglycemia all could play a contributory role. Although it is also uncertain that this deleterious effect could in part be reversed by correction of mild hypokalemia, the circumstantial evidence favoring treatment is reasonably strong (especially in patients with underlying heart disease) and the risks are relatively low, with hyperkalemia being unusual in patients without renal insufficiency or in the absence of combination therapy with potassium supplementation and a potassium-sparing diuretic.

Treatment of Hypokalemia

There are three ways in which diuretic-induced hypokalemia can be treated: dietary modification, potassium supplements, or potassium-sparing diuretics. Although many physicians begin by increasing the intake of potassium-rich foods such as oranges and bananas (the latter contain 2 to 2.5 mEq of potassium per inch) (56), there are two major problems with this regimen. First, the hypokalemia that occurs with diuretics is usually accompanied by metabolic alkalosis. This combined electrolyte disorder is best treated with potassium chloride (53). Bananas and oranges, however, have other anions (such as citrate and phosphate) (56), resulting in less effective potassium repletion (53). Second, supplying 40 to 60 mEq of potassium per day with fruits can provide between 350 and 600 calories (56), an undesirable effect in those patients who are overweight and in whom weight reduction can lead to a fall in blood pressure (84).

Thus, hypokalemia is best treated with some form of potassium chloride supplement (with more than 40 mEq per day usually being required) (68,93) or with a potassium-sparing diuretic such as amiloride. The latter may be preferable because it is easier to take and is also magnesium-sparing by enhancing distal magnesium reabsorption (60). Minimizing magnesium loss may be beneficial because hypomagnesemia can cause both arrhythmias and potassium depletion (25,104).

Correction of hypokalemia may have an additional benefit, producing a further reduction in blood pressure in some hypertensive patients (52,65). Increased urinary sodium loss either with potassium supplementation (33,65) or with potassium-sparing diuretics may account for at least part of the hypotensive effect.

RECOMMENDATIONS FOR DIURETIC USE

The preceding discussion has presented evidence concerning a possible long-term deleterious effect of diuretic therapy in some patients with mild hypertension. The inability to demonstrate these findings in earlier studies may have been related to the severity of the hypertension. Patients with moderate or severe diastolic hypertension are at much greater risk of cardiovascular complications, which can be reduced by 65 to over 90% with antihypertensive medications (110,111). In this setting, any adverse effect on therapy would be lost in the large benefit obtained from the associated fall in blood pressure. In comparison, the risk and subsequent benefits are much less in mild hypertension (71,91), allowing an unfavorable effect of therapy to be seen.

These observations, however, must be weighed against the proven antihypertensive efficacy of diuretic agents, which have been used in virtually every study evaluating the treatment of hypertension. When used as monotherapy, for example, thiazide diuretics have been shown to be as effective as, or even more effective than, either β-blockers or converting enzyme inhibitors in lowering the blood pressure (71,76, 113–115). This is especially true in blacks and in obese patients, who appear to be particularly responsive to diuretic therapy (30,74,76, 113,115).

At present, it is uncertain how to balance the positive and potentially negative effects of chronic diuretic therapy. Some physicians have elected to begin therapy with a different class of drugs such as a β-blocker or a converting enzyme inhibitor. Converting enzyme inhibitors, for example, are generally effective in all groups of patients (17,47,62,112,116), except in blacks when used as monotherapy (30,76). They also lack the metabolic side effects of the diuretics (121,123), and do not interfere with sympathetic function as do the sympatholytic agents, including the β-blockers. As a result, they are usually better tolerated than other antihypertensive agents and may be associated with an improved "quality of life" (17,47). It should be emphasized, however, that the long-term safety of these agents remains to be established.

With these considerations in mind, the following recommendations (which represent the opinion of the authors and not necessarily a general consensus) can be made regarding the use of diuretics in the patient with *uncomplicated essential hypertension:*

1. Thiazide-type diuretics are generally preferred, being somewhat more effective than the loop diuretics (4,83). The factors responsible for this difference are not well understood, but the shorter duration of action of the loop diuretics may allow sodium to be retained during the diuretic-free periods (4).
2. When used, thiazides should be given in the lowest effective dose, which is often 25 to 50 mg of hydrochlorothiazide or chlorthalidone per day (49,67,70,113). Although higher doses may be effective in some patients (49,113), they are associated with a greater incidence of metabolic complications (49), are more likely to produce symptomatic hypovolemia (particularly in elderly patients who frequently have decreased cardiovascular reserve) (95), and may increase the risk of coronary mortality (78). Hypokalemia should be treated if it occurs, with a potassium chloride supplement or preferably a potassium-sparing diuretic.
3. Thiazide-type diuretics remain the first-line agents of choice in blacks and in obese patients (30,74,76,113,115). It has been suggested that patients with low plasma renin levels are also more likely to respond to diuretic therapy. More recent studies, however, indicate that the plasma renin activity is of limited value, with the difference in efficacy between low and high renin groups being only a few millimeters of mercury (31,119).
4. Converting enzyme inhibitors may be used as first-line therapy in nonobese white patients. In this setting, adding a diuretic as a second drug (in doses as low as 25 mg per day) may be very effective (30,112). This combination has a synergistic effect, since the rise in angiotensin II that normally limits the drop in blood pressure seen with a diuretic (107,108) is now prevented by converting enzyme inhibition. Converting enzyme inhibitors have the added benefits of limiting the degree of diuretic-induced hypokalemia (due to the associated reduction in aldosterone release) and of preventing the diuretic-induced rise in plasma cholesterol levels by an unknown mechanism (121,123).
5. Nonsteroidal antiinflammatory drugs should be avoided if possible in hypertensive patients. These drugs inhibit the production of vasodilator prostaglandins and, in patients treated with diuretics, they can diminish renal perfusion (36), decrease the diuresis (12,26), and raise the systemic blood pressure by 5 to 10 mm Hg (81,98, 118,129). If one of these drugs has to be used, sulindac may be the safest because it has less or no effect on renal prostaglandin synthesis and therefore is less likely to exacerbate the hypertension (81,118, 129). The mechanism responsible for this relatively unique effect is incompletely understood (59,130).

Refractory Hypertension

Truly refractory hypertension is most often due to poor compliance with dietary or medical therapy or to a secondary cause such as renal artery stenosis (38). In some patients, however, volume expansion (due to underlying renal disease or to the sodium-retaining effects of drugs such as methyldopa, hydralazine, or minoxidil) may play an important role (23,38). To test for this possibility, the patient should be diuresed with a loop diuretic to "dry weight." This is defined as the point at which the blood pressure becomes normal or the patient develops symptoms (cramps, weakness, orthostatic dizziness) or signs (an otherwise unexplained rise in the blood urea nitrogen) of hypovolemia. Many "refractory" hypertensives will have a beneficial response to this intensive regimen, with recurrent volume expansion then being prevented by maintenance diuretic therapy (23,37,38). In addition to the direct effect of volume loss, the associated increase in renin release (which will limit the diuretic-induced fall in blood pressure) will make the patient more responsive to subsequent therapy with a converting enzyme inhibitor if another antihypertensive agent is required (37).

Hypertension in Renal Disease

Volume expansion also plays an important role in the hypertension associated with many acute and chronic renal diseases, particularly the glomerulopathies (1,87). As a result, diuretic therapy is frequently required for adequate blood pressure control. A loop diuretic is often necessary in those patients with a creatinine clearance below 20 to 25 ml/min, a setting in which a thiazide is unlikely to produce a diuresis (85) unless very high doses are given (the equivalent of 200 to 1,500 mg of hydrochlorothiazide in one study) (18).

REFERENCES

1. Acosta, J. H. (1982): Hypertension in chronic renal disease. *Kidney Int.*, 22:702–712.
2. Ames, R. P., and Hill, P. (1976): Elevation of serum lipid levels during diuretic therapy of hypertension. *Am. J. Med.*, 61:748–757.
3. Ames, R. P., and Peacock, P. B. (1984): Serum cholesterol during treatment of hypertension with diuretic drugs. *Arch. Intern. Med.*, 144:710–714.
4. Araoye, M. A., Chang, M. Y., Khatri, I. M., and Freis, E. D. (1978): Furosemide compared with hydrochlorothiazide. Long-term treatment of hypertension. *JAMA*, 240:1863–1866.
5. Ashouri, O. S. (1986): Severe diuretic-induced hyponatremia in the elderly. A series of eight patients. *Arch. Intern. Med.*, 146:1355–1357.
6. Ashraf, N., Locksley, R., and Arieff, A. I. (1981): Thiazide-induced hyponatremia associated with death or neurologic damage in outpatients. *Am. J. Med.*, 70:1163–1168.
7. Bennett, W. M., McDonald, W. J., Kuehnel, E., Harnett, M. N., and Porter, G. A. (1977): Do diuretics have antihypertensive properties independent of natriuresis? *Clin. Pharmacol. Ther.*, 22:499–504.
8. Benos, D. J. (1982): Amiloride: A molecular probe of sodium transport in tissues and cells. *Am. J. Physiol.*, 242:C131–C145.
9. Berglund, G., and Andersson, O. (1981): Beta-blockers or diuretics in hypertension? A six-year follow-up of blood pressure and metabolic side effects. *Lancet*, 1:744–747.
10. Blaustein, M. P. (1984): Sodium transport and hypertension. Where are we going? *Hypertension*, 6:445–451.
11. Boehringer, K., Weidmann, P., Mordasini, R., Schiffl, H., Bachmann, C., and Riesen, W. (1982): Menopause-dependent plasma lipoprotein alterations in diuretic-treated women. *Ann. Intern. Med.*, 97:206–209.
12. Brater, D. C. (1979): Analysis of the effect of indomethacin on the response to furosemide in man: Effect of dose of furosemide. *J. Pharmacol. Exp. Ther.*, 210:386–390.
13. Brown, M. J., Brown, D. C., and Murphy, M. B. (1983): Hypokalemia from beta-receptor stimulation by circulating epinephrine. *N. Engl. J. Med.*, 309:1414–1419.
14. Burg, M. B. (1982): Thick ascending limb of Henle's loop. *Kidney Int.*, 22:454–464.
15. Conway, J., and Lauwers, P. (1960): Hemodynamic and hypotensive effects of long-term therapy with chlorothiazide. *Circulation*, 21:21–27.
16. Corvol, P., Claire, M., Oblin, M. E., Geering, K., and Rossier, B. (1981): Mechanism of the antimineralocorticoid effects of spironolactones. *Kidney Int.*, 20:1–6.
17. Croog, S. H., Levine, S., Testa, M. A., Brown, B., Bulpitt, C. J., Jenkins, C. D., Klerman, G. L., and Williams, G. H. (1986): The effects of antihypertensive therapy on the quality of life. *N. Engl. J. Med.*, 314:1657–1664.
18. Dargie, H. J., Allison, M. E. M., Kennedy, A. C., and Gray, M. J. B. (1972): High dosage metolazone in chronic renal failure. *Br. Med. J.*, 4:196–198.
19. Dauber, T. R. (1980): *The Framingham Study. The Epidemiology of Atherosclerotic Disease*, Chapters 7 and 8. Harvard University Press, Cambridge.
20. de Carvalho, J. G. R., Dunn, F. G., Lohmoller, G., and Frohlich, E. D. (1978): Hemodynamic correlates of prolonged thiazide therapy: Comparison of responders and non-responders. *Clin. Pharmacol. Ther.*, 22:875–880.
21. de Wardener, H. E., and MacGregor, G. A. (1983): The relation of a circulating sodium transport inhibitor (the natriuretic hormone?) to hypertension. *Medicine*, 62:310–326.

22. Dirks, J. H., Cirksena, W. J., and Berliner, R. W. (1966): Micropuncture study of the effect of various diuretics on sodium reabsorption by the proximal tubules of the dog. *J. Clin. Invest.*, 45:1875–1885.
23. Dustan, H. P., Tarazi, R. C., and Bravo, E. L. (1972): Dependence of arterial pressure on intravascular volume in treated hypertensive patients. *N. Engl. J. Med.*, 286:861–866.
24. Dustan, H. P., Tarazi, R. C., Bravo, E. L., and Dart, R. A. (1973): Plasma and extracellular fluid volumes in hypertension. *Circ. Res.*, 32(*Suppl.* I):I73–I83.
25. Dyckner, T., and Wester, P. O. (1979): Ventricular extrasystoles and intracellular electrolytes before and after potassium and magnesium infusions in patients on diuretic treatment. *Am. Heart J.*, 97:12–18.
26. Favre, L., Glasson, P. H., Riondel, A., and Vallotton, M. B. (1983): Interaction of diuretics and non-steroidal anti-inflammatory drugs in man. *Clin. Sci.*, 64:407–415.
27. Favre, L., Glasson, P. H., and Vallotton, M. B. (1982): Reversible acute renal failure from combined triamterene and indomethacin. *Ann. Intern. Med.*, 96:317–320.
28. Fichman, M. P., Vorherr, H., Kleeman, C. R., and Telfer, N. (1971): Diuretic-induced hyponatremia. *Ann. Intern. Med.*, 75:853–863.
29. Friedman, P. A., and Hebert, S. C. (1987): Mechanism of action of diuretics. In: *Contemporary Issues in Nephrology, Vol. 17,* edited by B. M. Brenner and J. H. Stein. Churchill Livingstone, New York.
30. Freier, P. A., Wollam, G. L., Hall, W. D., Unger, D. J., Douglas, M. B., and Bain, R. P. (1984): Blood pressure, plasma volume, and catecholamine levels during enalapril therapy in blacks with hypertension. *Clin. Pharmacol. Ther.*, 36:731–737.
31. Freis, E. D., Materson, B. J., and Flamenbaum, W. (1983): Comparison of propranolol or hydrochlorothiazide alone for treatment of hypertension. II. Evaluation of the renin-angiotensin system, *Am. J. Med.*, 74:1029–1041.
32. Freis, E. D., Wanko, A., Schnaper, H. E., and Frohlich, E. D. (1960): Mechanism of the altered blood pressure responsiveness induced by chlorothiazide. *J. Clin. Invest.*, 39:1277–1281.
33. Fujita, T., and Sato, Y. (1983): Natriuretic and antihypertensive effects of potassium in DOCA-salt hypertensive rats. *Kidney Int.*, 24:731–739.
34. Gabow, P. A., Moore, S., and Schrier, R. W. (1979): Spironolactone-induced hyperchloremic acidosis in cirrhosis. *Ann. Intern. Med.*, 90:338–340.
35. Garcia-Filho, E., Malnic, G., and Giebisch, G. (1980): Effects of changes in electrical potential difference on tubular potassium transport. *Am. J. Physiol.*, 238:F235–F246.
36. Garella, S., and Matarese, R. A. (1984): Renal effects of prostaglandins and clinical adverse effects of nonsteroidal anti-inflammatory drugs. *Medicine*, 63:165–181.
37. Gavras, H., Waeber, B., Kershaw, G. R., Liang, C. S., Textor, C. S., Brunner, H. R., Tifft, C. P., and Gavras, I. (1981): Role of reactive hyperreninemia in blood pressure changes induced by sodium depletion in patients with refractory hypertension. *Hypertension*, 3:441–447.
38. Gifford, R. W., Jr., and Tarazi, R. C. (1978): Resistant hypertension: Diagnosis and management. *Ann. Intern. Med.*, 88:661–665.
39. Good, D. W., and Wright, F. S. (1979): Luminal influences on potassium secretion: Sodium concentration and flow rate. *Am. J. Physiol.*, 236:F192–F205.
40. Greenblatt, D. J., and Koch-Weser, J. (1973): Adverse reactions to spironolactone: A report from the Boston Collaborative Drug Surveillance Program. *JAMA*, 225:40–43.
41. Greger, R. (1985): Ion transport mechanisms in thick ascending limb of Henle's loop of mammalian nephron. *Physiol. Rev.*, 65:760–797.
42. Grimm, R. H., Leon, A. S., Hunninghake, D. B., Lenz, K., Hannan, P., and Blackburn, H. (1981): Effects of thiazide diuretics on plasma lipids and lipoproteins in mildly hypertensive men. A double-blind controlled trial. *Ann. Intern. Med.*, 94:7–11.
43. Harrington, J. T., Isner, J. M., and Kassirer, J. P. (1982): Our national obsession with potassium. *Am. J. Med.*, 73:155–159.
44. Havlik, R. J., and Feinleib, M. (1982): Epidemiology and genetics of hypertension. *Hypertension*, 4(*Suppl.* III):III-121–III-127.
45. Hebert, S. C., and Andreoli, T. E. (1984): Control of NaCl transport in the thick ascending limb. *Am. J. Physiol.*, 246:F745–F756.
46. Helderman, J. H., Elahi, D., Andersen, D. K., Raizes, G. S., Tobin, J. D., Shocken, D., and Andres, R. (1983): Prevention of the glucose intolerance of diuretics by maintenance of body potassium. *Diabetes*, 32:106–111.
47. Helgeland, A., Strommen, R., Hagelund, C. H., and Tretli, S. (1986): Enalapril, atenolol, and hydrochlorothiazide in mild to moderate hypertension. A comparative multicentre study in general practice in Norway. *Lancet*, 1:872–875.
48. Holland, O. B., Nixon, J. V., and Kuhnert, L. (1981): Diuretic-induced ventricular ectopic activity. *Am. J. Med.*, 70:762–768.
49. Hollifield, J. W., and Slaton, P. E. (1981): Thiazide diuretics, hypokalemia and cardiac arrhythmia. *Acta Med. Scand.*, 209(*Suppl.* 647):67–73.
50. Hropot, M., Fowler, N., Karlmark, B., and Giebisch, G. (1985): Tubular action of diuretics: Distal effects on electrolyte transport and acidification. *Kidney Int.*, 28:477–489.
51. Hypertension Detection and Follow-Up Program Cooperative Research Group (1984): The effect of antihypertensive drug treatment on mortality in the presence of resting electrocardiographic abnormalities at baseline: The HDFP experience. *Circulation*, 70:996–1003.
52. Kaplan, N. M., Carnegie, A., Raskin, P., Heller, J. A., and Simmons, M. (1985): Potassium supplementation in patients with diuretic-induced hypokalemia. *N. Engl. J. Med.*, 312:746–749.
53. Kassirer, J. P., Berkman, P. M., Lawrenz, D. R., and Schwartz, W. B. (1965): The critical role of

chloride in the correction of hypokalemic alkalosis in man. *Am. J. Med.*, 38:172–189.
54. Kelly, R. A., Wilcox, C. S., Mitch, W. E., Meyer, T. W., Souney, P. F., Rayment, C. M., Friedman, P. A., and Swartz, S. L. (1983): Response of the kidney to furosemide. II. Effect of captopril on sodium balance. *Kidney Int.*, 24:233–239.
55. Koeppen, B. M., Biagi, B. A., and Giebisch, G. (1983): Intracellular microelectrode catheterization of the rabbit cortical collecting duct. *Am. J. Physiol.*, 244:F35–F47.
56. Kopyt, N., Dalal, F., and Narins, R. G. (1985): Renal retention of potassium in fruit (letter). *N. Engl. J. Med.*, 313:582–583.
57. Kuller, L. H., Hulley, S. B., Cohen, J. D., and Neaton, J. (1986): Unexpected effects of treating hypertension in men with electrocardiographic abnormalities: A critical analysis. *Circulation*, 73:114–123.
58. Kunau, R. T., Jr., Weller, D. R., and Webb, H. L. (1975): Clarification of the site of action of chlorothiazide in the rat nephron. *J. Clin. Invest.*, 56:401–407.
59. Laffi, G., Daskalopoulos, G., Kronborg, I., Hsueh, W., Gentilini, P., and Zipser, R. D. (1986): Effects of sulindac and ibuprofen in patients with cirrhosis and ascites. An explanation for the renal-sparing effect of sulindac. *Gastroenterology*, 90:182–187.
60. Lau, K., Thomas, D., and Eby, B. (1986): Effects of amiloride on renal Mg handling: Evidence for enhanced transport in the distal tubule (*Abstr.*). *Kidney Int.*, 29:163.
61. Leren, P., and Helgeland, A. (1986): Coronary heart disease and treatment of hypertension: Some Oslo study data. *Am. J. Med.*, 80(Suppl. 2A):3–6.
62. Liberatore, S. M., and Botta, G. (1986): Treatment of essential aterial hypertension with captopril: Outpatient drug-supervision study with particular reference to elderly patients. *Cardiovasc. Rev. Rep.*, 7:29–43.
63. Linas, S. L., Peterson, L. N., Anderson, R. J., Aisenbrey, G. A., Simon, F. R., and Berl, T. (1979): Mechanism of renal potassium conservation in the rat. *Kidney Int.*, 15:601–611.
64. Lipid Research Clinics Program (1984): The Lipid Research Clinics Coronary Primary Prevention Trial results. I. Reduction in incidence of coronary heart disease. II. The relationship of reduction in incidence of coronary heart disease to cholesterol lowering. *JAMA*, 251:351–374.
65. MacGregor, G. A., Smith, S. J., Markandu, N. D., Banks, R. A., and Sagnella, G. A. (1982): Moderate potassium supplementation in essential hypertension. *Lancet*, 2:567–570.
66. Madias, J. E., Madias, N. E., and Gavras, H. P. (1984): Nonarrhythmogenicity of diuretic-induced hypokalemia. Its evidence in patients with uncomplicated hypertension. *Arch. Intern. Med.*, 144: 2171–2176.
67. Magee, P. F. A., and Freis, E. D. (1986): Is low-dose hydrochlorothiazide effective? *Hypertension*, 8(*Suppl.* II):II-135–II-139.
68. Maronde, R. F., Barr, J., Vlachakis, N. D., Spencer, C. A., and Chan, L. (1984): Oral potassium chloride and amiloride in hydrochlorothiazide-induced potassium loss. *Clin. Pharmacol. Ther.*, 36:431–435.
69. Maronde, R. F., Milgrom, M., Vlachakis, N. D., and Chan, L. (1983): Response of thiazide-induced hypokalemia to amiloride. *JAMA*, 249:237–241.
70. Materson, B. J., Oster, J. R., Michael, U. F., Bolton, S. M., Burton, Z. C., Stambaugh, J. E., and Morledge, J. (1978): Dose response to chlorthalidone in patients with mild hypertension: Efficacy of a lower dose. *Clin. Pharmacol. Ther.*, 24:192–198.
71. Medical Research Council Working Party (1985): MRC trial of treatment of mild hypertension: Principal results. *Br. Med. J.*, 291:97–104.
72. Medical Research Council Working Party on Mild to Moderate Hypertension (1981): Adverse reactions to bendrofluazide and propranolol for the treatment of mild hypertension. *Lancet*, 2:539–542.
73. Medical Research Council Working Party on Mild to Moderate Hypertension (1983): Ventricular extrasystoles during thiazide treatment: Substudy of MRC mild hypertension trial. *Br. Med. J.*, 287:1249–1253.
74. Meserli, F. H., Sundgaard-Riise, K., Reisin, E., Dreslinski, G., Dunn, F. G., and Frohlich, E. (1983): Disparate cardiovascular effects of obesity and arterial hypertension. *Am. J. Med.*, 74:808–812.
75. Morgan, D. B., and Davidson, C. (1980): Hypokalemia and diuretics: An analysis of publications. *Br. Med. J.*, 1:905–908.
76. Moser, M., and Lunn, J. (1982): Responses to captopril and hydrochlorothiazide in black patients with hypertension. *Clin. Pharmacol. Ther.*, 32:307–312.
77. Multiple Risk Factor Intervention Trial Research Group (1982): Risk factor changes and mortality results. *JAMA*, 248:1465–1477.
78. Multiple Risk Factor Intervention Trial Research Group (1985): Baseline resting electrocardiographic abnormalities, antihypertensive treatment, and mortality in the Multiple Risk Factor Intervention trial. *Am. J. Cardiol.*, 55:1–15.
79. Nordrehaug, J. E., Johannessen, K. A., and von der Lippe, G. (1985): Serum potassium concentration as a risk factor of ventricular arrhythmias early in acute myocardial infarction. *Circulation*, 71:645–649.
80. Nordrehaug, J. E., and von der Lippe, G. (1983): Hypokalemia and ventricular fibrillation in acute myocardial infarction. *Br. Heart J.*, 50:525–529.
81. Puddey, I. B., Beilin, L. J., Vandongen, R., Banks, R., and Rouse, I. (1985): Differential effects of sulindac and indomethacin on blood pressure in treated essential hypertensive subjects. *Clin. Sci.*, 69:327–336.
82. Puschett, J. B. (1986): Clinical pharmacologic implications in diuretic selection. *Am. J. Cardiol.*, 57:6A–13A.
83. Ram, C. V. S., Garrett, B. N., and Kaplan, N. M. (1981): Moderate sodium restriction and various diuretics in the treatment of hypertension. Effects on potassium wastage and blood pressure control. *Arch. Intern. Med.*, 141:1015–1019.
84. Reisin, E., Frohlich, E. D., Messerli, F. H., Dreslinski, G. R., Dunn, F. G., Jones, M. M., and Bat-

son, H. M. (1983): Cardiovascular changes after weight reduction in obesity hypertension. *Ann. Intern. Med.*, 98:315–319.

85. Reubi, F. C., and Cottier, P. T. (1961): Effects of reduced glomerular filtration rate on responsiveness to chlorothiazide and mercurial diuretics. *Circulation*, 23:200–210.
86. Ridgeway, N. A., Ginn, D. R., and Alley, K. (1986): Outpatient conversion of treatment to potassium-sparing diuretics. *Am. J. Med.*, 80:785–788.
87. Rodriguez-Iturbe, B., Baggio, B., Colina-Chourio, J., Favaro, S., Garcia, R., Sussana, F., Castillo, L., and Borsatti, A. (1981): Studies on the renin-aldosterone system in the acute nephritic syndrome. *Kidney Int.*, 19:445–453.
88. Rose, B. D. (1984): *Clinical Physiology of Acid Base and Electrolyte Disorders*, 2d ed., Chapter 13. McGraw-Hill, New York.
89. Rose, B. D. (1984): *Clinical Physiology of Acid Base and Electrolyte Disorders*, 2d ed., Chapter 16. McGraw-Hill, New York.
90. Rose, B. D. (1986): A new approach to disturbances in the plasma sodium concentration. *Am. J. Med.*, 81:1033–1040.
91. Rose, B. D. (1987): *Pathophysiology of Renal Disease*, 2d ed., Chapters 10 and 11. McGraw-Hill, New York.
92. Sansom, S. C., and O'Neil, R. G. (1985): Mineralocorticoid regulation of apical cell membrane Na^+ and K^+ transport of the cortical collecting duct. *Am. J. Physiol.*, 248:F858–F868.
93. Schwartz, A. B., and Swartz, C. D. (1974): Dosage of potassium chloride to correct thiazide-induced hypokalemia. *JAMA*, 230:702–704.
94. Shah, S., Khatri, I., and Freis, E. D. (1978): Mechanism of antihypertensive effect of thiazide diuretics. *Am. Heart J.*, 95:611–618.
95. Shannon, H., Wei, J. Y., Rosa, R. M., Epstein, F. H., and Rowe, J. W. (1986): The effect of age and sodium depletion on cardiovascular response to orthostasis. *Hypertension*, 8:438–443.
96. Sorgel, F., Ettinger, B., and Benet, L. Z. (1985): The true composition of kidney stones passed during triamterene therapy. *J. Urol.*, 134:871–873.
97. Spence, J. D., Wong, D. G., and Lindsay, R. M. (1985): Effects of triamterene and amiloride on urinary sediment in hypertensive patients taking hydrochlorothiazide. *Lancet*, 2:73–75.
98. Steiness, E., and Waldorff, S. (1982): Different interactions of indomethacin and sulindac with thiazides in hypertension. *Br. Med. J.*, 285:1702–1703.
99. Stokes, J. B. (1984): Sodium chloride absorption by the urinary bladder of the winter flounder. A thiazide-sensitive electrically neutral transport system. *J. Clin. Invest.*, 74:7–16.
100. Stokes, J. B. (1985): Mineralocorticoid effect on K^+ permeability of the rabbit cortical collecting tubule. *Kidney Int.*, 28:640–645.
101. Struthers, A. D., Murphy, M. B., and Dollery, C. T. (1985): Glucose tolerance during antihypertensive therapy in patients with diabetes mellitus. *Hypertension*, 7(*Suppl.* II):II95–II101.
102. Struthers, A. D., Whitesmith, R., and Reid, J. L. (1983): Prior thiazide diuretic treatment increases adrenaline-induced hypokalaemia. *Lancet*, 1:1358–1360.
103. Suki, W., Rector, F. C., Jr., and Seldin, D. W. (1965): The site of action of furosemide and other sulfonamide diuretics in the dog. *J. Clin. Invest.*, 44:1458–1469.
104. Swales, J. D. (1982): Magnesium deficiency and diuretics. *Br. Med. J.*, 285:1377–1378.
105. Szatalowicz, V. L., Miller, P. D., Lacher, J. W., Gordon, J. A., and Schrier, R. W. (1982): Comparative effect of diuretics on renal water excretion in hyponatremic oedematous disorders. *Clin. Sci.*, 62:235–238.
106. Tarazi, R. C., Dustan, H. P., and Frohlich, E. D. (1970): Long-term thiazide therapy in essential hypertension. Evidence for persistent alteration in plasma volume and renin activity. *Circulation*, 41:709–717.
107. van Brummelen, P., Man in't Veld, A. J., and Schalekamp, M. A. D. H. (1980): Hemodynamic changes during long-term thiazide treatment of essential hypertension in responders and nonresponders. *Clin. Pharmacol. Ther.*, 27:328–336.
108. Vaughan, E. D., Jr., Carey, R. M., Peach, M. J., Ackerly, J. A., and Ayers, C. R. (1978): The renin response to diuretic therapy: A limitation of antihypertensive potential. *Circ. Res.*, 42:376–381.
109. Velasquez, H., and Wright, F. S. (1986): Effect of diuretic drugs on Na, Cl, and K transport by rat renal distal tubule. *Am. J. Physiol.*, 250:F1012–F1023.
110. Veterans Administration Cooperative Study Group on Antihypertensive Agents (1967): Effects of treatment on morbidity in hypertension: Results in patients with diastolic blood pressure averaging 115 through 129 mm Hg. *JAMA*, 202:1028–1034.
111. Veterans Administration Cooperative Study Group on Antihypertensive Agents (1970): Effects of treatment on morbidity in hypertension. II. Results in patients with diastolic blood pressure averaging 90 through 114 mm Hg. *JAMA*, 213:1143–1152.
112. Veterans Administration Cooperative Study Group on Antihypertensive Agents (1982): Captopril: Evaluation of low doses, twice-daily doses, and the addition of diuretic for the treatment of mild to moderate hypertension. *Clin. Sci.*, 63(*Suppl.* 8):443s–445s.
113. Veterans Administration Cooperative Study Group on Antihypertensive Agents (1982): Comparison of propanolol and hydrochlorothiazide for the initial treatment of hypertension. I. Results of short-term titration with emphasis on racial differences in response. *JAMA*, 248:1996–2003.
114. Veterans Administration Cooperative Study Group on Antihypertensive Agents (1982): Comparison of propranolol and hydrochlorothiazide for the initial treatment of hypertension. II. Results of long-term therapy. *JAMA*, 248:2004–2011.
115. Veterans Administration Cooperative Study Group on Antihypertensive Agents (1983): Efficacy of nadolol alone and combined with bendroflumethazide and hydralazine for systemic hypertension. *Am. J. Cardiol.*, 52:1230–1237.

116. Veterans Administration Cooperative Study Group on Antihypertensive Agents (1984): Low-dose captopril for the treatment of mild to moderate hypertension. I. Results of a 14-week trial. *Arch. Intern. Med.,* 144:1947–1953.
117. Veterans Administration Cooperative Study Group on Antihypertensive Agents (1985): Propranolol or hydrochlorothiazide alone for the treatment of hypertension. IV. Effect on plasma glucose and glucose tolerance. *Hypertension,* 7:1008–1016.
118. Watkins, J., Abbott, E. C., Hensby, C. N., Webster, J., and Dollery, C. T. (1980): Attenuation of hypotensive effect of propranolol and thiazide diuretics by indomethacin. *Br. Med. J.,* 281:702–705.
119. Weber, M. A., and Drayer, J. I. (1984): Single-agent and combination therapy of essential hypertension. *Am. Heart J.,* 108:311–316.
120. Weidmann, P., Beretta-Piccoli, C., Meier, A., Keusch, G., Gluck, Z., and Ziegler, W. H. (1983): Antihypertensive mechanism of diuretic treatment with chlorthalidone. Complementary roles of sympathetic axis and sodium. *Kidney Int.,* 23:320–326.
121. Weidmann, P., Gerber, A., and Mordasini, R. (1983): Effects of antihypertensive therapy on serum lipoproteins. *Hypertension,* 5(*Suppl.* III):III-120–III-131.
122. Weinberg, M. S., Quigg, R. J., Salant, D. J., and Bernard, D. B. (1985): Anuric renal failure precipitated by indomethacin and triamterene. *Nephron,* 40:216–218.
123. Weinberger, M. H. (1983): Influence of an angiotensin converting-enzyme inhibitor on diuretic induced metabolic effects in hypertension. *Hypertension,* 5(*Suppl.* III):III-132–III-138.
124. Weinberger, M. H. (1986): Antihypertensive therapy and lipids: Paradoxical influences on cardiovascular disease risk. *Am. J. Med.,* 80(Suppl. 2A):64–70.
125. Weiner, I. M., and Mudge, G. H. (1985): Diuretics and other agents employed in the mobilization of edema fluid. In: *Goodman and Gilman's The Pharmacological Basis of Therapeutics,* 7th ed., edited by A. G. Gilman, L. S. Goodman, T. W. Rall, and P. Murad, pp. 887–907. Macmillan, New York.
126. Wilkinson, P. R., Issler, H., Hesp, R., and Raftery, R. E. (1975): Total body and serum potassium during prolonged thiazide therapy for essential hypertension. *Lancet,* 1:759–762.
127. Wilson, I. M., and Freis, E. D. (1959): Relationship between plasma and extracellular fluid volume depletion and the anti-hypertensive effect of chlorothiazide. *Circulation,* 20:1028–1036.
128. Winer, B. M., Lubbe, W. F., and Colton, T. (1968): Antihypertensive actions of diuretics: Comparative study of an aldosterone antagonist and a thiazide, alone and together. *JAMA,* 204:775–779.
129. Wong, D. G., Spence, J. D., Lamki, L., Freeman, D., and McDonald, J. W. D. (1986): Effect of nonsteroidal anti-inflammatory drugs on control of hypertension by beta blockers and diuretics. *Lancet,* 1:997–1001.
130. Zambraski, E. J., Chremos, A. M., and Dunn, M. J. (1984): Comparison of the effects of sulindac with other cyclooxygenase inhibitors on prostaglandin production and renal function in normals and chronic bile duct ligated dogs and swine. *J. Pharmacol. Exp. Ther.,* 228:560–566.

The Kidney in Hypertension, edited by Norman M. Kaplan, Barry M. Brenner, and John H. Laragh. Raven Press, New York © 1987.

Hypertensive Crises

C. Venkata S. Ram

Department of Internal Medicine, University of Texas Health Science Center, Southwestern Medical School, Dallas, Texas 75235-9030

Hypertensive crises constitute a group of medical conditions in which rapid blood pressure reduction is indicated to prevent serious complications. Although relatively uncommon in clinical practice, a hypertensive crisis should be promptly recognized and treated. Any form of hypertension may be associated with the development of hypertensive crisis, the chief determinant being the level of blood pressure rather than the etiology of hypertension. In certain situations, the abruptness with which the blood pressure rises seems to be more important than the absolute level of blood pressure in causing the hypertensive crisis, e.g., acute onset of hypertension in children with acute glomerulonephritis, and toxemia of pregnancy. In some other clinical situations, immediate reduction in blood pressure is indicated not so much because of its absolute level but because certain coexisting complications may make even moderate hypertension dangerous, e.g., acute aortic dissection, acute left ventricular failure.

Hypertensive crises are categorized into emergencies and urgencies (Tables 1 and 2). Hypertensive emergencies are conditions with poor prognosis unless the blood pressure is reduced rapidly, whereas hypertensive urgencies are conditions with less immediate danger but may ultimately deteriorate into emergencies if the blood pressure is not vigorously controlled.

ACCELERATED/MALIGNANT HYPERTENSION

The main difference between uncomplicated and accelerated/malignant hypertension is the presence of acute vascular lesions affecting the kidney and other target organs in the latter. Accelerated hypertension is characterized by the presence of severe retinopathy without papilledema—but with exudates, hemorrhages, arteriolar narrowing, and spasm. Malignant hypertension presumably is an extension of the accelerated form and is distinguished by the presence of papilledema. Both the accelerated and malignant forms of hypertension are associated with clinical evidence of severe vascular injury to the kidney and other target organs (1). Prior to the availability of effective antihypertensive therapy, malignant hypertension ran a short, fulminating course culminating in renal failure and death (2,3). With modern antihypertensive therapy, however, the prognosis has improved, with more than 90% of the treated patients surviving more than 5 years, and there is no difference in the course of those with accelerated or malignant disease, suggesting that the two be considered all part of the same process (4).

Pathogenesis

A key unanswered question concerning accelerated/malignant hypertension is what transforms a previously stable hypertensive state to a "malignant" course. The level of blood pressure, although a critical feature, does not explain the onset of malignant hypertension, as there is considerable overlap between the blood pressure levels in groups of patients with nonmalignant and malignant hypertension. Alterations in various vasoactive mechanisms—renin-angiotensin (5), catecholamines (6), vasopressin (7), kal-

Table 1. *Hypertensive emergencies*

Hypertensive encephalopathy
Acute aortic dissection
Pulmonary edema
Pheochromocytoma crisis
MAO[a] inhibitor + tyramine interaction
Intracranial hemorrhage
Eclampsia

[a]Monoamine oxidase.

likrein-kinin system (8), and hemostasis (9)—have been implicated in the genesis of malignant hypertension. Although there is no convincing evidence to link the vascular lesions of malignant hypertension to any of these derangements, renin-angiotensin levels are frequently high in malignant hypertension. The arteriolar lesions responsible for the clinical manifestations and course of malignant hypertension are found in many organs, including kidney, brain, heart, intestine, and pancreas (10,11).

The consequence of obstructive vascular lesions is a decrease in perfusion to the affected organs, with the kidney bearing the brunt of the damage. Two different renal lesions have been described in malignant hypertension: proliferative arteritis and fibrinoid necrosis. The combination of lesions is also referred to as hyperplastic arteritis, fibrinoid intimal hyperplasia, and musculomucoid intimal hyperplasia. Fibrinoid necrosis presumably results from the leakage of fibrin and other plasma elements into the arteriolar wall, resulting in obstruction, thus compromising the function of the organ involved—usually the kidney (12). The precise link between the blood pressure level and arteriolar lesions is not clearly established. It has been suggested that vascular permeability increases as a result of alternating contracted and dilated segments in the arterial vessels, and with the treatment of hypertension, these abnormal contractions and dilations are eliminated (1,13). A number of studies have demonstrated that the treatment of hypertension arrests or even reverses the arteriolar damage and paves the way for functional recovery.

What triggers the inappropriate and sustained release of renin in malignant hypertension? One hypothesis postulates an initial spontaneous sodium loss as the most likely cause (14,15). In experimental malignant hypertension, the lumen of the efferent renal arteriole remains unchanged, whereas the caliber of the afferent arteriole increases in size. Angiotensin sensitivity is enhanced in the afferent arteriole, whereas the efferent arteriole shows an increased sensitivity to both norepinephrine and angiotensin. This differential increases intraglomerular pressure and promotes natriuresis, which in turn stimulates the release of renin, vasopressin, the norepinephrine—and sets the vicious circle in motion. Initial weight loss, a phenomenon observed in malignant hypertension, may be due to the loss of salt and water (2,16). The course of malignant hypertension has been slowed down experimentally (17) and clinically (18) by administering a saline load. It appears, therefore, that the renin-angiotensin system may play an important role in the pathogenesis of most malignant hypertension. The renin-angiotensin system is obviously also involved in those whose hypertension is caused by renovascular disease. In one series, renal artery stenosis was detected in 35% of 123 patients with malignant hypertension (19). Cigarette smoking (20), immunological changes (21), and oral contraceptives (22,23) have also been implicated in the development of malignant hypertension.

Table 2. *Hypertensive urgencies*

Hypertension associated with coronary artery disease
Accelerated and malignant hypertension[a]
Severe hypertension in the kidney transplant patient
Postoperative hypertension
Uncontrolled hypertension in the patient who requires emergency surgery

[a]This condition is categorized as either hypertensive emergency or urgency.

Clinical Manifestations

Although the blood pressure in malignant hypertension is usually quite high, with diastolic levels often greater than 130 to 140 mm Hg, the height of the blood pressure alone is not the diagnostic criterion; it is the extent of vascular damage that determines the clinical picture and course. Headache with or without coexisting encephalopathy is the most common symptom that brings the patient to medical attention. Typically, the headache is occipital in location and more intense in the morning hours. Weight loss, as discussed earlier, may be prominent in some patients with malignant hypertension as a result of salt and water loss. A majority of patients with malignant hypertension report visual symptoms. Although blurring of vision is the most common complaint, temporary or permanent blindness can occur sometimes. Drowsiness and altered mental status are common in malignant hypertension and worsening of these symptoms may indicate progression to encephalopathy or cerebral hemorrhage.

Congestive heart failure can occur in patients with malignant hypertension as a direct consequence of left ventricular dysfunction or due to volume retention from associated renal insufficiency. Azotemia is one of the consistent features of malignant hypertension and may be associated with proteinuria. Without proper treatment, renal function deteriorates rapidly. Even with treatment, renal function may decline temporarily due to reduced renal perfusion. Although hypertension can result from chronic renal disease, renal failure in patients with malignant hypertension is a result rather than the cause of severe hypertension.

Anemia is a common finding in malignant hypertension. The degree of anemia may give a clue as to the proximate cause: Severe anemia suggests underlying chronic renal disease, whereas modest degrees may reflect microangiopathic hemolysis.

The diagnosis of accelerated/malignant hypertension can be made at the bedside on the basis of history and clinical examination. Simple investigations such as a chest X-ray, electrocardiogram, complete blood count, blood urea nitrogen, creatinine, electrolytes, and urinalysis are sufficient for the initial management of malignant hypertension.

Management

Patients with accelerated/malignant hypertension should be treated in the hospital, as the goal is not just to lower the blood pressure but to exclude reversible causes and monitor, stabilize, and reverse the damage to target organs. Ideally, the patients should be treated in an intensive care unit. However, those without significant target organ damage can be managed safely on the wards.

Although sodium restriction was successfully used to treat malignant hypertension three decades ago (24), sodium wasting, as discussed earlier, may be a feature of this condition. Therefore, sodium restriction is not necessary during the early treatment unless there is fluid overload. Similarly, the need for diuretic therapy must be individualized. Diuretic therapy may be needed to potentiate the hypotensive effects of potent vasodilators such as nitroprusside, diazoxide, and hydralazine; therefore, it is a common clinical practice to coadminister intravenous furosemide with these drugs.

Sodium nitroprusside is the drug of choice for immediate reduction of the blood pressure. The details of its use will be discussed later in this chapter. Thiocyanate, a product of nitroprusside metabolism, accumulates in patients with renal failure, and thiocyanate toxicity can occur in patients receiving high or prolonged infusions of nitroprusside. This is not a practical problem in patients receiving nitroprusside for periods less than 48–72 hr. Prompt reduction in blood pressure can also be accomplished by bolus injections or slow infusions of diazoxide or labetalol. Trimethapan has been found advantageous in patients with acute aortic dissection by virtue of its ability to decrease the force and velocity of left ventricular contraction. Once the blood pressure is stabilized, oral medications should be started.

Although parenteral therapy is widely used in the initial treatment of malignant hypertension, various oral therapies can also be successfully used. Captopril, minoxidil, clonidine, prazosin, labetalol, and nifedipine have all been used for initial treatment of malignant hypertension. The choice between oral and parenteral therapy depends on the treatment facility, condition of the patient, and coexisting complications.

Once the blood pressure is stabilized, long-term therapy must be initiated with appropriate agent(s) based on the renal, cardiac, and neurological status of the patient.

HYPERTENSIVE ENCEPHALOPATHY

Hypertensive encephalopathy is a serious, reversible complication of severe hypertension. Although encephalopathy occurs mainly in patients with malignant hypertension, it can also complicate acute hypertension of short duration. Despite its rarity, hypertensive encephalopathy should be quickly recognized and effectively treated, since it has a poor prognosis if untreated but is rapidly reversible with proper treatment. The clinical manifestations of hypertensive encephalopathy are precipitated by either the abrupt onset of hypertension in a previously normotensive individual (e.g., acute glomerulonephritis) or, more commonly, by poorly controlled chronic hypertension. Hypertensive encephalopathy occurs more frequently when the hypertension is complicated by renal insufficiency than when kidney function is normal (25).

The pathogenesis of hypertensive encephalopathy has been extensively studied, with divergent opinions. Normally, cerebral blood flow (CBF) remains relatively constant despite wide variations in systemic blood pressure. This constancy is accomplished by autoregulation of the CBF; by this process in the face of severe elevation in systemic blood pressure, cerebral arterioles constrict; with a fall in blood pressure, they dilate to maintain adequate CBF. In hypertensive encephalopathy, cerebral autoregulation is deranged such that CBF is adversely affected. It was originally proposed that in hypertensive encephalopathy, there is overregulation of cerebral circulation resulting in ischemia (26). Subsequent experimental work, however, suggested that hypertensive encephalopathy results not from overregulation but from a failure of vasoconstriction or a breakthrough of circulatory response, with a consequent increase in CBF, which results in cerebral edema (27). Which of these explanations is correct is immaterial in the management of hypertensive encephalopathy, as the syndrome resolves with prompt treatment irrespective of what the underlying pathogenetic mechanism may be.

Clinical Features

Salient manifestations of hypertensive encephalopathy are shown in Table 3. Severe, generalized headache is the usual initial clinical manifestation. Altered neurological function characterized by confusion, somnolence, and stupor may appear with or following the onset of headache. If the condition is not treated, progressive clouding of the sensorium occurs culminating in coma and death. Most patients are restless during the initial stages of the syndrome. Other clinical features may include projectile vomiting, visual disturbances ranging from blurring to frank blindness, and transient focal neurological deficits. Sometimes, especially in children, generalized or local seizures may dominate the clinical picture (28).

On clinical examination, the blood pressure is invariably elevated, but there is no arbitrary level of blood pressure above which encephalopathy is likely to occur. The fundi reveal arteriolar spasm with exudates/hemorrhages. Although papilledema is present in most patients with this complication, its absence does not exclude the diagnosis of hypertensive encephalopathy.

Diagnosis

When a patient with poorly controlled hypertension presents with severe headache, altered mental status, papilledema, and variable neurological deficits, the most likely diagnosis is hypertensive encephalopathy. Hypertensive

Table 3. *Clinical features of hypertensive encephalopathy*

Marked elevation of BP
Headache
Nausea, vomiting
Papilledema
Visual complaints
Transient neurological deficits (seizures)
Altered mental status, confusion

encephalopathy must be distinguished from other acute neurological complications of hypertension, such as cerebral infarction or hemorrhage and uremic encephalopathy (29). Meticulous evaluation of the patient should be carried out to consider these differential diagnoses. Finally, the possibility of reflex elevation of systemic blood pressure due to cerebral ischemia should be entertained in the differential diagnosis, as ischemia to the brainstem may reflexly increase the systemic blood pressure. The only definitive criterion to confirm the diagnosis of hypertensive encephalopathy is a prompt favorable response of the patient's condition to antihypertensive therapy.

Management

Once the diagnosis of hypertensive encephalopathy is made, the blood pressure should be lowered quickly to near normal levels. Rapid reduction in the blood pressure produces prompt and dramatic relief of symptoms of hypertensive encephalopathy. The patient should be preferably treated in an intensive care unit in order to monitor the response to therapy. The most important aspect of therapy is to prevent permanent neurological damage. The most useful and dependable drug in this situation is sodium nitroprusside. Specific details concerning this and other antihypertensive agents are discussed elsewhere. Although potent orally effective agents such as minoxidil, nifedipine, or captopril can control severe hypertension, parenteral drugs are preferred in treating a potentially lethal condition such as hypertensive encephalopathy.

Severe Hypertension With Cerebrovascular Accidents

A patient presenting with acute stroke and severe hypertension poses a therapeutic dilemma. When intracerebral pressure rises as a result of hemorrhage or thrombotic infarction, CBF may no longer be under normal autoregulation. Therefore, a reduction in the systemic blood pressure may conceivably further compromise CBF. On the other hand, persistent severe hypertension may worsen the stroke. In many patients with acute stroke, initial hypertension may resolve spontaneously within 48 hr (30). The need for blood pressure reduction in this setting should be individualized on the basis of the clinical course. If antihypertensive therapy is warranted, agents with short and rapid onset of action are to be preferred, so that harmful effects of a lower blood pressure can be reversed. Although there are no guidelines concerning the standard approach in managing these patients, drastic blood pressure reduction should be avoided. A safe therapeutic goal is to bring the diastolic level to no less than 100 mm Hg. Such a controlled reduction in blood pressure can only be accomplished with nitroprusside. Drugs with central mechanism of action, such as reserpine, clonidine, and methyldopa, should be avoided, as they may interfere with neurological evaluation of the patient.

ACUTE AORTIC DISSECTION

Hypertension is an important predisposing factor to the development of acute aortic dissection. The mortality from acute aortic dissection results not from the intimal tear itself but rather from the course taken by the dissecting hematoma, which may rupture anywhere along the aorta or which may obliterate blood supply to a major organ. Therefore, therapy should be implemented promptly, as soon as possible after the appearance of tear in order to arrest the disease. Aggressive and immediate treatment of hypertension is essential to the survival of the patient and to permit surgical treatment if needed.

Severe, persistent chest or abdominal pain is the most common symptom of acute aortic dissection. The precise location and radiation of the pain depends on the site and extent of the dissecting process. Hemoptysis, orthopnea, and dyspnea are sometimes present in patients with dissection of the thoracic aorta. Signs such as sudden loss of pulse in an extremity of sudden appearance of a new diastolic murmur should signal the possibility of acute dissection. Syncope, paralysis, and blindness may occur as a result of dissections involving the carotid and innominate vessels. Dissection of the abdominal aorta may cause a variety of gastrointestinal and genitourinary disturbances.

Diagnosis

The diagnosis of acute aortic dissection should be suspected in hypertensive patients with abrupt onset of pain, pulse deficits, and signs of circulatory compromise to a major organ (31). Obviously one has to consider in the differential diagnosis acute entities such as myocardial infarction, pulmonary embolism, cerebrovascular accidents, and surgical abdomen. The diagnosis is made by computed tomography or echocardiography and confirmed by digital or standard angiography.

Management

Initial management of both proximal and distal dissections should include measures to reduce the blood pressure and to relieve the pain. Once the patient's condition is stabilized, definitive therapy is undertaken. For most patients with proximal dissection (type I and II, class A) and for some with distal dissection (type II, class B), surgical repair of the aortic dissection and associated complications such as aortic regurgitation is indicated.

If the patient is hypertensive, blood pressure should be reduced rapidly to the lowest level tolerated by the patient, keeping in mind that the force and velocity of ventricular contraction (*dp*/*dt*) and the pulsatile flow determine the shearing force acting on the aortic wall (32). Therefore, blood pressure reduction should be accomplished with drugs that decrease, not increase, the *dp*/*dt*. In this context, trimethaphan, a ganglion blocking agent, is a rational choice, since it produces prompt and smooth reduction in the blood pressure to a desired level while blunting the sharpness of the pulse wave generated by the heart (33). The same goal can be achieved by the use of sodium nitroprusside and beta-blocker therapy. Drugs that stimulate the heart, e.g., diazoxide and hydralazine, should be avoided because of their adverse hemodynamic actions. Stated simply, medical management of acute aortic dissection should encompass the rational use of antihypertensive drugs that "sedate," not "whip," the heart. Once the blood pressure and clinical status of the patients are stabilized, definitive therapy (surgical or medical) should be planned without undue delay. Although the presenting manifestations of acute aortic dissection are ominous, the prospect of salvaging most patients warrants aggressive medical and surgical therapy.

ACUTE LEFT VENTRICULAR FAILURE

Acute left ventricular failure (pulmonary edema) in a hypertensive patient is an indication for prompt blood pressure reduction. The higher the blood pressure, the harder the ventricule must work. Therefore, decreasing the workload of the failing myocardium by reducing the systemic blood pressure improves the pump action of the heart. A failing heart demonstrates an increased end-diastolic fiber length, increased ventricular volume, and a reduced ejection fraction—factors that increase myocardial oxygen requirements. This could be particularly deleterious in patients with coexistent coronary artery disease. Prompt reduction of blood pressure with a balanced vasodilating agent such as nitroprusside is indicated in this circumstance (34). Sodium nitroprusside decreases both the pre- and afterload with restoration of myocardial function and cardiac output. Drugs that increase the cardiac work, such as hydralazine and diazoxide, should be avoided. Along with the treatment of hypertension, other measures for managing pulmonary edema should be instituted.

SEVERE HYPERTENSION ASSOCIATED WITH ISCHEMIC HEART DISEASE

Systemic hypertension increases myocardial oxygen consumption by increasing intraventricular pressure and left ventricular diameter. Patients with myocardial infarction and severe hypertension should therefore theoretically benefit from blood pressure reduction, but there are no conclusive data to prove that treatment is beneficial. Reduction of systemic blood pressure reduces the cardiac work, wall tension, and oxygen demand and may thus limit myocardial necrosis in the early phase of infarction (35). However, there are conflicting data in the literature about the value of reducing blood pressure (to reduce infarct size) in the absence of pulmonary congestion. Although hypertension usually precedes the onset of chest pain, a marked rise in blood pressure may follow the onset of coronary insufficiency. Therefore, an acute elevation of blood pressure in the setting of acute myocardial infarction may be transient and not harmful (36), but has been observed to increase the mortality rate and the incidence of cardiac failure in patients with severe systolic hypertension and acute myocardial infarction (37).

Reduction of systemic arterial pressure early in the course of acute myocardial infarction has been shown to protect the myocardium, as reflected by reduced release of CPK enzyme activity (35). Cautious treatment of hypertension in patients with acute myocardial infarction is therefore likely to be beneficial. Of the parenteral agents, sodium nitroprusside is widely used. Diazoxide should be avoided in this situation because of its adverse hemodynamic effects. It must be emphasized that the degree of blood pressure reduction should depend solely on the demonstration of beneficial hemodynamic response obtained in a given patient, and not on any predetermined level. Aortic diastolic pressure is a major determinant of coronary blood flow, and unnecessary reductions in the blood pressure could compromise an already critical situation.

MISCELLANEOUS CONDITIONS

Pheochromocytoma Crisis

Pheochromocytoma crisis presents with striking clinical features. Typically, the blood pressure is markedly elevated during the paroxysm, and the patient may have profound sweating, marked tachycardia, pallor (especially of the face), numbness, tingling, and coldness of the feet and hands. A single attack will last from a few minutes to hours and may occur as often as several times a day to once a month or less.

If pheochromocytoma is suspected, the alpha-adrenergic blocking drug, phentolamine, should be given in the dose of 5 to 10 mg intravenously, to be repeated in a few minutes if needed. An alternative to phentolamine would be sodium nitroprusside, but the former is more specific. A beta-blocking drug may be useful if the patient has a concomitant cardiac arrhythmia. Administration of beta-blocking agents should always be preceded by either phentolamine or phenoxybenzamine. If this is not done, beta-blockade can aggravate the unopposed alpha-mediated peripheral vasoconstriction. Labetalol, a combined alpha- and beta-receptor blocking drug, has also been successfully used in this condition.

Clonidine Withdrawal Syndrome

A syndrome mimicking pheochromocytoma crisis has been reported following abrupt discontinuation of the antihypertensive drug, clonidine (38). Clonidine exerts its antihypertensive effect by stimulating the alpha receptors in the brainstem, thus reducing peripheral sympathetic activity. When clonidine is abruptly discontinued, or even sometimes rapidly tapered, a specific syndrome has been noted with nausea, palpitations, anxiety, sweating, nervousness, and headache—along with marked elevation of the blood pressure. In some patients the blood pressure rises beyond the pretreatment level. The probable mechanism of the clonidine withdrawal syndrome is a sudden resurgence of sympathetic activity. The incidence of this peculiar syndrome is quite low, and in some there is only a rapid return of blood pressure toward the pretreatment level rather than an overshoot (39).

Symptoms of clonidine withdrawal can be relieved by reinstitution of clonidine. If there is marked elevation of blood pressure and the patient is experiencing severe and annoying symptoms—such as palpitations, chest discomfort, epigastric discomfort—intravenous administration of phentolamine or labetalol is recommended.

Hypertensive Crisis Associated with Drug and Food Interactions: Monoamine Oxidase Inhibitors

Patients receiving monoamine oxidase (MAO) inhibitors are at a risk of developing hypertensive crisis if they should also take drugs such as ephedrine or amphetamines, or foods containing high quantities of tyramine. In the presence of an inhibitor of MAO, tyramine and indirectly acting sympathetic amines escape oxidative degradation, enter the systemic circulation, and potentiate the actions of catecholamines. Sympathomimetic amines such as those contained in nonprescription cold remedies can also provoke this response.

The hypertensive attack occurs from 1 to 2 hr after intake of the offending agent, with an abrupt onset, and sometimes lasts up to several hours. Characteristically, the patient feels acutely ill with headache, sweating, and palpitations, and the blood pressure is often elevated to alarming levels. Manifestations of food/drug interaction with MAO inhibitors closely resemble those of pheochromocytoma. Immediate treatment is similar for both conditions.

Hypertensive Crisis in the Postoperative Period

Open heart operations and surgical manipulation of the carotid artery are sometimes followed by severe hypertension in the immediate postoperative period. Hypertension, even of moderate degree, may jeopardize the integrity of the vascular suture lines, so that it should be managed promptly with parenteral agents. Sodium nitroprusside is usually the agent of choice, though nerve blocks and other drugs may be effective.

Hypertensive Crisis in Quadriplegic Patients

Hypertensive crises have been reported in patients with transverse lesions of the spinal cord, usually above the origins of the thoracolumbar sympathetic neurons (40). Stimulation of dermatomes and muscles supplied by nerves below the injury may evoke severe hypertension, profound headache, and bradycardia. The blood pressure crisis is the result of excessive stimulation of sympathetic neurons, and the associated bradycardia is probably due to the excitation of the baroreceptor reflexes. Given the pathophysiological basis for such hypertensive reactions, these critical blood pressure elevations can be prevented by avoiding excessive stimulation of the susceptible portion of the dermatomes. Treatment is dictated by the severity of hypertension and the status of target organ function.

Hypertension Associated with Head Injury

Patients with head injury may present with marked elevation of blood pressure. The mechanism is likely complex, but may involve the medullary vasomotor centers, which, when rendered ischemic, may reflexly elevate the blood pressure. Increased intracranial pressure *per se* may induce certain cardiovascular changes resulting in hypertension. The dilemma is whether or not to lower the blood pressure under such circumstances. The same principles apply as discussed under the section dealing with cerebrovascular accidents.

Hypertensive Crisis Due to Systemic Vasculitis

Abrupt onset of severe hypertension has been known to occur as a complication of necrotizing vasculitis (41,42). The mechanism of hypertension has not been clearly delineated. Possible mechanisms include a direct increase in peripheral vascular resistance as a result of vasculitis, or as a result of activation of the renin-angiotensin system. Acute necrotizing vasculitis should be considered in young patients who develop hypertensive crisis.

Hypertensive Crisis Induced by Metoclopramide

This condition has been reported in previously normotensive subjects (43,44) and in patients with pheochromocytoma (45,46). The exact mechanism by which metoclopramide, a dopamine agonist, causes a hypertensive response is not known. It could sensitize the vascular endothelium to the pressor effects of catecholamines or cause a release of catecholamines from the adrenal medulla or adrenergic neurons.

MANAGEMENT OF HYPERTENSIVE CRISES

Patients with hypertensive crisis should be hospitalized. Whether or not they should be treated in the intensive care unit depends on the level of blood pressure and the extent of associated complications. Acute treatment of hypertension should be implemented with careful monitoring of blood pressure, cardiac, renal, and neurological functions. Drugs that can be administered parenterally to reduce the blood pressure are shown in Table 4. A major consideration in treating patients with hypertensive emergencies is the rapidity of onset and duration of action of the drug given. The physician must be aware of the pharmacological and hemodynamic actions of the drug to be used, since the aim is not just to lower the blood pressure but to do so with minimal adverse effects.

Parenteral Agents

Nitroprusside

Sodium nitroprusside is the most potent and valuable drug for the treatment of hypertensive crisis. Its hypotensive response occurs within seconds after infusion is started and disappears

Table 4. *Drugs for hypertensive emergencies*

Drug	Route and dose	Onset	Duration	Comments
Parenteral therapy				
Nitroprusside	i.v. infusion 0.25 8 μg/kg/min	Seconds	3–5 min	Thiocyanate toxicity may occur with prolonged (>48 hr) or high dose infusion (>15 μg/kg/min) (particularly in renal insufficiency)
Diazoxide	i.v. 50–150 mg q 5 min or as infusion of 7.5–30 mg/min	1–5 min	4–24 hr	Should not be used for patients with angina pectoris, myocardial infarction, dissecting aneurysm
Trimethaphan	i.v. infusion pump 0.5–5 mg/min	1–5 min	10 min	Drug of choice for treatment of aortic dissection
Labetalol	i.v. 2 mg/min or 20 mg q 10 min (can go to 80 mg doses); max cumulative dose 300 mg	5 min or less	3–6 hr	Prompt response. Can be followed by same drug taken orally
Hydralazine	i.m./i.v. 10–20 mg	10–30 min	2–4 hr	May precipitate angina, myocardial infarction
Acute oral therapy				
Nifedipine	10–20 mg p.o. or sublingual	5–15 min	3–5 hr	Generally good response. Short duration of action. Optimal dosage not standardized
Clonidine	p.o. 0.2 mg initial then 0.1 mg/hr, up to 0.8 mg total	$\frac{1}{2}$–2 hr	6–8 hr	Prominent sedation
Captopril	p.o. 6.5–25 mg	15 min	4–6 hr	Generally good, sometimes excessive response
Minoxidil	p.o. 5–10 mg	30–60 min	12–16 hr	Tachycardia, fluid retention.

almost as rapidly when the infusion is discontinued. Nitroprusside relaxes both the arteries and the veins, reducing systemic arterial and venous pressures along with systemic and pulmonary vascular resistances. The exact mechanism by which nitroprusside dilates the vasculature has not been firmly established. The cardiac output response is variable and depends on the preexisting hemodynamic status of the patient. In patients not in congestive heart failure, cardiac output usually falls; in patients with low output states, cardiac output consistently increases (47).

Because of its rapid onset of action and potency, nitroprusside infusion must be closely monitored by means of an infusion pump or a microdrop regulator, and intraarterial blood pressure recording. A safe initial dose is 0.3 μg/kg/min, and this can be increased every 5 min until the desired blood pressure level is obtained.

Once the desired effect of nitroprusside is achieved, the infusion usually can be maintained with minimal adjustment, but the blood pressure should be continuously monitored. Parenteral treatment of hypertensive crisis generally is needed for 12 to 48 hr, and the drug should be discontinued as soon as alternative modes of therapy have proven effective. Because of its short duration of action, the effects of stopping the therapy will be seen within a few minutes. If indicated, treatment can be resumed promptly. Hypotension is the most common side effect of nitroprusside therapy, a consequence of inadequate regulation of the infusion rate.

The immediate metabolic product of nitroprusside is cyanide, which is liberated by the direct combination of nitroprusside with the sulfhydryl groups in red cells and tissues. The circulating cyanide is rapidly converted in the liver to thiocyanate by the enzyme rhodanase or transsulfarase, which in turn is removed almost exclusively by the kidney with a half-life of approximately 1 week.

Cyanide toxicity from nitroprusside, although extremely rare, has occurred. Prophylactic infusion of hydroxycobalamin (Vit B_{12a}), 25 mg/hr, has been shown to decrease the cyanide concentration and tissue hypoxia resulting from nitroprusside infusion during surgery (47). Hydroxycobalamin has one cyanide radical less than cyanocobalamin and, therefore, allows cyanide to combine and form cyanocobalamin, which is then excreted in the urine.

Thiocyanate toxicity secondary to nitroprusside is uncommon and occurs only with high doses and in the presence of renal failure. Symptoms of thiocyanate toxicity include fatigue, nausea, anorexia, skin rashes, headaches, disorientation, and psychotic behavior. They tend to occur at plasma levels of 5 to 10 mg/dl, and levels greater than 20 mg/dl are dangerous. Therefore, during high-dose infusions of nitroprusside—and especially when renal function is impaired—periodic determinations of plasma thiocyanate levels are recommended; treatment should be interrupted when the thiocyanate level is close to 10 mg/dl. Monitoring of plasma thiocyanate levels is not mandatory as long as the patient's clinical status is closely assessed. Treatment of thiocyanate toxicity demands discontinuation of the drug and institution of dialysis.

Trimethaphan

Trimethaphan camsylate is a ganglion blocking agent. The hypotensive effect of trimethaphan is accompanied by a reduction in left ventricular ejection rate and cardiac output. These attributes make it a drug of choice for the medical treatment of acute aortic dissection. A rise in cardiac output may be seen in hypertensive patients with congestive heart failure, reflecting a reduction in the venous return induced by this drug, a property it shares with sodium nitroprusside. Trimethaphan has a rapid onset of action and its effects dissipate within a few minutes of discontinuation of the drug. The head of the bed should be elevated to augment the antihypertensive effect of this agent. Like nitroprusside, trimethaphan should be administered as a continuous intravenous drip, and constant monitoring is necessary, preferably in the intensive care unit. The usual starting dose of the drug should be 1 mg/min, titrated to obtain the desired blood pressure level. After prolonged infusion, tachphylaxis may result from intravascular volume expansion, which can be partially overcome by effective diuretic therapy.

The major disadvantage of trimethaphan is that it causes parasympathetic inhibition resulting in paralytic ileus, urinary retention, and mydriasis. These effects are particularly likely to occur when the drug is administered for more than a day or two. It is also recommended that the patient's respiratory status be monitored closely—particularly if large doses of trimethaphan are used—because of the remote possibility of respiratory depression by this drug.

Diazoxide

Diazoxide is a benzothiadizine derivative which, when given intravenously, has a direct relaxant effect on the vascular smooth muscle, causing a rapid fall in arterial blood pressure. The hypotensive effect of diazoxide is associated with striking increases in heart rate and cardiac output. Diazoxide has no effect on the capacitance vessels, and therefore the venous return to the heart is not impeded. Consequently there is an increase in cardiac output, which, in turn, may partly counteract the hypotensive effect of diazoxide (48).

Diazoxide has no direct effect on the myocardium, but reflex increases in the cardiac output and heart rate may pose a problem to patients with intrinsic cardiac disease. Expansion of plasma volume and edema formation occur during diazoxide therapy, partly because of its direct tubular antinatriuretic action.

Intravenous administration of diazoxide produces a rapid fall in blood pressure within 1 min, and the maximum effect is achieved within 2 to 5 min. The hypotensive effect of a single injection of diazoxide may last for 3 to 15 hr, but if there is no effect from the first injection, an additional dose can be given within 30 min. The previously recommended dose of diazoxide was 300 mg or 5 mg/kg given as a rapid intravenous injection. To be maximally effective, the dose should be injected rapidly—within 10 to 30 sec—to overcome protein binding of the drug.

Rapid injection of this relatively large single dose may cause hypotension with resultant myocardial and cerebral ischemia. Smaller bolus injections (49) and slow intravenous infusions (50) of diazoxide for the treatment of severe hypertension have been used in the hope of reducing the dangers of drastic and precipitous reduction in blood pressure. On the basis of these studies, it is suggested that minibolus injections of diazoxide (i.e., 50 mg given every 5 min) or 20- to 30-min infusions of 15 to 30 mg per minute can be effective in rapidly controlling severe hypertension while providing the advantage of ease of administration and relative freedom from side effects.

The most common side effects reported with diazoxide include nausea, vomiting, abdominal discomfort, sodium and water retention, and a sensation of warmth along the vein. The excessive hypotensive effect of diazoxide is particularly likely in patients who have had prior antihypertensive therapy.

To counteract fluid retention, 40 or 80 mg of furosemide must be given intravenously. The hyperglycemic effect of diazoxide rarely needs therapy, but blood glucose levels should be monitored—particularly in patients with impaired carbohydrate metabolism and with repeated injections of diazoxide.

Diazoxide is a powerful relaxant of uterine smooth muscle and may arrest labor when used in hypertensive crisis of eclampsia, but this inhibitory effect on the uterus can be easily reversed with oxytocin. The other important side effects of diazoxide include tachycardia and palpitations, which can be controlled by administration of a beta-adrenergic blocking agent such as propranolol.

Hydralazine Hydrochloride

The hypotensive action of hydralazine results from a direct relaxation of the vascular smooth muscle and is accompanied by reflex increases in stroke volume and heart rate, which can precipitate angina pectoris. Intramuscular or intravenous administration of hydralazine results in unpredictable but definite fall in blood pressure.

In the treatment of hypertensive emergencies, the initial dose should be 10 to 20 mg. The onset of the hypotensive effect occurs within 10 to 30 min and duration of action ranges from 3 to 9 hr. The dose and frequency of administration necessary to control the blood pressure are highly variable. The delayed onset and unpredictable degree of hypotensive effect present difficulties in titration. Nevertheless, hydralazine continues to be successfully employed in the treatment of severe hypertension—especially eclampsia. The sodium and water retention that occur with the use of this direct vasodilator can be overcome by the use of diuretic, and the reflex increases in the cardiac output and heart rate can be minimized by the administration of a beta-adrenergic blocking agent.

Labetalol

Labetalol is a combined alpha- plus beta-blocking drug that can be given parenterally (51,52) or orally (53) for the treatment of hypertensive crises. Intravenous labetalol administered in bolus injections or as slow infusion produces a prompt fall in blood pressure without inducing tachycardia. Patients treated with parenteral labetalol can be subsequently given the oral form for long-term management of hypertension. Due to its dual adrenergic blocking properties, labetalol is particularly indicated for acute treatment of hypertension associated with increased circulating catecholamines, e.g., pheochromocytoma, drug withdrawal hypertension, etc. It should be avoided in patients with congestive heart failure.

Phentolamine

Phentolamine, an alpha-receptor blocking agent, is specifically indicated for treating hypertensive crises associated with increased circulating catecholamines, e.g., pheochromocytoma crisis, certain cases of clonidine withdrawal syndrome, and crises resulting from MAO inhibitor and drug-food interaction. The hypotensive effect of a single intravenous bolus injection is short-lived and lasts less than 15 min.

Nitroglycerin

Nitroglycerin predominantly dilates the venous capacitance vessels, but higher infusion rates cause arterial dilation. Although there are no comparative data, nitroglycerin infusion may be particularly helpful in patients with severe hypertension with concomitant coronary artery disease (54).

Orally Effective Drugs

Certain orally effective antihypertensive drugs lower the blood pressure promptly and are useful in the management of hypertensive urgencies. Clinical experience suggests that these orally effective drugs can be conveniently used to lower the blood pressure in situations where parenteral drugs have been used in the past (55).

Minoxidil

This agent is a powerful direct vasodilator and has been successfully used in the treatment of refractory or severe hypertension. Because of its relatively rapid onset of action and sustained duration, this drug has been used for the treatment of hypertensive crises (56,57). Minoxidil in doses ranging from 2.5 to 10 mg can be given every 4 to 6 hr initially in the treatment of severe hypertension. It works best when given along with a diuretic, and an adrenergic blocker is necessary to counteract the reflex tachycardia.

Oral Clonidine

Clonidine, when given in incremental doses, has been shown to cause appreciable reduction in the blood pressure of patients presenting with severe hypertension (58). Although this form of therapy may be convenient, sedative effects of clonidine may alter the neurological function of patients presenting with severe hypertension.

Nifedipine

Nifedipine, a calcium channel blocker, given orally or sublingually, has been shown to reduce the blood pressure rapidly and may have an important place in the management of hypertensive crisis (59,60). Its major advantages are rapid onset of action and lack of CNS depression. It may cause reflex tachycardia. Since the duration of action of nifedipine is short, patients who receive this drug for hypertensive emergencies should be monitored for several hours to consider readministration of the drug. Nifedipine is an excellent choice for the management of hypertensive urgencies. For sublingual use, the capsule should be punctured and placed under the tongue for the content to be absorbed. If the patient can take oral medications, nifedipine can be given orally with equally satisfactory response. In contrast to clonidine therapy, nifedipine has been shown to preserve or increase CBF (61).

Converting Enzyme Inhibitors

Captopril, a converting enzyme inhibitor, has been found to be effective in the treatment of hypertensive crises (62). Captopril lowers the blood pressure promptly without causing tachycardia, and thus offers a distinct hemodynamic advantage over direct arteriolar dilators. High-renin states such as malignant hypertension associated with scleroderma renal crisis are particularly responsive to captopril (63). Enalaprilat, an intravenous converting enzyme inhibitor, has also been found to be effective in the treatment of hypertensive crises (64). Volume-depleted patients merit closer surveillance, as converting enzyme inhibition in this setting may cause profound hypotension.

Problems With Therapy

Renal Function

Accelerated/malignant hypertension and hypertensive encephalopathy are common in patients seen with the background of renal insufficiency. Effective control of hypertension under such circumstances may result in transient deterioration of renal function, and temporary dialysis may sometimes be necessary (65,66). Long-term treatment, however, is likely to stabilize or even improve renal function (67–69).

Cerebral Function and Effects of Acute Antihypertensive Therapy

Normally CBF is maintained within a safe margin despite wide variations in systemic blood pressure. However, CBF may be disrupted in certain hypertensive crises, e.g., hypertensive encephalopathy, and antihypertensive therapy may adversely influence cerebral circulation. Experimental data obtained from hypertensive rats suggest different antihypertensive drugs may have different effects on CBF. For example, diazoxide maintains the CBF fairly constant until systemic blood pressure falls to a very low level (70); hydralazine causes disruption of CBF independently of changes in systemic blood pressure (71); converting enzyme inhibitors (72) and nifedipine (61) appear to have a favorable impact on CBF. The relevance of these observations to humans remains to be determined.

Other Complications of Treatment

Treating extremely elevated blood pressure has its risks as well as its benefits. The complications of antihypertensive therapy usually result from hypotension and sometimes from the nature of therapy—such as diazoxide causing cardiac ischemia and nitroprusside causing thiocyanate toxicity. Some have noted worsening of neurological status following acute reduction in blood pressure (73–75). These complications can be avoided by careful evaluation of the patient and choosing an appropriate antihypertensive agent. In this respect, drugs with a short duration of action offer an advantage because unwanted hypotension can be quickly reversed by adjusting the dose of stopping the drug.

In patients recovering from acute cerebrovascular accident or hypertensive encephalopathy, centrally acting agents such as methyldopa or clonidine should not be used because of their sedative effects. One common error in managing hypertensive crises is to introduce oral drugs prematurely. Another error is the failure to monitor the standing blood pressure in a patient who has been receiving potent antihypertensive agents in the supine position.

SUMMARY

The most important immediate action in the management of hypertensive emergencies is to assess the patient's clinical state and to ascertain whether the patient's condition truly warrants emergency management. A patient with true hypertensive crisis ideally should be treated in any intensive care unit. The choice of oral versus parenteral drug depends on the urgency of the situation, as well as the patient's general condition. The level to which the blood pressure should be lowered varies with the type of hypertensive crisis and should be individualized. There is no predestined level for the goal of therapy. Complications of therapy, mainly hypotension and ischemic brain damage, have occurred in patients given multiple potent antihypertensive drugs in large doses without adequate monitoring. Such catastrophes can be minimized by gentle lowering of blood pressure and individualization of therapy.

A relatively asymptomatic patient who presents with severe hypertension, i.e., a diastolic blood pressure of 130 to 140 mm Hg, need not be treated with parenteral drugs. These patients should be managed on an individual basis and the usual course would be to intensify or alter the previous antihypertensive therapy.

After the resolution of hypertensive crisis, one should look into possible factors that might have contributed to the precipitous elevation of the blood pressure, such as nonadherence to prescribed therapy or the presence and/or progression of a secondary form of hypertension, such as renal artery stenosis.

REFERENCES

1. Kincaid-Smith, P. (1980): Malignant hypertension: Mechanisms and management. *Pharmacol. Ther.*, 9:245–269.
2. Kincaid-Smith, P., McMichael, J., and Murphy, E. A. (1958): The clinical course and pathology of hypertension with papilledema (malignant hypertension). *Q. J. Med.*, 105(New Series 27):117–153.
3. Keith, N. M., Wagener, H. P., and Parker, N. W. (1939): Some different types of essential hypertension: Their course and prognosis. *Am. J. Med. Sci.*, 197:332–343.
4. Kincaid-Smith, P. (1980): Malignant hypertension. *Cardiovasc. Rev. Rep.*, 1:42–50.
5. Giese, J. (1976): The renin angiotensin system and the pathogenesis of vascular disease in malignant hypertension. *Clin. Sci. Mol. Med.*, 51(*Suppl.* 3):19s–21s.
6. Constantinides, P., and Robinson, M. (1969): Ultrastructural injury of arterial endothelium II. Effects of vasoactive amines. *Arch. Pathol.*, 88:106–112.
7. Mohring, J., Mohring, B., Petri, M., and Haack, D. (1977): Vasopressor role of ADH in the pathogenesis of malignant DOC hypertension. *Am. J. Physiol.*, 232:F260–269.
8. Lee, T. C., Kushiro, T., Gassia, J. P., Girolami, J. P., Lupu, A. N., and Maxwell, M. H. (1979): The kallikrein-kinin system in blood pressure homeostasis. *Clin. Sci.*, 57:225s–258s.
9. Gavras, H., Oliver, N., Aitchison, J., et al. (1975): Abnormalities of coagulation and the development of malignant phase hypertension. *Kidney Int.*, 8:252–261.
10. Heptinstall, R. H. (1953): Malignant hypertension: A study of fifty-one cases. *J. Pathol. Bacteriol.*, 65:423–439.
11. Ljungquist, A. (1962): The intrarenal arterial pattern in essential hypertension. A micro-angiographic and histological study. *J. Pathol. Bacteriol.*, 84:313–325.
12. Ramos, O. (1984): Malignant hypertension: The Brazilian experience. *Kidney Int.*, 25:209–217.
13. Harington, M., Kincaid-Smith, P., and McMichael, J. (1959): Results of treatment in malignant hypertension: A seven year experience in 94 cases. *Br. Med. J.*, 2:969–980.
14. Gavras, H., Brunner, H. R., Laragh, J. H., et al. (1975): Malignant hypertension resulting from desoxycorticosterone acetate and salt excess. *Circ. Res.*, 36:300–309.
15. Mohring, J., Mohring, B., Peter, M., Haack, D., and Hackenthal, S. (1975): Studies on the pathogenesis of malignant course of hypertension in rats. *Kidney Int.*, 8:S174–S180.
16. Barraclough, M. A. (1966): Sodium and water depletion with acute malignant hypertension. *Am. J. Med.*, 40:265–272.
17. Mohring, J., Petri, M., Szokol, M., Haack, D., and Mohring, B. (1976): Effects of saline drinking on malignant course of renal hypertension in rats. *Am. J. Physiol.*, 230:849–857.
18. Kaneda, H., Yamauchi, T., Murata, T., Matsumoto, J., and Haruyama, T. (1980): Treatment of malignant hypertension with infusion of sodium chloride; a case report and a review. *Tohoku J. Exp. Med.*, 132:179–186.
19. Davis, B. A., Crook, J. E., and Vestel, L. E. (1979): Prevalence of renovascular hypertension in patients with Grade III or IV hypertensive retinopathy. *N. Engl. J. Med.*, 301:1273–1279.
20. Isles, C., Brown, J. J., Cumming, A. M. M., et al. (1979): Excess smoking in malignant-phase hypertension. *Br. Med. J.*, 1:579–581.
21. Gudbrandsson, T., Hansson, L., Herlitz, H., Lindholm, L., and Nilson, L. A. (1981): Immunological

changes in patients with previous malignant essential hypertension. *Lancet,* 1:406–480.
22. Dunn, F. G., Jones, J. V., and Fife, R. (1975): Malignant hypertension associated with use of oral contraceptives. *Br. Heart J.,* 37:336–338.
23. Zacherle, B. J., and Richardson, J. A. (1972): Irreversible renal failure secondary to hypertension induced by oral contraceptives. *Ann. Intern. Med.,* 77:83–85.
24. Kempner, W. (1944): Treatment of kidney disease and hypertensive vascular disease in rice diet. *NC Med. J.,* 5:125.
25. Ledingham, J. G. G. (1983): Management of hypertensive crisis. *Hypertension,* 5(*Suppl.* III):III114–III119.
26. Byrom, F. B. (1954): The pathogenesis of hypertensive encephalopathy and its relation to malignant hypertension. *Lancet,* 2:201–211.
27. Strandgaard, S., MacKenzie, E. T., Jones, J. V., and Harper, A. M. (1976): Studies on the cerebral circulation of the baboon in acutely induced hypertension. *Stroke,* 7:287–290.
28. Still, J. M., and Cottom, D. (1967): Severe hypertension in childhood. *Arch. Dis. Child.,* 42:34–39.
29. Ram, C. V. S. (1982): Hypertensive emergencies: Recognition and management. *Curr. Probl. Cardiol.,* 7:1–70.
30. Wallace, J. D., and Levy, L. L. (1981): Blood pressure after stroke. *JAMA,* 246:2177–2180.
31. Garrett, B. N., and Ram, C. V. S. (1984): Acute aortic dissection. *Cardiol. Clin.,* 2:227–238.
32. Prokop, E. K., Palmer, R. F., and Wheat, M. W. (1970): Hemodynamic forces in dissecting aneurysms. *Circ. Res.,* 27:121–127.
33. Wheat, M. W. (1973): Treatment of dissecting aneurysms of the aorta. Current status. *Prog. Cardiovasc. Dis.,* 16:87–101.
34. Cohn, J. N., and Burke, L. P. (1979): Nitroprosside. *Ann. Intern. Med.,* 91:752–757.
35. Shell, W. E., and Sobel, B. E. (1974): Protection of jeopardized ischemic myocardium by reduction of ventricular after load. *N. Engl. J. Med.,* 291: 481–486.
36. Gibson, T. C. (1978): Blood pressure levels in acute myocardial infarction. *Am. Heart J.,* 96:475–480.
37. Fox, K. M., Tomlinson, J. W., Portal, R. W., and Aber, C. P. (1975): Prognostic significance of acute systolic hypertension after acute myocardial infarction. *Br. Med. J.,* 3:128–130.
38. Hansson, L., Hunyor, S. N., Julius, S., and Hoober, S. W. (1973): Blood pressure crisis following withdrawal of clonidine. *Am. Heart. J.,* 85:605–610.
39. Ram, C. V. S., and Engelman, K. (1979): Abrupt discontinuation of clonidine therapy. *JAMA,* 242:2104–2105.
40. Naftchi, N. E., and Tuckman, J. (1979): Hypertensive crisis in spinal man. *Am. Heart J., 97:536–538.*
41. O'Connell, M. T., Kubrusly, D. B., and Fournier, A. M. (1985): Systemic necrotizing vasculitis seen initially as hypertensive crisis. *Arch. Intern. Med.,* 145:265–267.
42. Travers, R. L., Allison, D. J., Brettle, R. P., et al. (1979): Polyarteritis nodosa: Clinical and angiographic analysis of 17 cases. *Semin. Arthritis Rheum.,* 8:184–199.
43. Sheridan, C., Chandra, P., Jacinto, M., et al. (1982): Transient hypertension after high doses of metoclopramide. *N. Engl. J. Med.,* 307:1346.
44. Filibeck, D. J., Grimm, D., Forman, W. B., and Leidner, B. A. (1984): Metoclopramide-induced hypertensive crisis. *Clin. Pharmacol.,* 3:548–549.
45. Abe, M., Orita, Y., Nakashima, Y., and Nakamura, M. (1984): Hypertensive crisis induced by metoclopramide in patients with pheochromocytoma. *Angiology,* 35:122–128.
46. Agabiti-Rosei, E., Alicandri, C. L., and Corea, L. (1977): Hypertensive crisis in patients with pheochromocytoma given metoclopramide. *Lancet,* 1:600.
47. Cottrell, J. E., Casthely, P., Brodie, J. E., Patel, K., Klein, A., and Turndorf, H. (1978): Prevention of nitroprusside induced cyanide toxicity with hydroxycobalamin. *N. Engl. J. Med.,* 298:808–811.
48. Koch-Weser, J. (1976): Diazoxide. *N. Engl. J. Med.,* 296:1271.
49. Ram, C. V. S., and Kaplan, N. M. (1979): Individual titration of diazoxide dosage in the treatment of severe hypertension. *Am. J. Cardiol.,* 43:627–630.
50. Garrett, B. N., and Kaplan, N. M. (1982): Efficacy of slow infusion of diazoxide in the treatment of severe hypertension without organ hypoperfusion. *Am. Heart J.,* 103:390–394.
51. Lebel, M., Langlois, S., Belleau, L. J., and Grose, J. H. (1985): Labetalol infusion in hypertensive emergencies. *Clin. Pharmacol. Ther.,* 37:615–618.
52. Wilson, D. J., Wallin, J. D., Vlachakis, N. D., et al. (1983): Intravenous labetalol in the treatment of severe hypertension and hypertensive emergencies. *Am. J. Med.,* 75:95–102.
53. Ghose, R. R., Mathur, Y. B., Upadhyay, M., Morgan, W. D., and Khan, S. (1978): Treatment of hypertensive emergencies with oral labetalol. *Br. Med. J.,* 2:96.
54. Flaherty, J. T., Magee, P. A., Gardner, T. L., et al. (1982): Comparison of intravenous nitroglycerin and sodium nitroprusside for treatment of acute hypertension developing after coronary artery bypass surgery. *Circulation,* 65:1072–1077.
55. Ferguson, R. K., and Vlasses, P. H. (1986): Hypertensive emergencies and urgencies. *JAMA,* 255:1607–1613.
56. Bauer, J. H., and Alpert, M. A. (1980): Rapid reduction of severe hypertension with minoxidil. *J. Cardiovasc. Pharmacol.,* 2(*Suppl.*):S189–199.
57. Wood, B. C., Sharma, J. N., and Crouch, T. T. (1979): Oral minoxidil in treatment of hypertensive crisis. *JAMA,* 241:163.
58. Anderson, R. J., Hart, G. R., Crumpler, C. P., et al. (1981): Oral clonidine loading in hypertensive urgencies. *JAMA,* 246:848–850.
59. Haft, J. I., and Litterer, W. E., III (1984): Chewing nifedipine to rapidly treat hypertension. *Arch. Intern. Med.,* 144:2357–2359.
60. Beer, N., Gallego, I., Cohen, A., et al. (1981): Efficacy of sublingual nifedipine in the acute treatment of systemic hypertension. *Chest,* 79:571–574.
61. Bertel, O., Conen, D., Radu, E., et al. (1983): Nifedipine in hypertensive emergencies. *Br. Med. J.,* 286:19–21.

62. Biollaz, J., Waeber, B., and Brunner, H. R. (1983): Hypertensive crisis treated with orally administered captopril. *Eur. J. Clin. Pharmacol.*, 25:145–149.
63. D'Angelo, W. A., Lopez-Overjo, J. A., Saal, S. D., et al. (1980): Early versus late treatment of scleroderma renal crisis and malignant hypertension with captopril. *Arthritis Rheum.*, 23:664.
64. DiPette, D. J., Ferraro, J. C., Evans, R. R., and Martin, M. (1985): Enalaprilat, an intravenous angiotensin-converting enzyme inhibitor, in hypertensive crises. *Clin. Pharmacol. Ther.*, 38:199–204.
65. Barcenas, C. G., Eigenbrodt, E., Long, D. L., and Hull, A. R. (1976): Recovery from malignant hypertension with anuria after prolonged hemodialysis. *South Med. J.*, 69:1230–1233.
66. Adelman, R. D., and Russo, J. (1981): Malignant hypertension: Recovery of renal function after treatment with antihypertensive medications and hemodialysis. *J. Pediatr.*, 98:766–768.
67. Mitchell, H. C., Graham, R. M., and Pettinger, W. A. (1980): Renal function during long-term treatment of hypertension with minoxidil. *Ann. Intern. Med.*, 93:676–681.
68. Davidov, M., Mroczek, W., Gavrilovich, L., and Finnerty, F., Jr. (1975): Long term follow-up of aggressive medical therapy of accelerated hypertension with azotemia. *Angiology*, 26:396–407.
69. Cordingley, F. T., Jones, N. F., Wing, A. J., and Hilton, P. J. (1980): Reversible renal failure in malignant hypertension. *Clin. Nephrol.*, 14:98–103.
70. Barry, D. I., Jarden, J. O., Paulson, O. B., Graham, D. I., and Strandgaard, S. (1984): Cerebrovascular aspects of converting-enzyme inhibition I: Effect of intravenous captopril in spontaneously hypertensive and normotensive rats. *J. Hypertension*, 2:589–597.
71. Barry, D. I., Strandgaard, S., Graham, D. I., Braendstrup, O., Svendsen, U. G., and Bolwig, T. G. (1983): Effect of diazoxide-induced hypotension on cerebral blood flow in hypertensive rats. *Eur. J. Clin. Invest.*, 13:201–208.
72. Barry, D. I., Strandgaard, S., Graham, D. I., Svendsen, U. G., Braendstrup, O., and Paulson, O. B. (1984): Cerebral blood flow during dihydralazine-induced hypertensive rats. *Stroke*, 15:102–108.
73. Taylor, D., Ramsay, J., Day, S., and Dillon, M. (1981): Infarction of the optic nerve head in children with accelerated hypertension. *Br. J. Ophthalmol.*, 65:153–160.
74. Graham, D. I. (1975): Ischaemic brain damage of cerebral perfusion failure type after treatment of severe hypertension. *Br. Med. J.*, 4:739.
75. Singh, A., and Bedi, V. P. (1984): Transient paraplegia following sudden lowering of blood pressure. *J. Indian Med. Assoc.* 82:214–228.

The Kidney in Hypertension, edited by Norman M. Kaplan, Barry M. Brenner, and John H. Laragh. Raven Press, New York © 1987.

Medical Management of Renovascular Hypertension

Thomas G. Pickering

The New York Hospital-Cornell University Medical Center, Cardiovascular Center, New York, New York 10021

Although renovascular hypertension is the commonest curable form of hypertension, medical treatment still has an important role to play. It is needed in three different ways: first, in order to establish initial blood pressure control in patients who are subsequently going to undergo surgery or angioplasty; second, as maintenance therapy in those patients who are unwilling or unable to receive these more definitive forms of treatment; and third, in patients in whom surgery or angioplasty has failed to normalize blood pressure.

When the diagnosis of renovascular hypertension is made, it is necessary to decide what type of treatment should be recommended—medical, surgical, or angioplasty. This decision requires a careful consideration of the relative risks and benefits of each type of treatment, and ideally requires an understanding of the natural history of renovascular hypertension, which is reviewed below.

THE NATURAL HISTORY OF MEDICALLY TREATED RENOVASCULAR HYPERTENSION

For practical purposes, renovascular hypertension can be considered as being two distinct conditions, depending on whether the renal artery stenosis is due to fibromuscular dysplasia or atheroma. Fibromuscular dysplasia is typically diagnosed at a younger age than atheroma, and rarely progresses to complete occlusion of a renal artery or azotemia. Prospective studies of the progression of medically treated patients with this condition have been relatively few, largely because of the excellent results that can be obtained with surgery or angioplasty. Schreiber et al. (1) reported on a series of 75 patients who were followed for an average period of 45 months before undergoing surgery. Serum creatinine increased in only 2 patients (9%), and the size of the ischemic kidney decreased in 6 (27%). Sequential angiographic studies in these patients showed that in 33% the stenosis had become tighter, but none progressed to complete occlusion of the renal artery. In another earlier series, Meaney et al. (2) reported that 16% of patients showed a progression over an average follow-up period of 24 months. Most of these patients had medial fibroplasia, and it has been suggested that complete occlusion of the renal artery is more likely to occur when the stenosis is due to perimedial or intimal fibroplasia, which can be distinguished from the commoner medial fibroplasia by the arteriographic appearance (3), but is much less common.

In patients with atheromatous renal artery stenosis, the probability of progression is much higher. Wollenweber et al. (4) reported that 63% of patients followed for 28 months showed arteriographic progression, and Meaney et al. (2) reported it in 36% for a follow-up period of 32 months. Schreiber et al. (1) followed 85 patients for 52 months; during this period, 44% showed arteriographic evidence of progression of renal artery stenosis, and 16% progressed to complete occlusion of the renal artery. Elevation of serum creatinine and a diminished kidney size occurred in the majority of patients whose lesions progressed, but were uncommon in patients whose lesions remained static.

Thus, whatever the underlying etiology of the renovascular hypertension, the decision to treat it medically carries with it the risk of a progressive impairment of renal function. Although this risk is much smaller in patients with fibromuscular dysplasia, it is by no means negligible, particularly in view of the fact that such patients are typically young, with a prospect of many years before them.

COMPARISON OF MEDICAL TREATMENT WITH SURGERY AND ANGIOPLASTY

There have been no randomized clinical trials comparing the effects of the three different ways of managing renovascular hypertension, and there are unlikely to be any published in the near future. Although there have been several publications comparing the results of medical and surgical treatment, many of the earlier ones (5–7) are of little relevance today because of improvements in diagnostic criteria for renovascular hypertension, and also in the safety and effectiveness of both medical and surgical therapy. Thus, Owen's study (7), published in 1973, concluded that 57% of surgically treated patients were cured or improved, as compared to 34% in the medically treated group. This is in contrast to a more recent report by Zeck et al. (8), published in 1986, which gave corresponding figures of 90% and 86%. In none of these studies, however, were the medical and surgical groups comparable, so that they cannot really resolve the question as to which form of treatment is preferable.

One of the few attempts made to compare all three treatment modalities was recently reported by Greminger et al. (9) from a retrospective multicenter analysis of 202 patients. Approximately one-third were treated with surgery, one-third with angioplasty, and one third medically. Blood pressure control was similar in all three groups, although their baseline characteristics were dissimilar: The surgically treated group had the least severe disease, and the medically treated the most severe. The effects on renal function were not described.

Olin et al. (10) analyzed the effects of the three treatment modalities in 50 elderly patients (whose average age was 70 years) with atheromatous renovascular hypertension. The surgical group fared best, with improved blood pressure control in 90% and deterioration of renal function over an 18-month follow-up in only 19%. There was a 4% operative mortality. Angioplasty improved the blood pressure in 43%, and renal function deteriorated in 25%. Medical therapy controlled the blood pressure in 67% of patients, and in 50% renal function got worse.

Dean et al. (11) randomly allocated patients to medical or surgical treatment, and have reported on a series of 41 patients who were treated medically for 28 months. All had atheromatous renal artery stenoses. During the follow-up period, 12% developed a complete occlusion of the renal artery, and 37% a decrease of renal size of more than 10%; 25% showed a greater than 50% increase of their serum creatinine. Whether or not the renal artery stenosis progressed did not appear to be related to the degree of blood pressure control. This trial is still in progress, so no information is available as to the comparative outcome of medically and surgically treated patients.

Hunt et al. (12) compared medical and surgical treatment in 214 patients followed for 7 to 14 years. Their results are shown in Table 1, but must be interpreted with caution because patients were not randomly allocated to the two treatment modalities; thus 100 of the patients were treated medically for only 3 months, and subsequently had surgery because of failure to control the blood pressure or a deterioration of renal function. The proportions of atheromatous and fibromuscular patients who required surgery by these criteria were identical (46% and 47%). Both survival and blood pressure control were clearly better in the surgical groups, and the fibromuscular patients fared better than those with atheroma. It should be pointed out, however, that this study was done at a time when angiotensin converting enzyme inhibitors were

Table 1. *Comparison of medical and surgical treatment (7-year follow-up data) in renovascular hypertension*[a]

	Atheroma		Fibromuscular dysplasia	
	Medical	Surgical	Medical	Surgical
Survivors	48%	78%	80%	95%
BP cured	0%	45%	0%	65%
BP controlled (on meds)	71%	48%	86%	27%
BP poorly controlled	29%	3%	14%	7%

[a]Data from ref. 12.

not available, and there is evidence that these agents may lower blood pressure to the same extent as surgery.

Factors that might influence the decision as to which treatment modality is appropriate for an individual patient are listed in Tables 1 to 3, with fibromuscular dysplasia and atheroma being considered separately. Several points can be made: First, the costs and risks associated with surgery and angioplasty are initially much greater than with medical treatment, but, if the procedures are successful, may be much lower over the long term. Thus, in younger patients with fibromuscular dysplasia, who if treated medically might require treatment over 40 years, the case for definitive interventional treatment is overwhelming. The majority of these patients can be expected to have their hypertension permanently cured by angioplasty, at relatively little risk and expense. We have performed follow-up arteriograms 5 years after angioplasty in such patients, and have frequently been unable to detect any residual stenosis.

In older patients with atheromatous stenoses, the advantages of interventional therapy over medical treatment are much less clear-cut. In the first place, the cure rate for either surgery or angioplasty is much lower (13). There may be three reasons for this: First, in many patients it is possible that the hypertension is not wholly renovascular in origin. Essential hypertension may itself cause acceleration of the formation of atheromatous plaques, in the renal arteries as elsewhere. Grim (14) reported that 84% of patients with atheromatous renal artery stenosis had a positive family history of hypertension, and suggested that this implied that the hypertension was originally essential, with the renal artery stenosis being secondary. We have observed that the majority of such patients are smokers (15), which could further accelerate the development of a stenosis. Revascularization of the ischemic kidney may not fully normalize the blood pressure of such patients, therefore. Second, the duration of the hypertension is often longer, so that there may be nephrosclerosis of the contralateral kidney, which also contributes to a lack of reversibility of the hypertension (16). And third, the atheromatous lesion may progress.

Table 2. *Cost-benefit analysis of three different types of treatment of renovascular hypertension due to fibromuscular dysplasia*

	Medical	Surgical	Angioplasty
Costs			
Financial	Low (but cumulative)	High	Moderate
Risk associated with treatment	Low (side effects)	Low	Low
Risks to renal function	20% deteriorate	Low	Low
Benefits			
Probability of cure	0	70%	70%
Probability of BP improvement	95%	25%	25%

Table 3. *Cost-benefit analysis of three different types of treatment of renovascular hypertension due to atheroma (focal or diffuse)*

	Medical	Surgical	Angioplasty
Costs			
Financial	Low (but cumulative)	High	Moderate
Risks associated with treatment	Low (side effects)	Low (focal) Moderate-high (diffuse)	Low (focal) Low-moderate (diffuse)
Risks to renal function	50% deteriorate	Low	Low
Benefits			
Probability of cure	0%	40% (focal)	30% (focal)
Probability of BP improvement	95%	45% (focal) 45% (diffuse)	60% (focal)

In addition to the lower probability of success from either surgery or angioplasty in patients with atheromatous stenoses, the risks associated with the procedures are correspondingly higher (17). In many patients, the atheroma is not confined to the renal arteries, but may also involve the coronary and cerebral circulation, so that the risk of perioperative coronary or cerebral infarction is increased. Finally, with surgery that involves inserting grafts into the aorta, or with angioplasty, there is a risk of provoking cholesterol emboli in patients with diffuse atheroma.

One of the main limitations of medical therapy is, of course, the risk of continued deterioration of renal function. Against this, it must be remembered that surgical treatment sometimes includes nephrectomy, although revascularization is clearly the preferred form of treatment. Thus, in two recently published series (8,14), 41% and 16% of patients with atheromatous stenosis eventually required nephrectomy. In some other series this rate may be as low as 4% (18).

PRINCIPLES FOR THE MEDICAL TREATMENT OF RENOVASCULAR HYPERTENSION

In most respects, the principles for the medical treatment of renovascular hypertension are the same as those for essential hypertension. There are two important factors that need special consideration, however. First, in the majority of patients plasma renin activity is high; and second, the maintenance of adequate perfusion of the ischemic kidney is profoundly influenced by the renin-angiotensin system. Special attention, therefore, needs to be given to drugs that lower blood pressure as a result of interfering with the renin-angiotensin system. In animal models of renovascular hypertension, the two dominant mechanisms responsible for maintaining the hypertension appear to be increased activity of the renin-angiotensin-aldosterone system and sodium retention (19,20). The former predominates in two-kidney, one-clip hypertension (analogous to unilateral renal artery stenosis in humans), and the latter in one-kidney, one-clip models (analogous to bilateral renal artery stenosis in humans). The principal differences between these two models are summarized in Table 4. In general, the degree of renin dependency becomes less the longer the hypertension is maintained. Thus, in the one-clip, one-kidney rat, plasma renin activity may return to normal levels in the chronic phase of hypertension, and acute administration of captopril has little effect. Despite this, however, a prolonged infusion of captopril may still lower blood pressure to normal levels (21). That both mechanisms are important has been demonstrated by experiments in which one-clip, one-kidney hypertensive animals have been studied under different conditions of sodium balance: When they are sodium repleted, the blood pressure shows little change during blockade of the renin-an-

Table 4. *Changes in experimental Goldblatt hypertension*

	1-clip, 1-kidney	1-clip, 2-kidney
Human equivalent	Bilateral stenosis	Unilateral stenosis
PRA[a]	Normal	Raised (less in chronic phase)
Plasma volume	Raised	Normal
Exchangeable Na	Raised	Normal
Plasma NE[b]	Raised	Raised
AII[c] antagonist effect on BP	Little change	Falls (less in chronic phase)

[a]Plasma renin activity; [b]norepinephrine; [c]angiotensin II.

giotensin system (by angiotensin converting enzyme inhibitors), but when sodium depleted, blood pressure falls markedly (22).

It is not clear to what extent the parallel situation exists in human renovascular hypertension, but it seems likely that it does. There is very little published data comparing the relative contributions of renin and volume to the hypertension of patients with unilateral and bilateral renal artery stenosis, perhaps because the latter are often too sick to study in the unmedicated state. Bianchi et al. (23) compared plasma renin concentration and plasma volume in patients with essential and renovascular hypertension, and in patients with parenchymal renal disease. Renin levels were higher in renovascular hypertension than in essential hypertension, but there was no difference between patients with unilateral and bilateral renal artery stenosis. Patients with bilateral renal parenchymal disease did not have high renins. That there may be a similar reciprocal relationship between renin and volume that was observed in the animal studies is suggested by their finding that renovascular patients with high renins tended to have normal plasma volumes, whereas those with normal renins had high plasma volumes.

We have recently observed different hemodynamic patterns in unilateral and bilateral renal artery stenosis (24). Patients with bilateral stenoses tend to have higher cardiac outputs and more dilated left ventricles than those with unilateral stenoses, both of which would be consistent with a greater volume load associated with bilateral renal artery stenosis.

CHOICE OF MEDICATIONS FOR THE TREATMENT OF RENOVASCULAR HYPERTENSION

The effectiveness of medical therapy for renovascular hypertension has been increasing progressively over the years. Treatment based on the use of diuretics, hydralazine, methyldopa, and guanethidine may give satisfactory control of blood pressure in only about 40% of patients (6,7); with the addition of beta-blockers, about 75% can be controlled (25). Finally, the recent introduction of angiotensin converting enzyme inhibitors has increased this figure to nearly 90% (26).

DIURETICS

Although thiazide diuretics are often used as the initial treatment of patients with essential hypertension, their role in renovascular hypertension is relatively minor. They are most effective in patients with low renin hypertension, and in patients with very high renins, such as occur in renovascular hypertension, they may occasionally cause a paradoxical rise of blood pressure (27). The same effect has been observed with sodium depletion in one-clip, one-kidney Goldblatt hypertensive rats (28). There is also an increased risk of hypokalemia.

Sodium retention may be a feature of patients with bilateral renal artery stenosis, and in such patients loop diuretics such as furosemide may be used in an adjunctive role, but excessive use may exacerbate azotemia. Potassium-sparing diuretics are generally contraindicated in patients with renal disease.

PRAZOSIN

This agent is an alpha-adrenergic blocker which is a vasodilator and causes little change in renal blood flow or glomerular filtration rate, even in patients with advanced renal disease (29). It also has little effect on plasma renin activity (30). It appears to be well tolerated in patients with renovascular hypertension, although no formal studies have been published.

VASODILATORS

Hydralazine can be used in conjunction with beta-blockers and diuretics in patients with renovascular hypertension, and appears to have no adverse effect on renal function (31). Minoxidil is much more potent, but also requires the concomitant use of a beta-blocker and a loop diruetic. It has been reported to delay the progressive decline of renal function in patients with parenchymal renal disease (32), but must be used with caution in renovascular hypertension.

BETA-BLOCKERS

The majority of patients with renovascular hypertension have normal or high renin levels, and there is abundant evidence that all of the clinically available beta-blockers lower plasma renin activity, and that this is the most important mechanism by which they lower blood pressure (25). Most beta-blockers decrease renal blood flow and glomerular filtration rate in patients with essential hypertension (33,34), and may occasionally produce azotemia (35), but nadolol has been reported to be an exception to this: Renal blood flow may be maintained despite a decreased cardiac output (36,37). This has been attributed to a selective decrease in renal vascular resistance, possibly at the efferent arteriole, because filtration fraction falls (38).

Although the mechanism by which they inhibit renin release is by blockade of the sympathetic beta-adrenergic receptors, it has been demonstrated that they lower renin in patients with renovascular hypertension as well as essential hypertension, although often not to the same degree (39).

ANGIOTENSIN CONVERTING ENZYME INHIBITORS

The introduction of angiotensin converting enzyme (ACE) inhibitors represented a major advance for both the diagnosis and medical management of patients with renovascular hypertension. In our experience, a single-dose captopril test may be the best screening test for identifying the presence of renovascular disease (40).

There can be little question that ACE inhibitors are the most powerful antihypertensive agents in such patients. Although other mechanisms have occasionally been implicated, it is generally agreed that inhibition of angiotensin II formation is the most important mechanism by which they lower blood pressure, so that the response to them identifies a renin-dependent component of an individual patient's hypertension. The acute blood pressure response to an ACE inhibitor is proportional to the baseline plasma renin activity, and patients with renovascular hypertension may show a bigger response than those with essential hypertension (41). Following the acute response there may be a transient return of blood pressure toward pretreatment levels despite maintenance of therapy, with a subsequent further fall. This has been labeled a triphasic response. The long-term but not the acute response of blood pressure to captopril has been found to be a good predictor of the response to successful surgical revascularization (42,43). In patients with essential hypertension, captopril produces a natriuresis and an insignificant change of plasma volume, but the natriuresis may be absent in patients with renovascular hypertension, and plasma volume increases (44).

Captopril is largely excreted by the kidneys, and because many of its effects are dose dependent, the dosage should be reduced in patients with impaired renal function. Side effects include skin rash, loss of taste, neutropenia,and proteinuria. The latter has been seen mainly in patients with conditions where the hypertension is secondary to a systemic disease such as scleroderma or lupus (45), and is not particularly a problem in patients with renovascular hypertension. These side effects are less pronounced with enalapril.

Greminger et al. (46) examined the effects of switching two groups of patients (with essential or renovascular hypertension) from standard triple therapy (a diuretic, propranolol, and hydralazine) to captopril, on which they were followed for 3 years. Captopril lowered blood pressure to the same extent in both groups. Serum creatinine was unchanged in the patients with essential hypertension, but increased progressively in the renovascular group. This increase was most marked in patients with an initially high plasma renin activity or bilateral renal artery stenosis.

Enalapril has also been used for the long-term treatment of patients with renovascular hypertension. Tillman et al. (47) reported on 20 patients treated for an average of 19 months; 15 had unilateral renal artery stenosis and 5 bilateral stenoses. Blood pressure was effectively controlled with enalapril monotherapy, and serum creatinine rose by approximately 20%. In only one patient was there an excessive rise, and the average changes were no greater in the patients with bilateral stenoses than unilateral stenosis. The renal artery stenosis progressed in 5 of the patients, and proteinuria, when present, tended to improve.

Franklin and Smith (48) reported the results of a multicenter trail comparing enalapril and hydrochlorothiazide with standard triple therapy (hydrochlorothiazide, timolol, and hydralazine) in 75 patients with renovascular hypertension. Blood pressure control was satisfactory in 96% of the enalapril group, and 82% of the triple therapy group. An inadequate blood pressure response in the latter was related to the presence of bilateral renal artery stenosis, a very tight unilateral stenosis, or impaired renal function. Renal function declined in 20% of the enalapril group, but in only 3% of the triple therapy group. This was not because of the better control of blood pressure with enalapril, because it was seen in some patients whose blood pressure did not fall. The decline in renal function was not due to any decrease of renal blood flow, which actually tended to increase in all patients.

In patients with normal kidneys, ACE inhibitors may increase renal blood flow and glomerular filtration rate (GFR) (49). In patients with bilateral renal artery stenosis, or with a stenosed renal artery and a solitary kidney, treatment with ACE inhibitors may sometimes cause a dramatic increase in the serum creatinine and blood urea nitrogen (50). Renal artery occlusion has also been reported (51) to have developed in a small number of patients after treatment with captopril for relatively short periods (13–21 weeks). The same phenomenon has been observed in one-clip, one-kidney Goldblatt hypertensive rats (52). It has been suggested that this occurs because of the loss of the effect of angiotensin on the efferent glomerular arterioles, which serves to maintain GFR in the presence of renal ischemia. This cannot be the entire reason, however, because we have observed the same phenomenon in patients with renovascular hypertension treated with minoxidil, and Textor et al. (53) have shown that a nitroprusside infusion in patients with bilateral renal artery stenosis caused a marked reduction in GFR. Indeed, these authors have used this test as a diagnostic tool to investigate whether there is functional ischemia of both kidneys. Successful revascularization of one kidney results in a preservation of GFR during such acute hypotension. Ying et al. (54) have also observed that azotemia may be precipitated by a variety of antihypertensive medications. This phenomenon appears to be specific to renovascular hypertension, because it is rarely seen in patients with azotemia due to nephrosclerosis (55).

THE RENIN-ANGIOTENSIN SYSTEM AND THE CONTROL OF INTRARENAL HEMODYNAMICS IN RENOVASCULAR HYPERTENSION

The clinical observation that ACE inhibitors may cause a deterioration of renal function in some patients with renovascular hypertension can be accounted for by animal studies that have demonstrated the important effects of angiotensin on intrarenal hemodynamics. All of the components of the renin-angiotensin system, that is, renin, angiotensin I, converting enzyme, and angiotensin II, are present within the kidney, particularly in the region of the juxtaglomerular apparatus, and the concentrations of renin and angiotensin II are greater in renal lymph than in the renal vein (56). One of the most important intrarenal effects of angiotensin II is to decrease renal blood flow, with a smaller decrease of GFR. Thus, filtration fraction increases (57). It has been proposed that these changes are brought about by a vasoconstriction of both afferent and efferent arterioles, with the predominant effect being on the latter. Another important effect of angiotensin II is to cause contraction of glomerular mesangial cells, which tends to reduce glomerular filtration. This effect can be blocked by ACE inhibitors and by calcium antagonists such as verapamil (58). Thus, in the normal kidney, particularly when renin levels are high, angiotensin blockade increases renal blood flow, with less consistent changes of GFR (59). In patients with essential hypertension, angiotensin blockade with drugs such as enalapril does not result in any change of glomerular filtration rate or renal blood flow, presumably because renal vascular resistance falls (38).

CLONIDINE

The administration of clonidine may produce an acute reduction of blood pressure in patients with renovascular hypertension, which occurs without any reduction of plasma renin activity but is associated with a decreased plasma norepinephrine (60).

CALCIUM ANTAGONISTS

The role of calcium antagonists in the treatment of renovascular hypertension is somewhat controversial. Numerous animal studies have shown that calcium antagonists tend to increase renal blood flow. In contrast to most other vasodilators, they may also increase GFR (61). In humans, one study reported that nifedipine and verapamil had no effect on creatinine clearance in normal subjects and patients with essential hypertension (62), although nifedipine produced a natriuresis. In another (63), it was reported that acute administration of nifedipine increased renal blood flow and GFR in patients with essential hypertension, but not in patients with chronic glomerulonephritis. Huang (64) studied the effects of verapamil on blood pressure and renal function in one-clip, two-kidney hypertensive rats. Verapamil lowered blood pressure and increased GFR and sodium excretion in the contralateral kidney, but decreased both in the ischemic kidney. These effects were very similar to those of captopril, which when added to the verapamil produced no further effects. It is possible that calcium and angiotensin interact at a common receptor site.

This finding raises the possibility that calcium antagonists might have the same deleterious effect on renal function that has been observed with ACE inhibitors in patients with renovascular hypertension, particularly when the stenosis is bilateral. We have treated many such patients with calcium antagonists without observing this phenomenon, however. There is one report, by Diamond et al. (65), of four elderly male patients with renal failure of varying etiology (including bilateral renal artery stenosis in one) whose renal function was adversely affected by nifedipine. This was reversible when the nifedipine was discontinued and was independent of any effect on blood pressure. It has also been reported that calcium antagonists may prevent the renal vasoconstriction that occurs in response to radiocontrast dyes (66).

CONCLUSIONS

Medical therapy is required for virtually all patients with renovascular hypertension at some stage of their disease. In each patient, a decision has to be made as to whether an attempt should be made to cure the hypertension by surgery or angioplasty, or to continue with medical therapy indefinitely. This decision does not depend so much on how well the blood pressure can be controlled, because with the advent of ACE inhibitors virtually all patients with renovascular hypertension can have adequate blood pressure control. Rather, it depends on the adverse effects (both financial and medical) of the different forms of treatment, and in particular on their effect on renal function.

For the young patient with renovascular hypertension due to fibromuscular dysplasia, there can be little doubt that angioplasty is the preferred treatment, and that medical treatment plays only a secondary role. In older patients with atheromatous renovascular hypertension, the benefits of surgery and angioplasty are much less clear-cut. In the first place, many of these patients may have underlying essential hypertension, so that the blood pressure is less likely to be improved by the intervention. In the second, the risks associated with the procedures are correspondingly higher. Nevertheless, the atheromatous lesion is likely to progress, and revascularization of an ischemic kidney is one of the few effective means of reversing chronic azotemia. And it is in precisely this group of patients where the most powerful form of medical treatment, the ACE inhibitors, must be used with the greatest caution.

When medical treatment is decided on, ACE inhibitors are usually the first line of treatment. There is no question that their specific action on the renin-angiotensin system makes them the most potent agents available for renovascular hypertension. Over the long term, however, it is possible that they may in some patients contribute to the decline of renal function, and if this is suspected, other antihypertensive agents should be used, or revascularization attempted.

REFERENCES

1. Schreiber, M. J., Pohl, M. A., and Novick, A. C. (1984): The natural history of atherosclerotic and fibrous renal artery disease. *Urol. Clin. North Am.*, 2:383–392.
2. Meaney, T. F., Dustan, H. P., and McCormack, L. J. (1968): Natural history of renal artery disease. *Radiology*, 91:881–887.
3. Goncharenko, V., Gerlock, A. J., Shaff, M. L., and Hollifield, S. W. (1981): Progression of renal artery fibromuscular dysplasia in 42 patients as seen on angiography. *Radiology*, 139:45–51.
4. Wollenweber, J., Sheps, S. G., and David, D. G. (1968): Clinical course of atherosclerotic renovascular disease. *Am. J. Cardiol.*, 21:60–71.
5. Shapiro, A. P., Perez-Stable, E., and Scheib, E. T. (1969): Renal artery stenosis and hypertension. *Am. J. Med.*, 47:175–193.
6. Dustan, A. P., Page, I. H., Poutasse, E. F., and Wilson, L. (1963): An evaluation of treatment of hypertension associated with occlusive renal arterial disease. *Circulation*, 27:1018–1027.
7. Owen, K. (1973): Results of surgical treatment in comparison with medical treatment of renovascular hypertension. *Clin. Sci.*, 45:955–985.
8. Zech, P., Finaz de Villaine, J., Pozet, N., Sassard, J., Vincent, M., Labeeuw, M., Collard, M., and Hadj-Aissa, A. (1986): Surgical versus medical treatment in renovascular hypertension. *Nephron*, 44(*Suppl.* 1):105–108.
9. Greminger, P., Lüscher, T. F., Züber, J., Kuhlmann, U., Schneider, E., Siegenthaler, W., Largiader, F., and Vetter, W. (1986): Surgery, transluminal dilatation and medical therapy in the management of renovascular hypertension. *Nephron*, 44(Suppl. 1):36–39.
10. Olin, J. W., Vidt, D. G., Gifford, R. W., and Novick, A. C. (1985): Renovascular disease in the elderly: An analysis of 50 patients. *J. Am. Coll. Cardiol.*, 5:1232–1238.
11. Dean, R. H., Kieffer, R. W., Smith, B. M., Oates, J. A., Nadeau, J. H. J., Hollifield, J. W., and DuPont, W. D. (1981): Renovascular hypertension. Anatomic and renal function changes during drug therapy. *Arch. Surg.*, 116:1408–1414.
12. Hunt, J. C., and Strong, C. G. (1973): Renovascular hypertension. Mechanisms, natural history and treatment. In: *Hypertension Manual*, edited by J. H. Laragh, pp. 509–536. Yorke, New York.
13. Pickering, T. G., Sos, T. A., and Laragh, J. H. (1984): Role of balloon dilatation in the treatment of renovascular hypertension. *Am. J. Med.*, 77:61–66.
14. Grim, C. E., Yune, H. Y., Donohue, J. P., Weinberger, M. H., Dilley, R., and Klatte, E. C. (1986): Renal vascular hypertension. Surgery vs dilatation. *Nephron*, 44(*Suppl.* 1):96–100.
15. Nicholson, J. P., Teichman, S. L., Alderman, M. H., Sos, T. A., Pickering, T. G., and Laragh, J. H. (1983): Cigarette smoking and renovascular hypertension. *Lancet*, 765–766.
16. Pickering, T. G., Sos, T. A., Vaughan, E. D., Case, D. B., Sealey, J. E., Harshfield, G. A., and Laragh, J. H. (1984): Predictive value and changes of renin secretion in patients undergoing successful renal angioplasty. *Am. J. Med.*, 76:398–404.
17. Sos, T. A., Pickering, T. B., Sniderman, K., Saddekni, S., Case, D. B., Silane, M. F., Vaughan, E. D., and Laragh, J. H. (1983): Percutaneous transluminal renal angioplasty in renovascular hypertension due to atheroma or fibromuscular dysplasia. *N. Engl. J. Med.*, 309:274–279.
18. Dean, R. H. (1986): Comparison of medical and surgical treatment of renovascular hypertension. *Nephron*, 44(Suppl. 1):101–104.
19. Freeman, R. H., Davis, J. O., and Seymour, A. A. (1982): Volume and vasoconstriction in experimental renovascular hypertension. *Fed. Proc.*, 41:2409–2414.

20. Brunner, H. R., Kirschman, J. E., Sealey, J. E., ana Laragh, J. H. (1971): Hypertension of renal origin: Evidence for two different mechanisms. *Science*, 174:1344–1346.
21. Wallace, E. C. H., and Morton, J. J. (1984): Chronic captopril infusion in two-kidney, one-clip rats with normal plasma renin concentration. *J. Hypertension*, 2:285–289.
22. Seymour, A. A., Davis, J. O., Freeman, R. H., DeForrest, J. M., Rowe, B. P., Stephens, G. A., and Williams, G. M. (1981): Sodium and angiotensin in the pathogenesis of experimental renovascular hypertension. *Am. J. Physiol.*, 240:H788–792.
23. Bianchi, G., Campolo, L., Vegato, A., Pietra, V., and Piazza, U. (1970): The value of plasma renin concentration *per se*, and in relation to plasma and extracellular fluid volume in diagnoses and prognosis of human renovascular hypertension. *Clin. Sci.*, 39:559–576.
24. Vensel, L. A., Devereux, R. B., Pickering, T. G., Herrold, E. M., Borer, J. S., and Laragh, J. H. (1986): Cardiac status and function in renovascular hypertension produced by unilateral and bilateral renal artery stenosis. *Am. J. Cardiol.*, 58:575–582.
25. Bühler, F. R., Laragh, J. H., Vaughan, E. D., Brunner, H. R., Gavras, H., and Baer, L. (1973): Antihypertensive action of propranolol. Specific antirenin responses in high and normal renin forms of essential, renal, renovascular, and malignant hypertension. *Am. J. Cardiol.*, 32:511–522.
26. Case, D. B., Atlas, S. A., Marion, R. M., and Laragh, J. H. (1982): Long-term captopril in renovascular and essential hypertension. *Am. J. Cardiol.*, 49:1440–1446.
27. Baer, L., Parra-Carrillo, J. Z., Radichevich, I., and Williams, G. S. (1977): Detection of renovascular hypertension with angiotensin II blockade. *Ann. Intern. Med.*, 86:257–260.
28. Seymour, A. A., Davis, J. O., Freeman, R. H., DeForrest, J. M., Rowe, B. P., Stephens, G. A., and Williams, G. M. (1980): Hypertension produced by sodium depletion and unilateral nephrectomy: A new experimental model. *Hypertension*, 2:125–129.
29. Curtis, J. R., and Bateman, F. J. A. (1975): Use of prazosin in management of hypertension in patients with chronic renal failure and in renal transplant recipients. *Br. Med. J.*, 4:432–434.
30. Letcher, R. L., Chien, S., and Laragh, J. H. (1979): Changes in blood viscosity accompanying the response to prazosin in patients with essential hypertension. *J. Cardiovasc. Pharmacol.*, 1(*Suppl.*)S8–20.
31. Judson, W. E., Hollander, W., and Wilkins, R. W. (1957): The effect of exercise in the supine position on cardiovascular and renal function hypertensive patients before and during chronic and oral hydralazine therapy. *J. Lab. Clin. Med.*, 49:672–683.
32. Pettinger, W. (1980): Minoxidil and the treatment of severe hypertension. *N. Engl. J. Med.*, 303:922–926.
33. Sullivan, J. M., Adams, D. F., and Hollenberg, N. K. (1976): Beta-adrenergic blockade in essential hypertension. *Circ. Res.*, 39:532–536.
34. Ibsen, H., and Sederberg-Olsen, P. (1973): Changes in glomerular filtration rate during long-term treatment with propranolol in patients with arterial hypertension. *Clin. Sci.*, 44:129–134.
35. Warren, D. J., Swainson, C. P., and Wright, N. (1974): Deterioration in renal function after beta-blockade in patients with chronic renal failure and hypertension. *Br. Med. J.*, 2:193–194.
36. Textor, S. L., Fouad, R. M., Bravo, E. L., Tarazi, R. C., Vidt, D. G., and Gifford, R. W. (1982): Redistribution of cardiac output to the kidneys during oral nadolol administration. *N. Engl. J. Med.*, 307:601–605.
37. Hollenberg, N. K., Adams, D. F., McKinstry, D. N. Williams, G. H., Boruchi, L. J., and Sullivan, J. M. (1979): Beta-adrenoceptor blocking agents and the kidney: Effect of nadolol and propranolol on the renal circulation. *Br. J. Clin. Pharmacol.*, 7(*Suppl.* 2):219s–225s.
38. O'Connor, D. T., Mosley, C. A., Cervenkia, J., and Bernstein, K. N. (1984): Contrasting renal haemodynamic response to the angiotensin converting enzyme inhibitor enalapril and the beta-adrenergic antagonist metoprolol in essential hypertension. *J. Hypertension*, 2(*Suppl.* 2):89–92.
39. Salvetti, A., Sassano, P., Poli, L., Pedrinelli, R., and Arzilli, F. (1977): The effect of beta-adrenergic blockade on patterns of urinary sodium excretion, blood pressure and plasma renin activity in patients with essential and renovascular hypertension. *Eur. J. Clin. Invest.*, 7:331–336.
40. Muller, F. B., Sealey, J. E., Case, D. B., Atlas, S. A., Pickering, T. G., Pecker, M. S., Preibisz, J. J., and Laragh, J. H. (1986): The captopril test for identifying renovascular disease in hypertensive patients. *Am. J. Med.*, 80:633–644.
41. Case, D. B., Atlas, S. A. Laragh, J. H., Sealey, J. E., Sullivan, P. A., and McKinstry, D. N. (1978): Clinical experience with blockade of the renin-angiotensin-aldosterone system by an oral converting enzyme inhibitor (SQ 14,225, captopril) in hypertensive patients. *Prog. Cardiovasc. Dis.*, 21:195–206.
42. Staessen, J., Bulpitt, C., Fagard, R., Lijnen, A., and Amery, A. (1983): Long-term converting-enzyme inhibition as a guide to surgical curability of hypertension associated with renovascular disease. *Am. J. Cardiol.*, 51:1317–1322.
43. Atkinson, A. B., Brown, J. J., Cummings, A. M. M., Fraser, R., Lever, A. F., Leckie, B. J., Morton, J. J., and Robertson, J. I. S. (1982): Captopril in renovascular hypertension: Long-term use in predicting surgical outcome. *Br. Med. J.*, 284:689–692.
44. Aldigier, J. C., Plouin, P. F., Guyere, T. T., Thibonnier, M., Corvol, P., and Menard, J. (1982): Comparison of the hormonal and renal effects of captopril in severe essential and renovascular hypertension. *Am. J. Cardiol.*, 49:1447–1459.
45. Case, D. B., Atlas, S. A., Mouradian, J. A., Fishman, R. A., Sherman, R. L., and Laragh, J. H. (1980): Proteinuria during long-term captopril therapy. *JAMA*, 244:346–349.
46. Greminger, P., Vetter, H., Steurer, J., Siegenthaler, W., and Vetter, W. (1986): Captopril and kidney function in renovascular and essential hypertension. *Nephron*, 44(*Suppl.* 1):91–95.

47. Tillman, D. M., Malatino, S. L., Cumming, A. M. M., Hedsman, G. P., Leckie, B. J., Lever, A. F., Morton, J. J., Webb, D. J., and Robertson, J. I. S. (1984): Enalapril in hypertension with renal artery stenosis: Long-term follow-up and effects on renal function. *J. Hypertension,* 2(*Suppl.* 2):93–100.
48. Franklin, S. S., and Smith, R. D. (1986): A comparison of enalapril plus hydrochlorothiazide with standard triple therapy in renovascular hypertension. *Nephron,* 44(*Suppl.* 1):73–82.
49. Hollenberg, N. K., Swartz, S. L., Passan, D. R., and Williams, G. A. (1979): Increased glomerular filtration rate after converting enzyme inhibition in essential hypertension. *N. Engl. J. Med.,* 301:9–12.
50. Hricik, D. E., Browning, P. J., Kapelman, R., Groorno, W. E., Madias, N. E., and Dzau, V. J. (1983): Captopril-induced functional renal insufficiency in patients with bilateral renal-artery stenosis or renal-artery stenosis in a solitary kidney. *N. Engl. J. Med.,* 308:373–376.
51. Hoefnagels, W. H. L., and Thien, T. (1986): Renal artery occlusion in patients with renovascular hypertension treated with captopril. *Br. Med. J.,* 292:24–25.
52. Bengis, R. G., and Coleman, T. G. (1979): Antihypertensive effect of prolonged blockade of angiotensin formation in benign and malignant one- and two-kidney Goldblatt hypertensive rats. *Clin. Sci.,* 57:53–62.
53. Textor, S. C., Novick, A. C., Tarazi, R. C., Linas, V., Vidt, D. G., and Pohl, M. (1985): Critical perfusion pressure for renal function in patients with bilateral atherosclerotic renal vascular disease. *Ann. Intern. Med.,* 102:308–314.
54. Ying, C. Y., Tifft, C. P., Gavras, H., and Chobanian, A. V. (1984): Renal revascularization in the azotemic hypertensive patient resistant to therapy. *N. Engl. J. Med.,* 311:1070–1075.
55. Omvik, P., Tarazi, R. C., and Bravo, E. L. (1980): Regulation of sodium balance in hypertension. *Hypertension,* 2:515–523.
56. Navar, L. G., and Rosivall, L. (1984): Contribution of the renin-angiotensin system to the control of intrarenal hemodynamics. *Kidney Int.,* 25:857–868.
57. Rosivall, L., and Navar, L. G. (1983): Effects on renal hemodynamics of intra-arterial infusions of angiotensins I and II. *Am. J. Physiol.,* 245:F181–187.
58. Brenner, G. M., Schor, N., and Ichikawa, I. (1982): Role of angiotensin II in the physiologic regulation of glomerular filtration. *Am. J. Cardiol.,* 49:1430–1433.
59. Kimbrough, H. M., Vaughan, E. D., Jr., Carey, R. M., and Ayers, C. R. (1977): Effect of intrarenal angiotensin II blockade on renal function in conscious dog. *Circ. Res.,* 40:174–178.
60. Mathias, C. J., Wilkinson, A., Lewis, P. S., Peart, W. S., Sever, P. S., and Snell, M. E. (1983): Clonidine lowers blood pressure independently of renin suppression in patients with unilateral renal artery stenosis. *Chest,* 83s:357s–359s.
61. Loutzenhiser, R., and Epstein, M. (1985): Effects of calcium antagonists on renal hemodynamics. *Am. J. Physiol.,* 249:F619–629.
62. Leonetti, G., Cuspidi, C., Sampieri, L., Terzoli, L., and Zanchetti, A. (1982): Comparison of cardiovascular, renal and humoral effects of acute administration of two calcium channel blockers in normotensive and hypertensive subjects. *J. Cardiovasc. Pharmacol.,* 4:S319–324.
63. Yokoyama, A., and Kaburagi, T. (1983): Clinical effects of intravenous nifedipine on renal function. *J. Cardiovasc. Pharmacol.,* 5:67–71.
64. Huang, W. C. (1986): Effects of verapamil alone and with captopril on blood pressure and bilateral renal function in Goldblatt hypertensive rats. *Clin. Sci.,* 70:453–460.
65. Diamond, J. R., Cheung, J. Y., and Fang, L. S. T. (1984): Nifedipine-induced renal dysfunction. Alterations in renal hemodynamics. *Am. J. Med.,* 77:905–909.
66. Bakris, G. L., and Burnett, J. C. (1985): A role for calcium in radiocontrast-induced reductions in renal hemodynamics. *Kidney Int.,* 27:465–468.

The Kidney in Hypertension, edited by Norman M. Kaplan, Barry M. Brenner, and John H. Laragh. Raven Press, New York © 1987.

Surgical Management of Renovascular Hypertension

Andrew C. Novick

Department of Urology, Cleveland Clinic Foundation, Cleveland, Ohio 44106

There are currently three therapeutic options available for patients with renovascular hypertension: medical therapy, surgical therapy, and percutaneous transluminal angioplasty (PTA). Multiple factors must be weighed in determining whether medical or interventive management is more appropriate for a given patient. These include the causal relationship of renovascular disease to hypertension, the adequacy of blood pressure control with medical therapy, the natural history of untreated renovascular disease with particular regard for the risk of sustaining impaired renal function, the medical condition of the patient, and the known results of surgical therapy and PTA in various clinical subgroups.

There are two main categories of renal artery disease, atherosclerosis and fibrous dysplasia, which account for approximately 60% and 40% of all such lesions, respectively (1). There are three different varieties of fibrous arterial disease (intimal fibroplasia, medial fibroplasia, and perimedial fibroplasia), each with distinctive histologic and angiographic features and each with a different biologic history. Other unusual disorders that can cause renovascular hypertension include an arterial aneurysm, arteriovenous fistula, neurofibromatosis, extrinsic obstruction of the renal artery, the middle aortic syndrome, and renal artery thrombosis or embolism.

It is important to differentiate between renovascular disease and renovascular hypertension, since lesions of the renal artery do not always result in hypertension. The diagnosis of renovascular disease depends on angiographic demonstration of a lesion in the renal artery or its branches, whereas the diagnosis of renovascular hypertension can be confirmed only in retrospect and connotes permanent relief of hypertension after surgical therapy or PTA. In our experience, the most useful clinical assessments for establishing the diagnosis of renovascular hypertension are a positive rapid-sequence intravenous pyelogram, a systolic/diastolic abdominal bruit, a short (<5 years) duration of hypertension, and the finding on angiography of a high-grade stenotic lesion involving the renal artery (2–4). Lateralization to the affected kidney (≥2:1) with differential renal vein plasma renin assays and/or a depressor response to angiotensin II inhibition strongly support the presence of renin-dependent hypertension but these tests must be interpreted with caution when they are negative (5). By considering all of these factors in the aggregate, patients with renovascular hypertension can be identified with a high degree of accuracy.

INDICATIONS FOR SURGICAL TREATMENT

A randomized controlled study to compare the efficacy of medical versus surgical therapy for renovascular hypertension has never been performed. The best available data are from Hunt et al., who enrolled 214 patients with this disease in a prospective trial during the 1960s (6).

Of these, 100 patients underwent operation and 114 patients were treated medically. After 7 to 14 years of follow-up, 16% of the surgically treated patients had died compared to 40% of those treated medically. Myocardial infarction, cerebrovascular accidents, and end-stage renal failure were more commonly observed in the medical group compared to the surgical group. Furthermore, hypertension was cured or improved in more than 90% of the surgical survivors. Although current medical therapy for hypertension is clearly more effective than that employed during the era of this trial, these data nonetheless support the value of restoring normal renal arterial blood flow in properly selected patients.

Fibrous Dysplasia

In patients with fibrous dysplasia, the need for surgical treatment is guided by the specific type of disease based on angiographic findings and the associated natural history (7). Medical management of hypertension is the preferred initial treatment for patients with medical fibroplasia, since loss of renal function from progressive obstruction is uncommon with this disease. Surgical treatment in the latter category is reserved for patients whose blood pressure is difficult to control with multiple-drug antihypertensive therapy. Conversely, renal artery stenosis due to intimal fibroplasia or perimedial fibroplasia generally progresses and often eventuates in ischemic renal atrophy. Furthermore, these lesions tend to occur in younger patients and cause hypertension that is extremely difficult to control. Early surgical revascularization in these groups is therefore indicated both to preserve renal function and to minimize the need for long-term antihypertensive medication.

Atherosclerotic

In patients with atherosclerotic renovascular hypertension, the indications for surgical therapy are more restrictive due to their older age and the frequent presence of extrarenal vascular disease. In this group, more vigorous attempts at medical management are warranted and multiple-drug regimens that control the blood pressure are often the preferred approach, particularly in patients with generalized atherosclerosis. Surgical therapy is best reserved for patients whose hypertension cannot be adequately controlled or wherein renal function is threatened by advanced vascular disease (7). The latter designation applies to patients with bilateral high-grade arterial stenosis or with arterial stenosis involving a solitary kidney. In such patients, since the consequences of progressive atherosclerotic renovascular disease are particularly grave, surgical revascularization warrants stronger consideration for the dual purpose of improving blood pressure control and preserving renal function (8).

Aneurysms

Renal artery aneurysms may require surgical treatment when they are the cause of significant hypertension or to obviate the risk of rupture (9,10). The latter is of greatest concern with aneurysms that are larger than 2 cm in diameter and noncalcified, particularly when they occur in premenopausal females because of the predisposition for aneurysmal rupture during pregnancy. Saccular aneurysms are the most common type and they can cause hypertension through several mechanisms. These include compression or displacement of the renal artery or its branches with resulting ischemia, aneurysmal erosion into a renal vein with formation of an arteriovenous fistula, mural thrombus formation within the aneurysm with peripheral renal embolization, and the association of some aneurysms with stenosing fibrous renal artery disease. Saccular aneurysms may also cause hypertension, in the absence of any of the above mechanisms, through relative renal ischemia caused by the turbulent flow of blood as it passes through the aneurysmally dilated arterial segment.

PREOPERATIVE CONSIDERATIONS

It is important to accurately define the general medical condition of the patient, since this will determine the risk of undertaking surgical treatment. Most patients with renal arterial fibrous dysplasia are young and otherwise healthy, and the operative risk is minimal in this group. In patients with atherosclerotic renovascular disease, evidence of generalized atherosclerosis should be carefully sought. Particularly important are a history of angina pectoris, congestive heart failure, myocardial infarction, transient ischemic attacks, cerebrovascular accidents, or intermittent claudication. On physical examination, careful attention should be paid to the presence of carotid bruits, focal neurologic deficits suggesting a prior cerebral infarct, third and fourth heart sounds, precordial left ventricular heave, arterial pulsations in the extremities, and the presence of an aortic aneurysm on examination of the abdomen.

The preoperative evaluation should include a thorough search for coronary artery disease, because this has been the leading cause of operative mortality following surgical treatment for atherosclerotic renovascular disease (11). In addition to a careful history, physical examination, and electrocardiogram, all operative candidates in this category should undergo a cardiac stress test. If any of the latter assessments suggest the presence of coronary artery disease, our policy is to then perform coronary cine angiography and left ventriculography (12). Coronary artery bypass grafting is recommended for patients with significant correctable coronary artery disease before renal revascularization. Patients with either mild to moderate or advanced but compensated coronary artery disease can safely undergo renal revascularization without prior coronary artery bypass grafting. For patients with severe noncorrectable coronary artery disease, major operative intervention for renovascular disease carries a significantly increased risk and is best deferred except for the most dire of circumstances.

Cerebrovascular accident has also been a major operative complication of renal revascularization in patients with atherosclerosis, albeit a less common complication than myocardial infarction. The approach to patients whose history or examination suggests the presence of extracranial cerebrovascular disease is analogous to that employed for patients with suspected coronary artery disease. In such patients, carotid arteriography is obtained preoperatively, and if significant occlusive disease is found, endarterectomy is recommended before renal revascularization (12).

In patients with renovascular hypertension and bilateral renal artery stenosis, our policy is to revascularize the kidney with angiographically more severe arterial stenosis or higher renal vein renin levels, or both. Bilateral simultaneous revascularization increases the risk of operation and is also unnecessary, since most patients with bilateral disease will experience relief of hypertension from unilateral revascularization. Contralateral repair is reserved for patients with persistent hypertension postoperatively and when repeat renal vein renin assays lateralize to the unoperated side.

SURGICAL METHODS OF TREATMENTS

Nephrectomy

Total or partial nephrectomy is rarely done today, since it is now possible to achieve successful renovascular reconstruction in most cases. These operations are occasionally indicated in patients with renal infarction, severe arteriolar nephrosclerosis, severe renal atrophy, and noncorrectable renovascular lesions. Nephrectomy may also be indicated in the elderly, poor surgical risk patient with a normal contralateral kidney or following a failed revascularization procedure, where extensive renal hilar fibrosis precludes satisfactory secondary revascularization.

It is also appropriate to emphasize that angiographic demonstration of complete renal artery occlusion does not necessarily imply a nonsalvable kidney. With gradual renal artery occlusion, although renal function may be severely impaired, renal viability can be maintained by the development of collateral arterial supply from ureteral, lumbar, adrenal, capsular, or mesenteric vessels. The most important clinical assessments suggesting a salvable kidney in this setting are angiographic demonstration of retrograde renal artery filling from collateral vascular supply and an intraoperative renal biopsy showing intact glomeruli with minimal vascular sclerosis. When the latter are present, revascularization can allow both control of hypertension and improvement in overall renal function (13,14).

Aortorenal Bypass

Although a variety of renal revascularization procedures are available for treating renovascular hypertension, aortorenal bypass with autogenous saphenous vein or arterial grafts is the preferred method in most cases (Fig. 1). Although excellent clinical results have been obtained with both types of bypass grafts (15–17), long-term studies of aortorenal saphenous vein grafts have shown a large number of dilated grafts on follow-up angiography (18). The clinical significance of these observations remains uncertain, since most of these patients continue to be normotensive with excellent renal function. Nevertheless, these findings have led to preferential use of arterial autografts when these are available. The viscoelastic properties of arterial grafts, unlike the saphenous vein, match those of the renal artery, and postoperative graft dilation has not been observed. We have used the hypogastric and splenic arteries as free bypass grafts with cure or improvement of hypertension in 96% of patients postoperatively (17); similar results have been reported by other authors with aortorenal arterial grafts (16). Currently, aortorenal bypass with a synthetic material is indicated only when autogenous vascular grafts are not available, and polytetrafluoroethylene is the preferred synthetic graft in these cases (19).

Revascularization is more complicated when vascular disease extends into the branches of the renal artery or when reconstruction is required for a kidney supplied by multiple renal arteries.

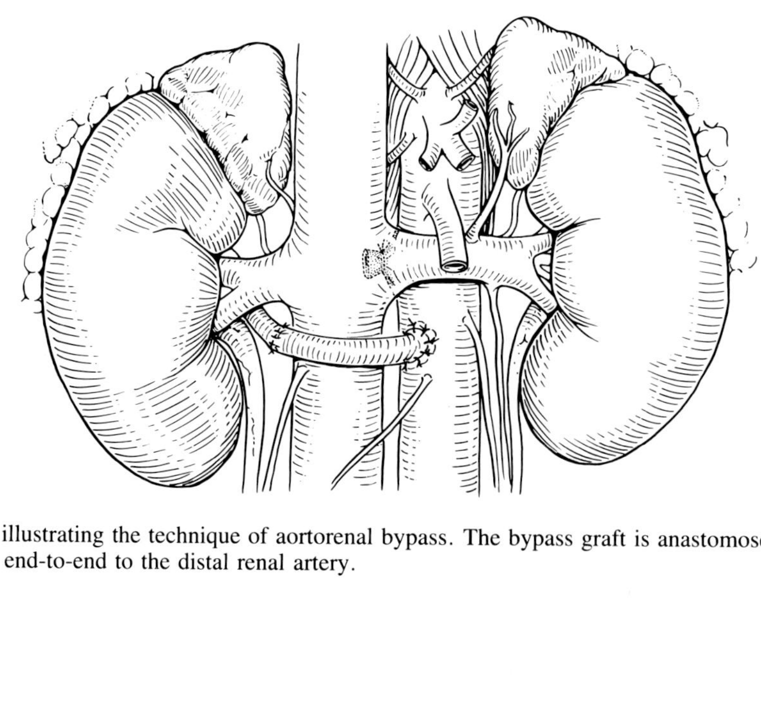

FIG. 1. Sketch illustrating the technique of aortorenal bypass. The bypass graft is anastomosed end-to-side to the aorta and end-to-end to the distal renal artery.

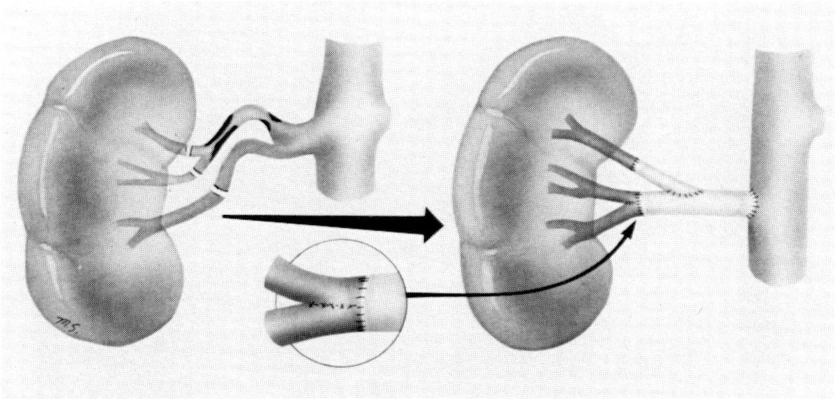

FIG. 2. Method of *in situ* branch renal arterial reconstruction with a double-armed branched aortorenal bypass graft anastomosed end-to-end to one branch and end-to-end to two conjoined branches (right kidney).

Recently developed microvascular techniques now enable successful revascularization *in situ* with an aortorenal bypass operation when the diseased renal vessels are located outside the hilus of the kidney (20). The most useful technique for *in situ* revascularization of multiple segmental renal arteries is aortorenal bypass with a branched autogenous vascular graft (21) (Fig. 2). Extracorporeal branch arterial repair and autotransplantation are indicated only when preoperative angiography demonstrates intrarenal extension of renovascular disease.

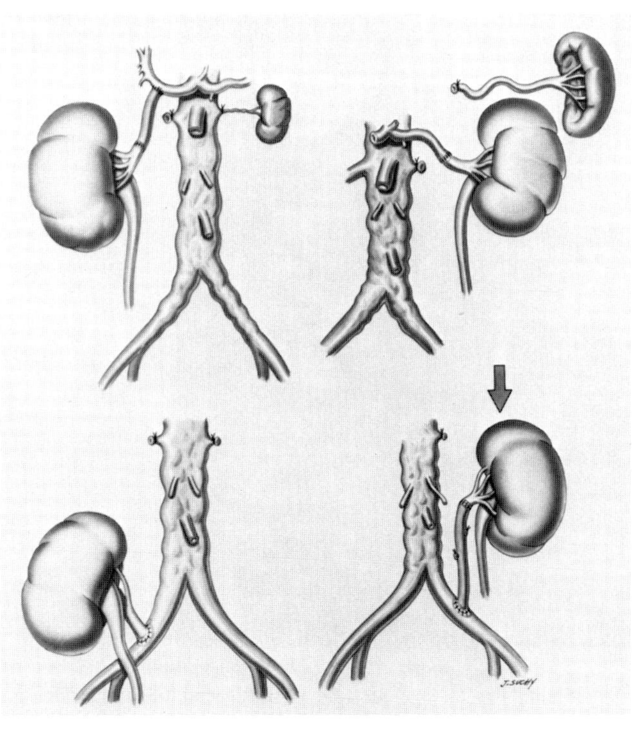

FIG. 3. Methods of renal revascularization for patients with a surgically difficult aorta. These include hepatorenal bypass (*top left*), splenorenal bypass (*top right*), autotransplantation (*bottom left*), and iliorenal bypass (*bottom right*).

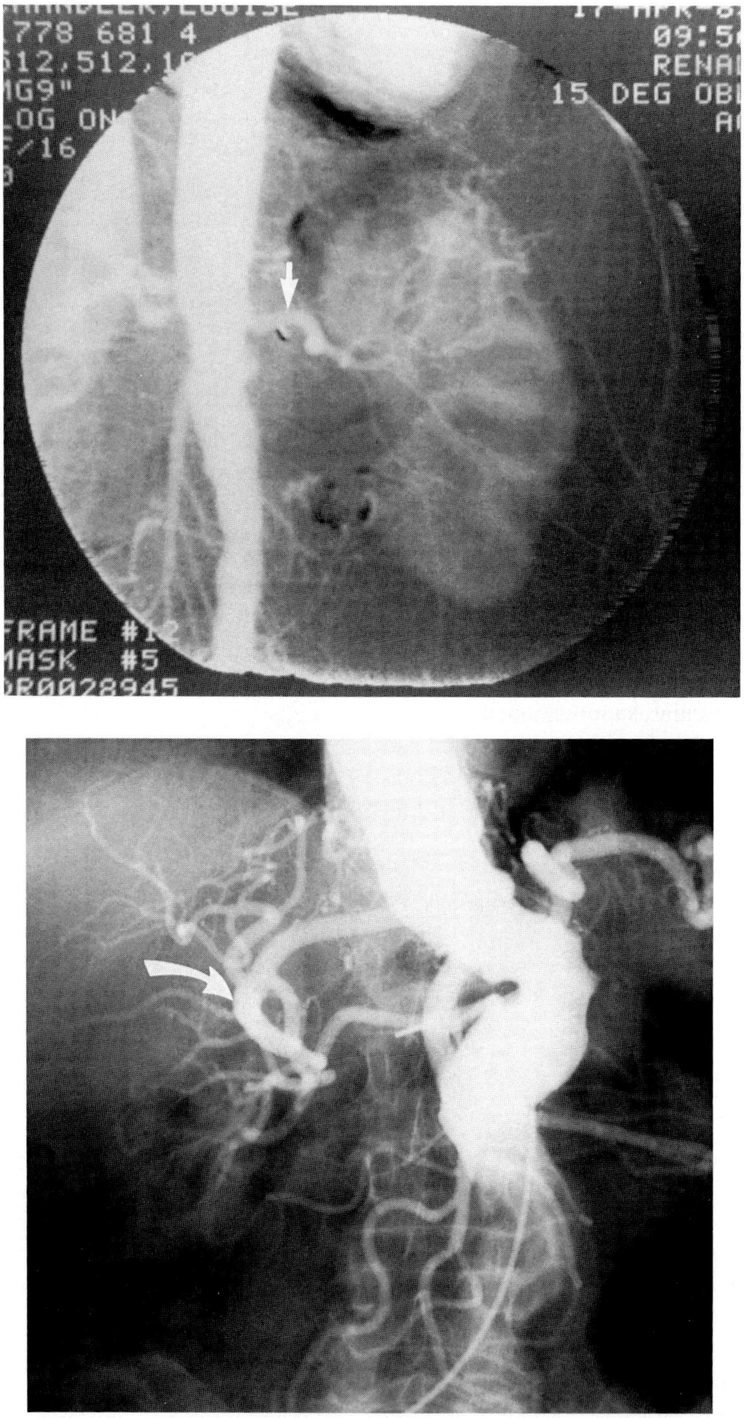

A

B

FIG. 4. A: Digital subtraction angiogram in a patient who underwent splenorenal bypass demonstrates a patent anastomosis (*arrow*). **B**: Digital subtraction angiogram in a patient who underwent hepatorenal bypass with *arrow* indicating the interposition saphenous vein graft.

Techniques in the Surgically Difficult Aorta

In some patients with renal artery disease, severe atherosclerosis or a previous operation on the abdominal aorta may preclude safe performance of aortorenal bypass. These patients present difficult clinical problems, since they frequently present with intractable hypertension and failing renal function, and may possess only a solitary functioning kidney. Fortunately, alternative methods of revascularization are available that may be safely and effectively employed in such patients (22) (Fig. 3).

Splenorenal bypass provides an excellent method of performing left renal revascularization when preoperative aortography with selective celiac angiography demonstrates a healthy splenic artery. The advantages of this procedure are that it can be carried out in untouched vascular tissues at a distance from the aorta, and it involves performance of only a single vascular anastomosis (23) (Fig. 4A). Since the liver receives dual vascular supply from the hepatic artery and portal vein, hepatorenal saphenous vein bypass represents the optimum method of achieving right renal revascularization in such patients (24) (Fig. 4B). In unusual cases, when aortography reveals an enlarged superior mesenteric artery, mesenterorenal bypass has been performed (25) (Fig. 5). Unfortunately, this artery either will usually be of normal calibre or will itself be involved in the disease process. Finally, renal autotransplantation or iliorenal bypass may be employed to treat renovascular hypertension in patients with severe aortic atherosclerosis when both good flow through the aorta and disease-free iliac vessels are present (26) (Fig. 6).

Complete excision of the aorta and replacement with a prosthesis may be done but, when combined with renal revascularization, has been associated with operative mortality rates ranging from 6% to 30% (27–29). This approach should therefore be limited to patients with an abdominal aortic aneurysm or symptomatic aortoiliac occlusive disease. Transaortic endarterectomy is also an extensive operation with a significant potential morbidity, and the techniques described above are more effective and less hazardous.

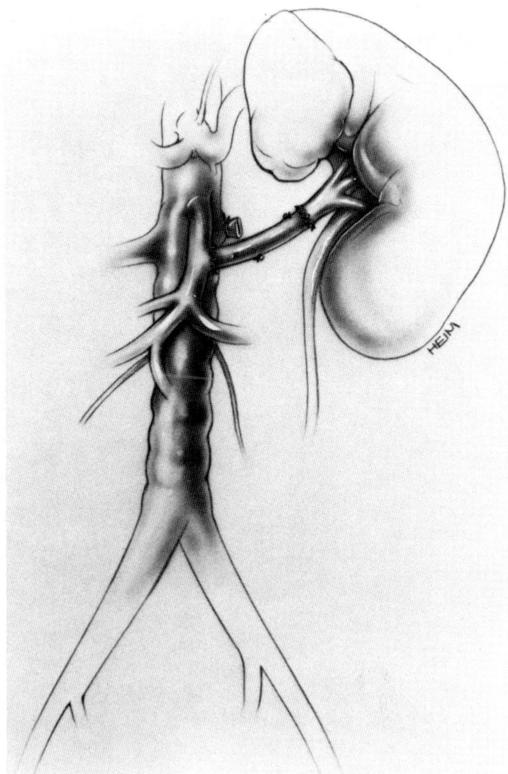

FIG. 5. Sketch illustrating technique of superior mesenterorenal bypass with an interposition saphenous vein graft.

Extracorporeal Microvascular Renal Revascularization and Autotransplantation

Extracorporeal microvascular repair and autotransplantation are indicated in patients with extensive branch renal artery disease where intrarenal vascular extension precludes a satisfactory *in situ* repair (30). Prior to the advent of extracorporeal surgery, such patients would have been considered either inoperable or candidates for

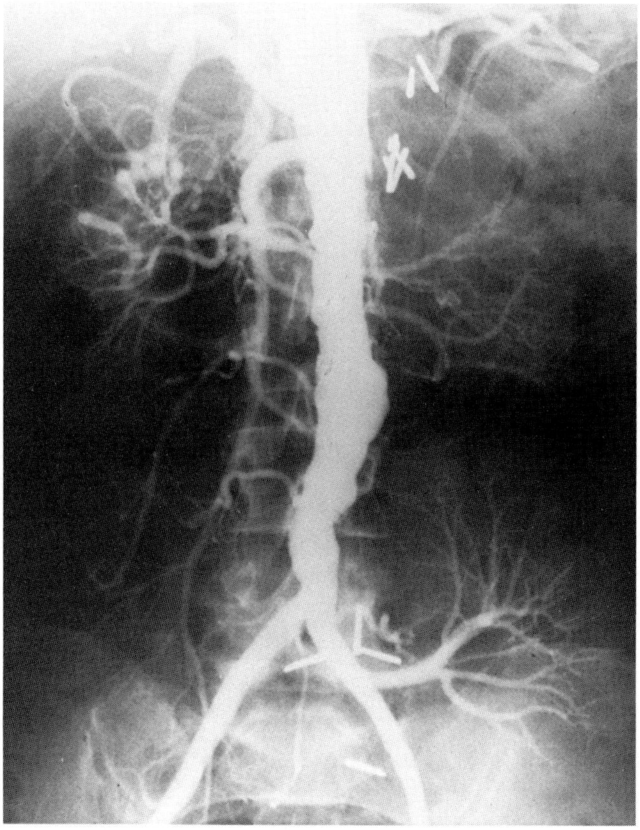

FIG. 6. Arteriogram in a patient with severe aortic atherosclerosis who underwent autotransplantation of the left kidney demonstrates a patent anastomosis of the left renal artery to the left common iliac artery.

nephrectomy. The advantages of performing extracorporeal revascularization include optimum exposure and illumination, a bloodless surgical field, greater protection from prolonged renal ischemia, and more facile employment of microvascular techniques and optical magnification. The removed kidney is flushed with an intracellular electrolyte solution and is then submerged in ice slush saline to maintain hypothermia. Under these conditions, the kidney can safely tolerate periods outside the body far in excess of those required to perform even the most complex arterial repair. Extracorporeal revascularization is accomplished with a branched autogenous vascular graft of the hypogastric artery, saphenous vein, or inferior epigastric artery. The repaired kidney is then autotransplanted to the iliac fossa, using the same technique as in renal allotransplantation (Fig. 7).

RESULTS OF SURGICAL TREATMENT

In evaluating the results of surgical treatment for renovascular hypertension, patients are considered cured if the blood pressure is 140/90 mm Hg or less with a minimum follow-up interval of 6 months postoperatively. Patients are considered improved if they have shown a reduction in diastolic pressure of 15 mm Hg or more, or are normotensive on medication. Failures are those who do not qualify for either of the aforementioned categories.

A

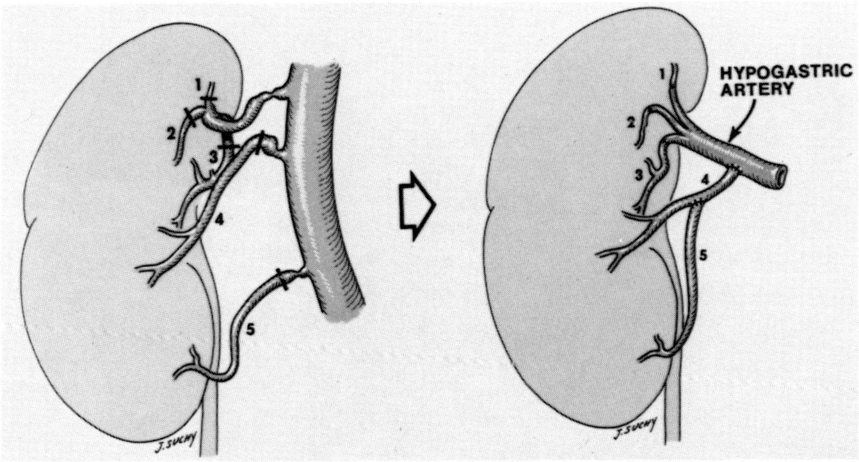

B

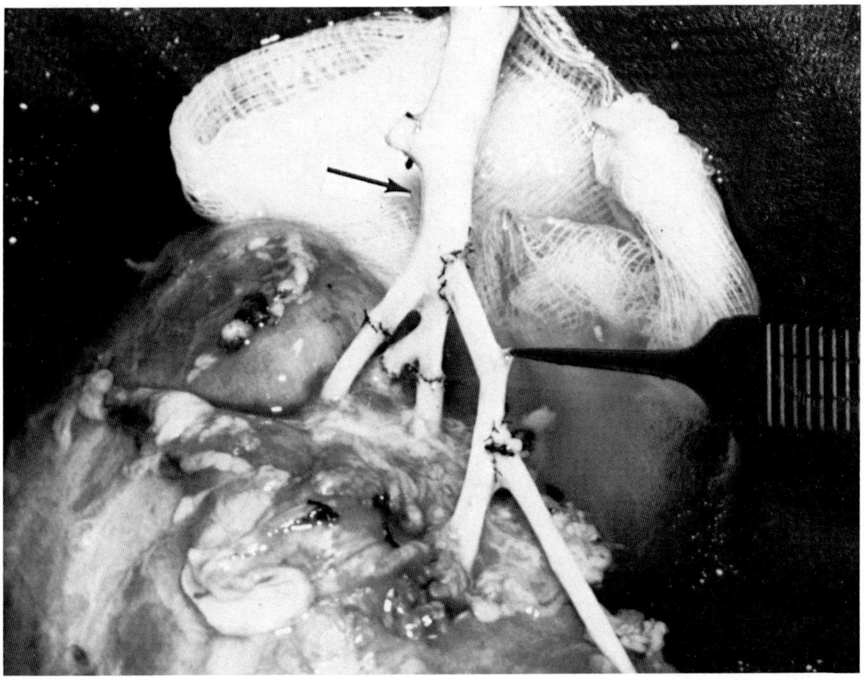

FIG. 7. A: Sketch illustrating preoperative extent of renal artery disease (left) and completed extracorporeal repair with branched hypogastric arterial graft (right). **B**: Operative photograph of completed extracorporeal revascularization of five segmental branches. The three diseased upper branches were repaired with branched graft of the hypogastric artery. The middle and lower renal arteries were anastomosed end-to-side into the graft and adjacent branch, respectively. **C**: Sketch of revascularized kidney following autotransplantation into the iliac fossa. **D**: Postoperative arteriogram of autotransplant demonstrates patency of all five revascularized segmental arteries. (Reproduced from the *Journal of Urology* with permission of Williams & Wilkins Co., Baltimore, MD.)

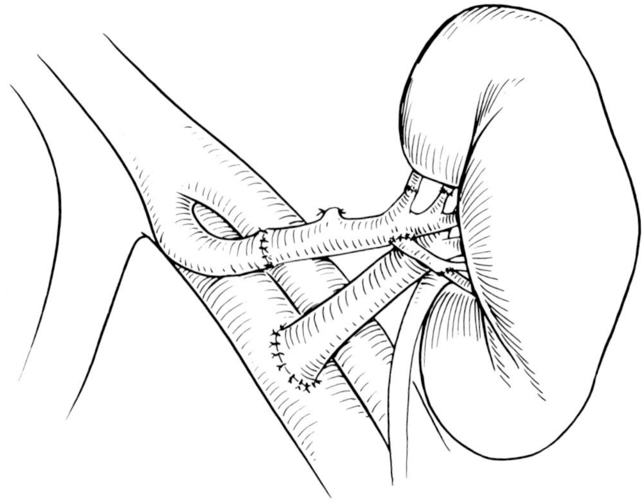

C

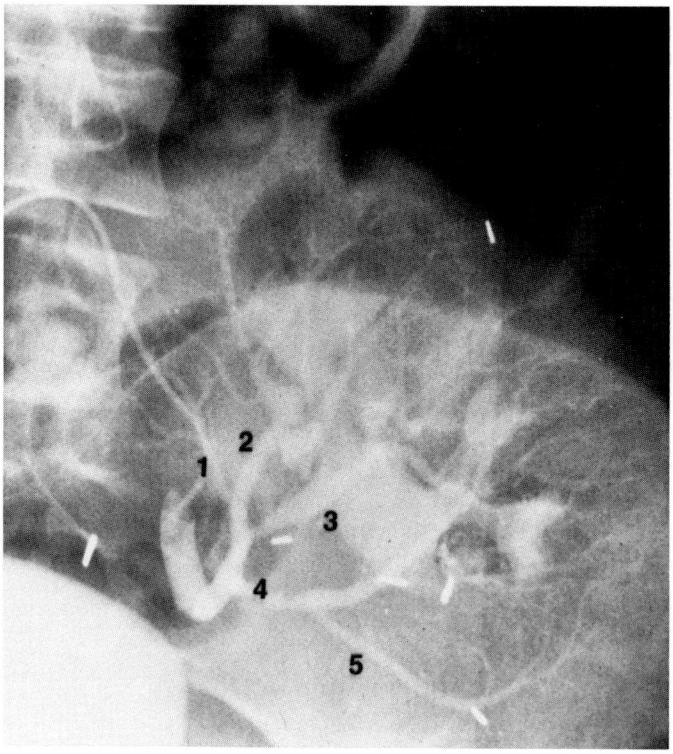

D

FIG. 7. *Continued*

Table 1. *Surgical revascularization technique for renal artery disease at the Cleveland Clinic (1975–84)*

	Atherosclerosis (n = 254)	Fibrous dysplasia or aneurysm (n = 126)
Aortorenal bypass	138	82
Splenorenal bypass	42	4
Hepatorenal bypass	29	0
Iliorenal bypass	19	0
Autotransplantation	8	1
Aortic replacement	11	0
Ex vivo repair and autotransplantation	0	37
Other	7	2

The results of surgical treatment for renovascular hypertension must also be viewed within the context of the pathologic diagnosis. Several major referral centers have reported long-term cure or improvement of hypertension following renal revascularization in approximately 90% of patients with fibrous dysplasia (15–17,31). Less satisfactory results have traditionally been obtained in patients with atherosclerotic renovascular hypertension. For example, in the National Cooperative Study, operative therapy yielded no improvement in blood pressure control for 37% of patients with atherosclerotic disease (32). Nevertheless, more recently, refinements in establishing a preoperative diagnosis of renin-mediated hypertension and an enhanced technical efficacy of vascular reconstruction have led to improved surgical results in this category. There are now reports from several groups of 85% to 90% cure or improvement rates following renal revascularization for atherosclerotic renovascular hypertension (12,33,34).

We have recently reviewed the Cleveland Clinic experience with surgical revascularization (SR) for renal artery disease (RAD) from January 1975 to December 1984 (35). During this 10-year period, a total of 380 SR operations were performed in 361 patients with RAD; 19 patients underwent simultaneous or staged bilateral SR. The cause of RAD was atherosclerosis in 241 patients, fibrous dysplasia in 104 patients, and an arterial aneurysm in 16 patients. The indication for SR in all patients with fibrous dysplasia or an aneurysm was to treat severe renovascular hypertension. The indications for SR in patients with atherosclerotic RAD were treatment of renovascular hypertension in 80 patients, preservation of renal function in 61 patients, and both control of hypertension and preservation of renal function in 100 patients.

The 380 SR operations performed in these 361 patients are listed in Table 1. Operative mortality was 2.1% in patients with atherosclerotic RAD and 0% in patients with fibrous dysplasia or an aneurysm. Postoperative thrombosis or stenosis of the repaired renal artery occurred following 17 or 380 SR operations (4.5%). Hypertension was cured or improved postoperatively in 91.7% of patients with atherosclerotic RAD and 93% of patients with fibrous dysplasia or an aneurysm (Table 2). Postoperative renal function was improved or stable in 88.8% of patients with atherosclerosis who underwent SR to preserve renal function. These data illustrate the excellent clinical results that continue to be achieved with surgical revascularization in

Table 2. *Results of surgical revascularization for renovascular hypertension at the Cleveland Clinic (1975–84)*

	Number patients	Postoperative blood pressure: Cured	Improved	Failed	Follow-up (months)
Atherosclerosis	180	55 (31%)	110 (61%)	15 (8%)	6–117
Fibrous dysplasia	104	66 (63%)	31 (30%)	7 (7%)	10–115

properly selected patients with renal artery disease.

REFERENCES

1. Novick, A. C. and Stewart, B. H. (1979): Surgical treatment of renovascular hypertension. *Curr. Probl. Surg.*, 16.
2. Hughes, J. S., Dove, H. G., Gifford, R. W., and Feinstein, A. R. (1977): Non-invasive predictors of surgical cure of renovascular hypertension. *Clin Res*, 25:265.
3. Eipper, D. F., Gifford, R. W., Stewart, B. H., Alfidi, J. R., McCormack, L. J., and Vidt, D. G. (1976): Abdominal bruits in renovascular hypertension. *Am. J. Cardiol.*, 13:48.
4. Hughes, J. S., Dove, H. G., Gifford, R. W., and Feinstein, A. R. (1981): Duration of blood pressure elevation in accurately predicting surgical cure of renovascular hypertension. *Am. Heart J.*, 101:408.
5. Novick, A. C., Fouad, F. M., Textor, S.C., et al. (1983): Predictive value of angiotensin II blockade with $(SAR^1THR^8)A_{II}$ in renovascular hypertension. *J. Urol.*, 129:7.
6. Hunt, J. C., Steps, S. G., Harrison, H. G., Strong, C. G., and Bernatz, P. E. (1947): Renal and renovascular hypertension. A reasoned approach to diagnosis and management. *Arch. Intern. Med.*, 133:988.
7. Schreiber, M. J., Pohl, M. A., and Novick, A. C. (1984): The natural history of atherosclerotic and fibrous renal artery disease. *Urol. Clin. Am. North*, 11:383.
8. Novick, A. C., Pohl, M. A., Schreiber, M. J., Gifford, R. W., and Vidt, D. G. (1983): Renal revascularization for preservation of kidney function in patients with atherosclerotic renovascular disease. *J. Urol.*, 129:907.
9. Poutasse, E. F. (1975): Renal artery aneurysms. *J. Urol.*, 113:433.
10. Novick, A. C. (1982): Renal artery aneurysm and arteriovenous malformation. In: *Vascular Problems in Urologic Surgery*, edited by A. C. Novick and R. A. Straffon. Saunders Publishing Co., Philadelphia.
11. Franklin, S. S., Young, J. D., Maxwell, M. H., Foster, J. S., Palmer, J. M., Cerny, J., and Varady, P. D. (1975): Operative morbidity and mortality in renovascular disease. *JAMA*, 231:1148.
12. Novick, A. C., Straffon, R. A., Stewart, B. H., Gifford, R. W., and Vidt, D. G. (1981): Diminished operative morbidity and mortality following revascularization for atherosclerotic renovascular disease. *JAMA*, 246:749.
13. Schefft, P., Novick, A. C., Stewart, B. H., and Straffon, R. A. (1980): Renal revascularization in patients with total occlusion of the renal artery. *J. Urol.*, 124:184.
14. Libertino, J. A., Zinman, L., Breslin, D. J., Swinton, N. W., and Legg, M. A. (1980): Renal artery revascularization: Restoration of renal function. *JAMA*, 244:1340.
15. Ernst, C. B., Stanley, J. C., Marshall, F. F., et al. (1972): Autogenous saphenous vein aortorenal autografts: A ten-year experience. *Arch. Surg.*, 150:855.
16. Stoney, R. J., Deluccia, N., Ehrenfeld, W. K., et al. (1981): Aortorenal arterial autografts: Long-term assessment. *Arch. Surg.*, 116:1416.
17. Novick, A. C., Straffon, R. A., and Stewart, B. H. (1977): Autogenous arterial grafts in the treatment of renal artery stenosis. *J. Urol.*, 118:919.
18. Stanley, J. C., Ernst, C. B., and Fry, W. J. (1973): Fate of 100 aortorenal vein grafts: Characteristics of late graft expansion, aneurysmal dilatation, and stenosis. *Surgery*, 74:931.
19. Khauli, R. B., Novick, A. C., and Coseriu, G. V. (1984): Renal revascularization with polytetrafluoroethylene grafts. *Cleve. Clin. Q.*, 51:365.
20. Novick, A. C. Straffon, R. A., and Stewart, B. H. (1980): Surgical management of branch renal artery disease: *In situ* versus extracorporeal methods of repair. *J. Urol.*, 123:311.
21. Streem, S. B., and Novick, A. C. (1982): Aortorenal bypass with a branched saphenous vein graft for *in situ* repair of multiple segmental renal arteries. *Surg. Gynecol. Obstet.*, 155:855.
22. Novick, A. C., Stewart, B. H., Straffon, R. A., and Banowsky, L. H. (1977): Renal revascularization in patients with atherosclerosis or a previous operation on the abdominal aorta. *Surg. Gynecol. Obstet.*, 144:211.
23. Novick, A. C., Banowsky, L. H., Stewart, B. H., and Straffon, R. A. (1977): Splenorenal bypass in the treatment of stenosis of the renal artery. *Surg. Gynecol. Obstet.*, 144:891.
24. Chibaro, E. A., Libertino, J. A., and Novick, A. C. (1984): Use of the hepatic circulation for renal revascularization. *Ann. Surg.*, 199:406.
25. Khauli, R. B., Novick, A. C., Coseriu, G. V., Beven, E. G., and Hertzer, N. R. (1985): Superior mesenterorenal bypass for renal revascularization with infrarenal aortic occlusion. *J. Urol.*, 133:188.
26. Novick, A. C., and Banowsky, L. H. (1979): Iliorenal saphenous vein bypass: Alternative for renal revascularization in patient with surgically difficult aorta. *J. Urol.*, 122:243.
27. Foster, J. H., Dean, R. H., Pinkerton, J. A., and Rhamy, R. K. (1973): Ten years' experience with the surgical management of renovascular hypertension. *Ann. Surg.*, 177:755.
28. Gomes, M., and Bernatz, P. E. (1970): Aortoiliac occlusive disease: Extension cephalad to origin of renal arteries, with considerations and results. *Arch. Surg.*, 101:161.
29. Shahian, D. M., Najafi, H., Javid, H., Hunter, J. A., Goldin, M. D., and Monson, D. O. (1980): Simultaneous aortic and renal artery reconstruction. *Arch. Surg.*, 115:1491.
30. Novick, A. C. (1981): Management of intrarenal branch arterial lesions with extracorporeal microvascular reconstruction and autotransplantation. *J. Urol.*, 126:150.
31. Lankford, N. S., Donahue, J. P., Grim, C. E., et al. (1979): Results of surgical treatment of renovascular hypertension. *J. Urol.*, 122:439.

32. Foster, J. H., Maxwell, M. H., Franklin, S. S., et al. (1975): Renovascular occlusive disease: Results of operative treatment. *JAMA*, 231:1043.
33. Foster, J. H., Dean, R. H., Pinkerton, J. A., and Rhamy, R. K. (1973): Ten years' experience with the surgical management of renovascular hypertension. *Ann. Surg.*, 177:755.
34. Buda, J. A., Baer, L., Parra-Carillo, J. Z., et al. (1976): Predictability of surgical response in renovascular hypertension. *Arch. Surg.*, 111:1243.
35. Novick, A. C., Ziegelbaum, M., Vidt, D. G., Gifford, R. W., Pohl, M. A., and Goormastic, M. (1987): Trends in revascularization for renal artery disease: Ten years experience. *JAMA*, 257:498.

The Kidney in Hypertension, edited by Norman M. Kaplan, Barry M. Brenner, and John H. Laragh. Raven Press, New York © 1987.

Percutaneous Transluminal Renal Artery Angioplasty

D. E. Schwarten

St. Vincent Hospital and Health Care Center, Indianapolis, Indiana 46260

Dotter and Judkins' report (1) of the treatment of atherosclerosis using percutaneous transluminal angioplasty (PTA) was met with guarded enthusiasm by angiographers and with little or no enthusiasm by most other physicians. The difficulties associated with the technique employed by Dotter and Judkins and the inherent limitations of their system were overcome with the development of Gruntzig's "rigid balloon" angioplasty catheter (2). The catheter was constructed in such a way that would allow it to track over a guidewire or pass through a guiding catheter to access a variety of vessels for percutaneous transluminal angioplasty of atherosclerotic and other pathologic entities. The balloon catheter not only offers versatility but also avoids the undesirable shear forces associated with passage of the Dotter type angioplasty system through occluded or stenotic vessels. The shear forces produce a significantly greater amount of intimal trauma and are felt to be responsible for a high incidence of restenosis.

Although Dotter's original concept of successful angioplasty resulting from compression of the atherosclerotic material was initially supported by Gruntzig, it was subsequently shown by Castenada-Zuniga (3) and independently by Fogarty (4) that compression plays only a very small role in a successful angioplasty procedure in the atherosclerotic vessel. The predominant mechanism is disruption of the plaque at its junction with the intima and media with the creation of a cleft in the intima and media. During dilatation the media and adventitia are, in fact, stretched beyond their normal caliber.

PATIENT SELECTION FOR PERCUTANEOUS TRANSLUMINAL RENAL ANGIOPLASTY FOR THE MANAGEMENT OF RENOVASCULAR HYPERTENSION

Patients should be selected for PTA for management of renovascular hypertension on the basis of not only clinical but also anatomic criteria.

Anatomic Indications for PTA

Renal Artery Nonostial Atherosclerosis

The vast majority of patients with renovascular hypertension will exhibit an atherosclerotic lesion within the first 2.0 cm of the renal artery. These patients constitute, on anatomic grounds alone, nearly ideal candidates for balloon angioplasty (Fig. 1A,B).

Fibrous Dysplastic Lesions of the Renal Artery

Within this group of diverse disorders, medial fibroplasia constitutes the largest single group and is ideally suited for PTA. This process usually involves the mid to distal portions of the main renal artery and may extend into renal artery branches (Fig. 2A–C). Branch renal ar-

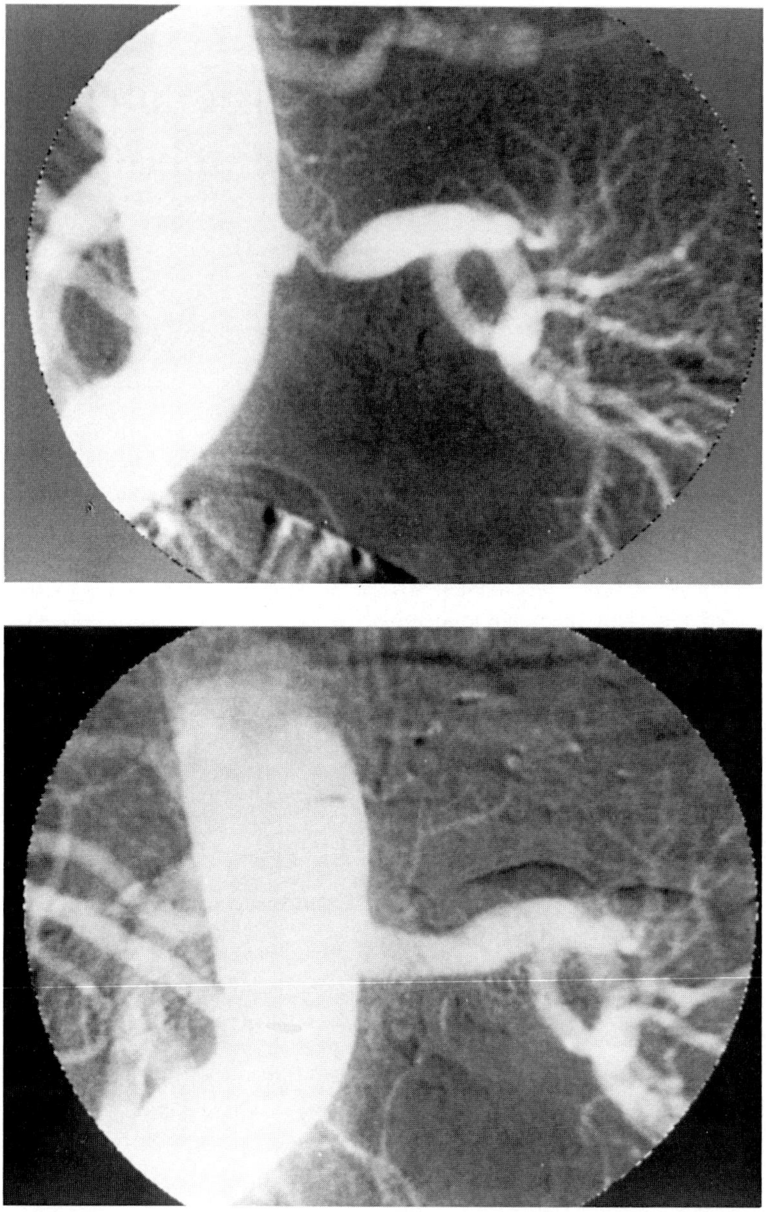

A

B

FIG. 1. A: A high-grade proximal atherosclerotic renal artery stenosis ideally suited for renal angioplasty. **B**: Postangioplasty appearance of minimal residual stenosis.

tery involvement does not preclude angioplasty in the hands of an experienced angiographer. On the contrary, branch renal artery lesions may be more effectively and certainly more easily managed using a small balloon catheter than an operative approach.

Inactive Arteritis

Inactive arteritis is a distinctly unusual cause for renovascular hypertension. There have been case reports of successful renal angioplasty in this group of patients. (6)

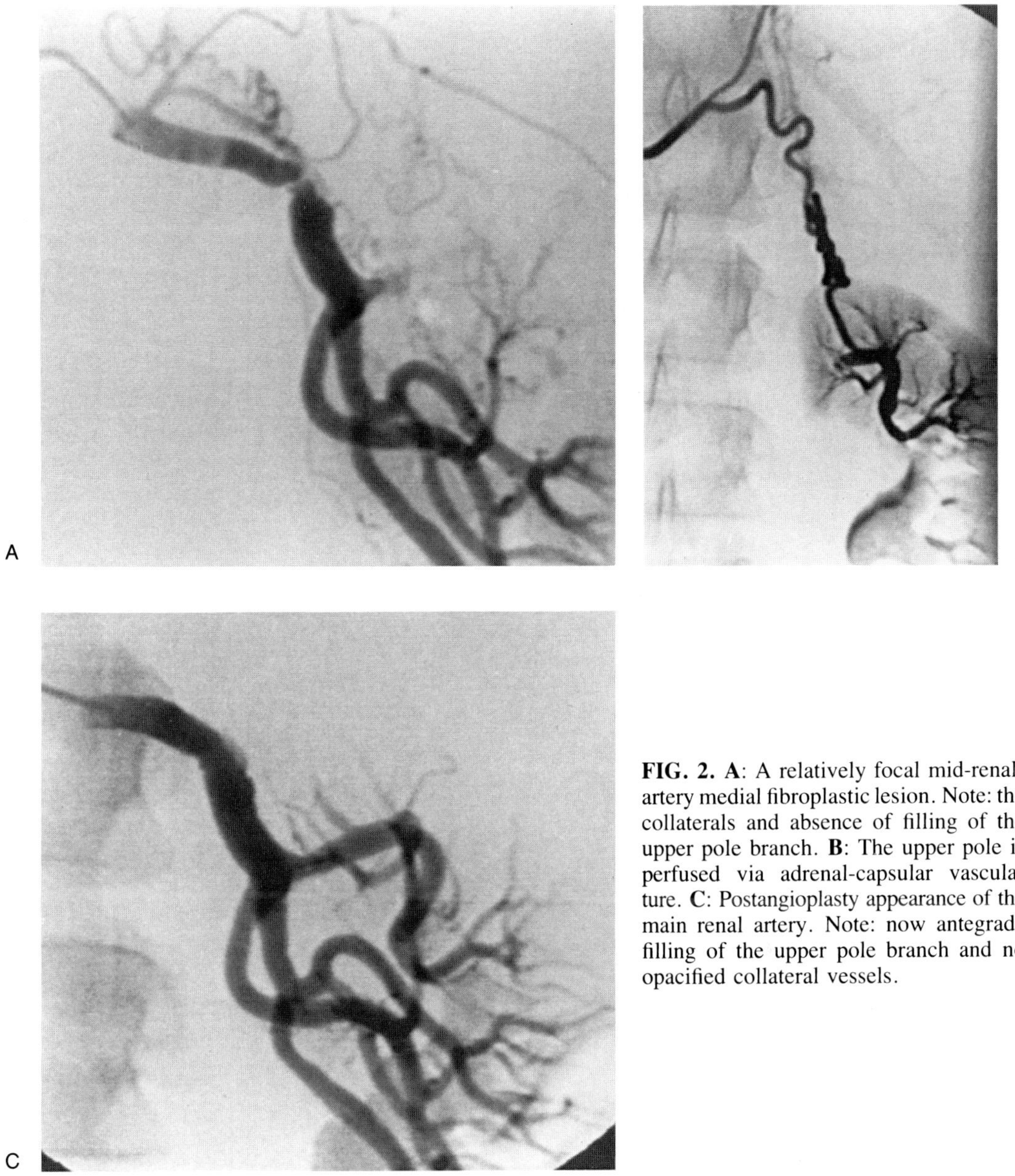

FIG. 2. A: A relatively focal mid-renal-artery medial fibroplastic lesion. Note: the collaterals and absence of filling of the upper pole branch. **B**: The upper pole is perfused via adrenal-capsular vasculature. **C**: Postangioplasty appearance of the main renal artery. Note: now antegrade filling of the upper pole branch and no opacified collateral vessels.

Recurrent Stenosis Following an Initially Successful PTA

One of the advantages of PTA is the ease with which the procedure can be repeated in the event of recurrent or new disease. The primary success rate with recurrent stenoses approximates that achieved with initial attempts, and the long-term patency rates likewise approximate those achieved with initial angioplasty.

Anastomotic Stenoses in Previously Operated Patients

These patients may be optimal candidates for PTA, particularly if native vasculature was used

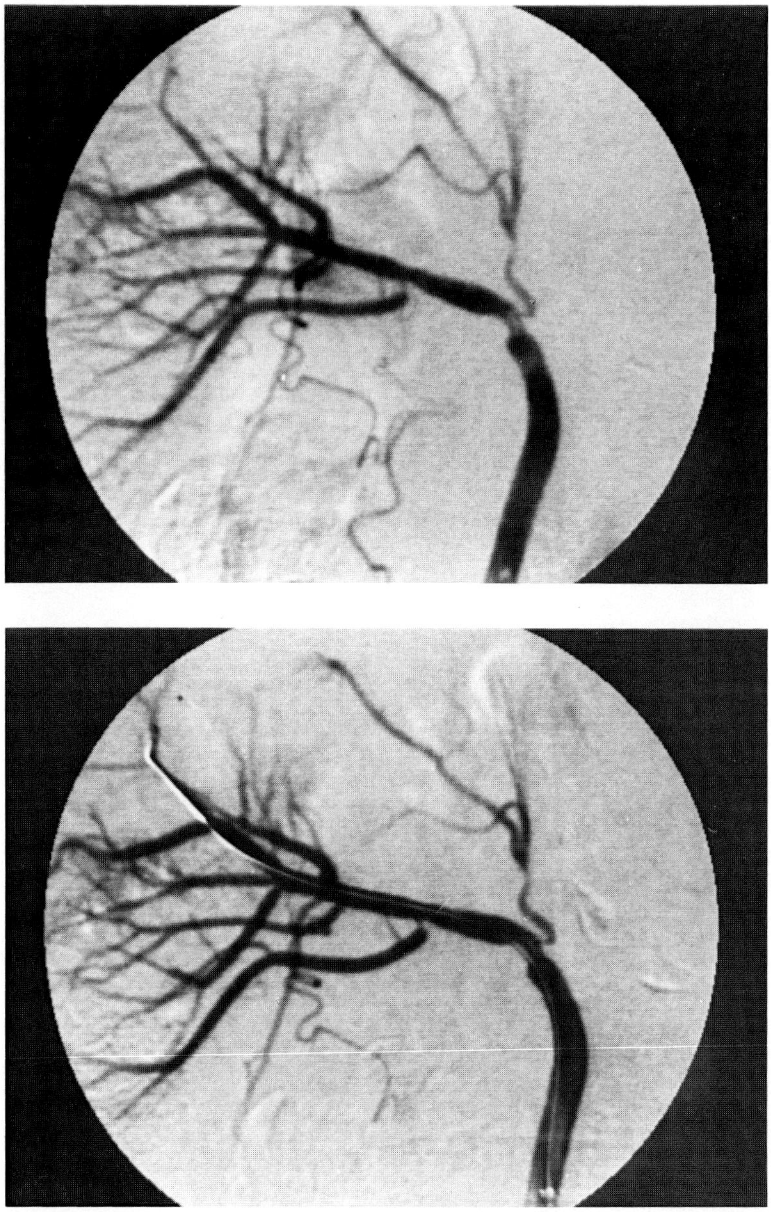

A

B

FIG. 3. A: Distal anastomotic stenosis in a patient with a reverse saphenous vein bypass graft. Note the presence of a branch stenosis. No attempt was made to angioplasty the branch lesion. The angioplasty was performed for preservation of renal function. **B**: Postangioplasty appearance of the anastomotic site with a 0.018″ guidewire remaining in the vessel prior to procedural completion.

as the bypass conduit (Fig. 3A,B). The lesions, if they represent endothelial proliferation due to a clamp injury adjacent to the anastomotic site, will frequently be rigid but will yield, in most cases, to polyethylene balloons, and almost all will yield to "mylar" type balloon materials at very high pressures, thus avoiding the need for what may be a relatively high-risk complex reoperation.

Anatomic Contraindications to PTA

Ostial Atherosclerosis

Atherosclerosis is most commonly a systemic process involving the cerebral, coronary, abdominal aortic, and peripheral vasculature. When the abdominal aorta is severely involved by atherosclerotic disease, large aortic plaques may compromise the orifice of the renal artery, giving the appearance of a renal artery stenosis. These large plaques are, in fact, aortic disease masquerading as renal artery disease and are unlikely to be successfully dilated with a balloon catheter (7). This is an unfortunate circumstance not only on anatomic grounds but usually on clinical grounds because of the diffuse nature of the disease process and other organ involvement. We consider this to be a relative contraindication rather than an absolute contraindication to renal angioplasty and will attempt angioplasty in patients with ostial lesions, as occasionally success will be forthcoming and surgery avoided. If angioplasty is unsuccessful or felt to be unwarranted, a variety of operative procedures are available to negate adverse effects of the diffusely diseased abdominal aorta (splenorenal, hepatorenal, etc., bypass procedures).

Bifurcation Stenoses

These lesions are considered to be a relative contraindication to PTA. If the stenosis involves both vessels of the bifurcation and only one vessel is entered with a guidewire and catheter system, there is an approximately 20% risk of occlusion of the other branch at the bifurcation because of a non-colinear intimal-medial fracture. In the hands of an experienced angiographer who is able to cannulate both branch vessels, this risk is avoided and this anatomy does not preclude angioplasty, since both vessels can be preserved.

Mural Thrombus

The presence of mural thrombus is a relative contraindication to renal angioplasty. Fresh thrombus, if within the area of manipulation of catheter, will most likely embolize distally during the angioplasty procedure. Preparatory thrombolysis in the hands of individuals experienced with the use of thrombolytic agents may permit lysis of the thrombus and visualization of an underlying stenosis suitable for PTA.

CLINICAL INDICATIONS FOR PERCUTANEOUS TRANSLUMINAL ANGIOPLASTY FOR THE MANAGEMENT OF RENOVASCULAR HYPERTENSION

The presence of hypertension requiring medical management with confirmatory renin data supporting the functional significance of a renovascular lesion is the preeminent clinical indication for PTA. Moderate to severe hypertension requiring multiple drug therapy preferably with confirmatory renin data is likewise a strong clinical indication for PTA. Severe hypertension that is difficult to control, requiring multiple drug therapy in the presence of a arteriographically documented unilateral 75% or greater atherosclerotic renal artery stenosis, is indication for PTA with or without confirmatory renin data.

The preservation of renal function, despite reasonable blood pressure control on medication, is a clinical indication for PTA in the presence of atherosclerosis. Minimal, if any, blood pressure response is likely to be expected in this subgroup of patients, as will be discussed later in this chapter.

CLINICAL CONTRAINDICATIONS TO PERCUTANEOUS TRANSLUMINAL RENAL ANGIOPLASTY

Lack of Angiographer Experience with Renal Angioplasty

Renal angioplasty is not a simple procedure. It cannot be adeptly performed with reasonable primary success rates and low complication rates by all angiographers who occasionally pass catheters for diagnostic studies. Some experience with angioplasty in general is necessary before it is appropriate to undertake renal angioplasty, and extensive experience with renal angioplasty is necessary for managing complex or distal renal artery lesions or branch stenoses.

Lack of a Suitable Surgeon

The lack of a cooperative, experienced urologic or vascular surgeon within the hospital and available to perform emergency revascularization within a reasonable time frame relative to the timing of the renal angioplasty procedure makes it unjustifiable to perform a renal angioplasty procedure. Without such support, in the event of complication, nephrectomy will likely be the inevitable outcome.

Active Arteritis

Laboratory evidence of an active arteritis is considered to be an absolute contraindication to renal angioplasty.

PREPARATION OF THE PATIENT FOR PERCUTANEOUS TRANSLUMINAL ANGIOPLASTY FOR THE CONTROL OF RENOVASCULAR HYPERTENSION

Most angiographers do not routinely admit patients to the hospital and are not facile in the management of patients with complex medical problems. Although there are institutions in which interventional radiologists have established what are essentially clinical services, in most situations the preparation and postangioplasty care of the patient with renovascular hypertension will be a cooperative effort, leaning heavily on the skills of an internist/nephrologist to manage the patient's antihypertensive medications, fluids, and electrolyte balance. Katzen (8) has shown that these patients are generally severely volume-depleted and require vigorous hydration to avoid the potential complications of a severe postangioplasty hypotension, fluid and electrolyte imbalance, and contrast-induced acute renal failure. The latter problem is likely to be significantly reduced by the wide availability of isoosmolar nonionic contrast agents.

Long-acting oral and parenteral antihypertensive medications should be discontinued at an appropriate time prior to angioplasty commensurate with the length of activity of the drug. If blood pressure control is a significant problem with the patient off long-acting agents, the use of titratable agents, such as nitroprusside, may be necessary in the periangioplasty period.

CARE OF THE PATIENT POSTANGIOPLASTY FOR RENOVASCULAR HYPERTENSION

Following angioplasty, patients are prone to development of wide swings in blood pressure. Approximately 30% of patients who undergo a successful renal angioplasty procedure will experience a transient increase in blood pressure in the time period 1 to 5 hr postangioplasty (G. K. McLean, *unpublished data*). It is important to recognize that this phenomenon may occur and not administer potent long-acting antihypertensive medications to these patients for what may be only a brief hypertensive episode. The administration of a potent vasodilator, for example, may well result in a patient 2 hr later being severely hypotensive. This phenomenon is more noticeable the more profoundly renin-dependent the patient was prior to angioplasty. Therefore, in the postangioplasty period, the patient who has undergone a successful uncomplicated procedure should be followed in a nursing unit familiar with management of post-renal-angioplasty patients. The patient should be kept at bedrest for a longer period than the routine angioplasty patient or a patient who has simply undergone a diagnostic angiographic procedure, and these patients should be more vigorously hydrated than the other groups mentioned.

Some patients who undergo an anatomically successful uncomplicated renal angioplasty procedure may not promptly exhibit a blood pressure decrease. Blood pressure may remain elevated for a period of several days or even 1 or 2 weeks postangioplasty only to slowly fall over a period of several days within that time frame. The development of the above-mentioned transient systolic hypotension phenomenon or the failure of the pressure to respond to the angioplasty procedure may concern the physicians involved enough that they may consider that the freshly angioplastied vessel, with an intimal-medial cleft, may have thrombosed following the concluding arteriogram which had documented a patent vessel. If a vessel has been documented to be patent with only a modest intimal-medial cleft post-PTA, it is highly unlikely that abrupt closure will occur. In the absence of objective signs of renal ischemia, particularly in the absence of flank or back pain, repeat aortography is probably not warranted. Some patients do exhibit mild flank discomfort postangioplasty in the presence of a widely patent renal artery. The mechanism responsible for this is not known with certainty but probably relates to distention of the kidney/renal capsule. The investigation of this patient, or the patient with persistent or more severe hypertension following angioplasty, might be carried out using digital techniques or computed tomographic (CT) scanning. The presence of persistent back/flank pain postangioplasty is an indication for a CT scan of the kidney to exclude the presence of retroperitoneal blood.

THE TECHNIQUE OF RENAL ANGIOPLASTY

The majority of renal angioplasty procedures can be performed from the femoral artery. With the array of catheters available today, it is uncommon to be forced to use the axillary approach and its attendant additional risks, even in a patient with a relatively caudally angulated renal artery. The procedure is performed using the usual Seldinger or modified Seldinger technique. Most angiographers prefer to use a precurved diagnostic selective catheter to engage the renal artery and then use a single guidewire or a series of guidewires to pass the renal artery stenosis and place the balloon catheter within the lesion for angioplasty. The procedure is usually a relatively simple two-step procedure for atherosclerotic lesions in the proximal portion of the main renal artery, and for fibroplastic lesions involving the main renal artery alone (9).

Fibroplastic lesions, or other lesions involving the distal portion of the main renal artery, its bifurcation, or branch vessel lesions, are considerably more complex to manage, but with experience even these lesions can successfully be managed, particularly with the availability of the extremely small low-profile balloon catheters originally devised for use within the coronary vasculature (5). These catheters have been modified by almost all balloon angioplasty catheter manufacturers to facilitate their use within renal branch vasculature (Fig. 4A,B).

There is considerably more to the technique of renal angioplasty than simply manipulating catheters and guidewires to effect the desired anatomic result. The catheters and guidewires induce vasospasm in a high percentage of patients with fibromuscular disease and an unexpectedly high percentage of patients with atherosclerotic disease (10). Vasospasm may involve only small terminal branch vessels but has also been observed to involve the main renal artery, and it is now generally accepted that prophylactic renal artery nitroglycerin is valuable, as is prophylactic oral or sublingual nifedipine, particularly in female patients with medial fibroplasia (11).

There is some dissent as to the value of systemic anticoagulation during angioplasty of main renal artery lesions, but we believe systemic heparinization during the procedure is worthwhile for a number of reasons. In atherosclerotic patients in the postangioplasty period, it is almost uniformly agreed that small doses (80–325

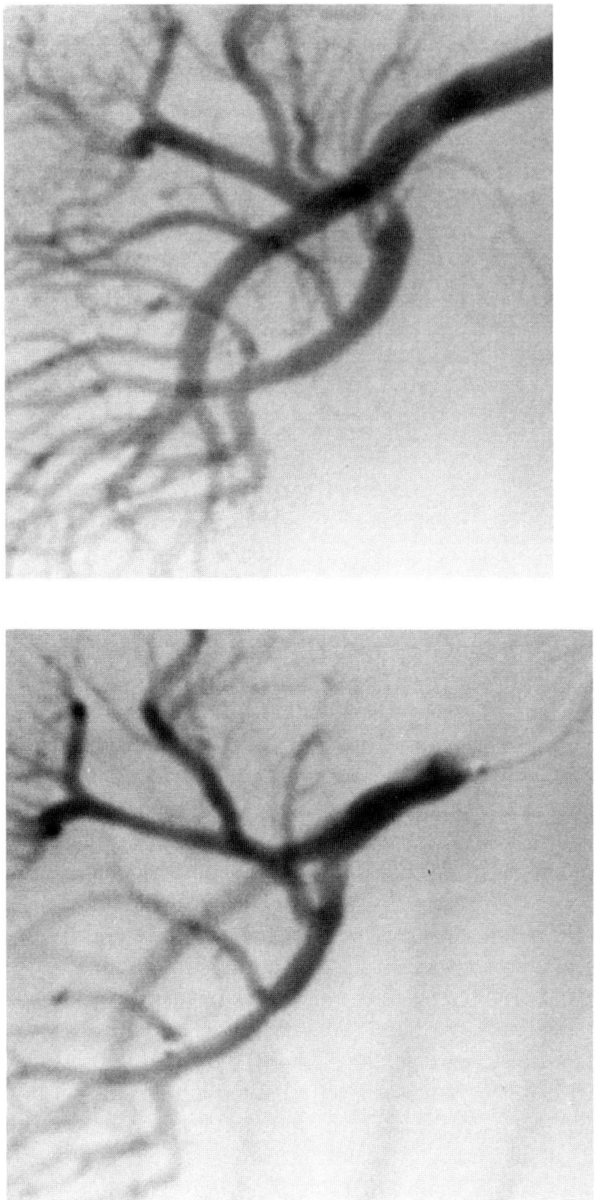

A

B

FIG. 4. A: Focal branch stenosis in a patient with severe renovascular hypertension. **B**: Successful angioplasty performed using a low-profile balloon derived from those designed for coronary arteries. Note the focal spasm in a more distal branch, which was easily relieved with a 100-μ bolus of intraarterial nitroglycerin.

mg/day) of aspirin are valuable in reducing the likelihood of restenosis. The value of dipyridamole is less clearly defined, but it is our habit to place patients with atherosclerosis on aspirin and dipyridamole indefinitely following a successful procedure in an atherosclerotic renal artery. Patients treated with fibroplastic lesions do not receive long-term antiplatelet therapy.

RESULTS OF RENAL ANGIOPLASTY FOR MANAGEMENT OF RENOVASCULAR HYPERTENSION

The results of renal angioplasty in terms of the primary success rate, the long-term patency rate, and favorable blood pressure response are all dependent on the initial pathology.

The management of medial fibroplasia with PTA provides almost uniformly good results. In our series of approximately 100 patients, we have yet to fail to cross and successfully dilate a medial fibroplastic lesion, nor have we seen a recurrent stenosis at the angioplasty site with a follow-up period of 6 months to 8 years (12). Tegtmeyer has concluded that percutaneous transluminal angioplasty is the treatment of choice for patients with medial fibroplasia (13). In his series, he had only one patient with a recurrent stenosis, which was easily redilated. B. T. Katzen's results (*personal communication*) parallel those of Tegtmeyer.

In nonostial atherosclerosis, primary success rates of 93% to 98% have been reported, and patency rates of 81% to 93% with follow-up periods of 3 to 6 years have been reported (14). It is generally accepted that recurrent disease in atherosclerotic patients will occur within the first year following angioplasty, and if a recurrent stenosis is not developed within that time period it is unlikely that recurrent disease will develop at the angioplasty site.

Clearly, the above data are at some significant variance with the data presented by Grim on the anatomic results of percutaneous transluminal angioplasty (15). This now dated, small series of 12 patients that reported a 100% restenosis rate within 1 year appears to be an anomaly.

Blood pressure response to a revascularization procedure is the ultimate measurement of success or failure if the procedure was performed for the management of renin-mediated secondary hypertension. Tegtmeyer reported his results and related blood pressure change to the etiology of the stenosis (16). He found that among patients with a renal artery stenosis of atherosclerotic etiology, 23% were considered cured of their hypertension and 71% were considered improved based on criteria defined by the cooperative study of renovascular hypertension (a 94% blood pressure benefit rate). Follow-up time in this group of patients ranged from 1 month to 6 years. Among patients with fibrous dysplasia as the etiology for the renal artery stenosis, 37% were cured and 63% improved, with follow-up time of 2 to 51 months. Colapinto (17) and B. T. Katzen (*personal communication*) have observed similar results. We have observed, among 373 patients who have undergone renal angioplasty for atherosclerotic lesions considered to be causing secondary hypertension, an 85% 2-year patency rate and an 80% cure or improvement rate in blood pressure as defined by National Cooperative Study guidelines. Among the 111 patients with medial fibroplasia, we have observed a 100% 2-year patency rate and a 93% beneficial blood pressure response.

COMPLICATIONS OF RENAL ANGIOPLASTY

Between 1978 and 1986, I have performed 433 renal angioplasty procedures and have yet to have a patient require emergency or urgent surgical intervention as the result of a complication at the renal angioplasty site. One patient required repair of a femoral artery thrombosis, and 10 patients developed transient contrast-induced acute renal failure. No groin hematoma has required surgical intervention. Tegtmeyer (16) reports 12 major complications in 166 renal artery dilatations. Six of these patients experienced exacerbation of chronic renal insufficiency secondary to contrast. Four patients required surgery following angioplasty; one for a ruptured renal artery, one for distal microembolization, one for popliteal artery embolization, and one patient died of a cerebral hemorrhage several hours after correction of bilateral renal artery stenoses. Other series with high complication rates have been collected and reported, but clearly, with meticulous care, gentle technique, and considerable experience, renal angioplasty is a low-risk, high-yield procedure.

The complications related to contrast-induced nephrotoxicity have almost all occurred in patients with preexisting compromised renal function, and as previously noted, with the availability of isoosmolar nonionic contrast agents and the widespread use of digital imaging to minimize contrast volumes, this complication is likely to significantly decrease in incidence.

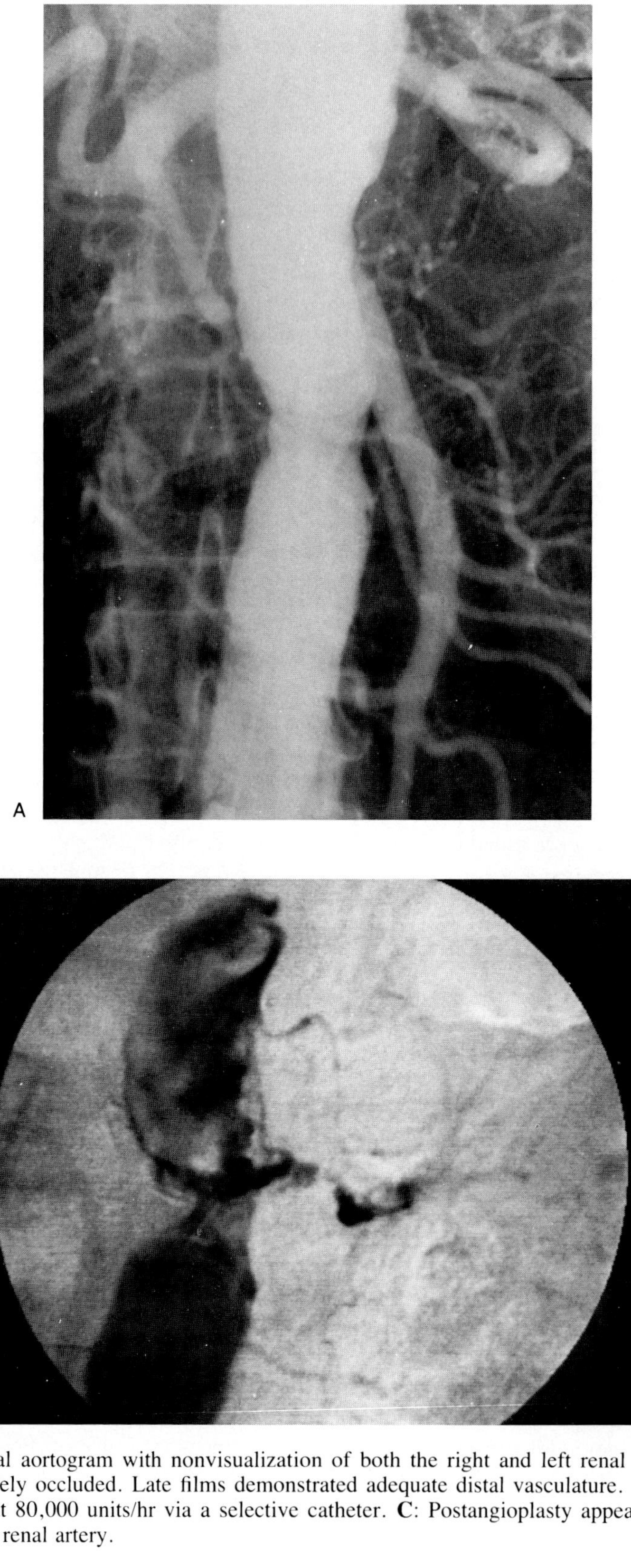

FIG. 5. A: Abdominal aortogram with nonvisualization of both the right and left renal arteries. The left renal artery is subacutely occluded. Late films demonstrated adequate distal vasculature. **B**: One hour into a urokinase infusion at 80,000 units/hr via a selective catheter. **C**: Postangioplasty appearance of the successfully dilated main renal artery.

C 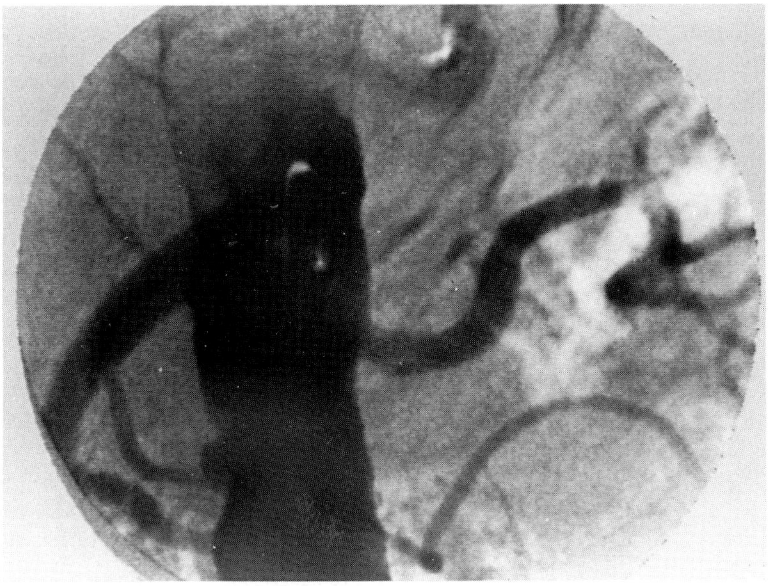

FIG. 5. *Continued*

PERCUTANEOUS TRANSLUMINAL ANGIOPLASTY FOR THE PRESERVATION OF RENAL FUNCTION

Renal angioplasty is being performed not only for the management of renovascular hypertension but also for the preservation of renal function. Schreiber (18) reported on the evolution of the atherosclerotic process in 85 patients with sequential angiographic follow-up studies and found 37 of the 85 patients (44%) exhibited a progressive renal artery narrowing, including 14 patients (16%) who progressed to complete occlusion with mean angiographic follow-up time of 52 months and a mean clinical follow-up of 87 months. The clinical follow-up revealed a decrease both in overall renal function and in the size of the involved kidney. These changes occurred despite little or no change in blood pressure and/or blood pressure medication requirements.

Novick (19) reported on 51 patients revascularized for mild to moderate chronic renal insufficiency. He was able to demonstrate improvement in renal function in 34 patients (67%), no change in 14 patients (20%), and deterioration in renal function in 3 patients (6%). Beginning in 1983, we undertook to perform angioplasty in a group of patients similar to those reported by the group at Cleveland Clinic and have compiled data on 32 patients who had mild to moderate chronic renal insufficiency with admission serum creatinines ranging from 2.0 to 3.1 with a mean of 2.7. All patients had kidneys 9.0 cm in length or greater. Fifteen patients had bilateral renal artery stenoses of 75% or greater. Seventeen patients had greater than 75% unilateral renal artery stenosis with a single functioning kidney. Angioplasty was performed on these patients using dilute contrast material and digital imaging to avoid the induction of more profound renal failure with excessive contrast volumes. Using this technique, as little as 25 cc of contrast was used for a complete procedure. The maximum dose utilized was 65 cc. The results using the same criteria as Novick were similar to those achieved with surgical revascularization. Twenty-three patients were improved; seven patients exhibited no change, and two patients were worse, with an observed follow-up time of 1 to 24 months. Lastly, we have undertaken urgent angioplasty in a small number of patients with known renal artery atherosclerotic disease who were admitted to the hospital for an acute event (e.g., acute pulmonary edema, acute myocardial infarction). These patients, on admission, had serum creatinines consistent with their known mild to moderate chronic azotemia. During the first 24 to 48 hr postadmission there were profound elevations in serum creatinine levels. At angiography, they were found to have complete renal artery occlusion, for which urokinase thrombolysis was undertaken, and in all cases (10 patients), thrombolysis was successful in revealing an underlying high-grade renal artery stenosis, which was subjected to angioplasty with an anatomically successful outcome (Fig. 5A–C). Each patient promptly exhibited a return of serum creatinine to admission levels (20).

CONCLUSION

The efficacy of renal angioplasty has been debated since its introduction by Gruntzig (21). The evidence is mounting that angioplasty is the procedure of choice for the correction or control of anatomically suitable renovascular hypertension and for the correction of atherosclerotic lesions that jeopardize renal function.

ACKNOWLEDGMENTS

I am indebted to the efforts of Connie Busick, R.T., Kathlyn Davis, R.T., Daniel Latimer, R.T., Margaret Schaffer, R.T., and Richard Werner, R.T., for their daily assistance and encouragement in the Cardiovascular Laboratory, and to Anna Prince for her considerable efforts in aiding in the preparation of this manuscript.

REFERENCES

1. Dotter, C. T., and Judkins, M. P. (1964): Transluminal treatment of arteriosclerotic obstruction. *Circulation,* 30:654–670.
2. Gruntzig, A., and Hopff, M. (1974): Perkutane Rekanalisation chronischer arterieller Verschlusse mit einem neuen Dilatations Katheter: Modifikation der Dotter Technik. *Dtsch. Med. Wschr.,* 99:2505.
3. Castenada-Zuniga, W. R., Formanek, A., Tadavarthy, M., et al. (1980): The mechanism of angioplasty. *Radiology,* 135:565–571.
4. Fogarty, T. J., and Chen, A. K. (1981): Adjunctive intraoperative arterial dilatation: Simplified instrumentation and technique. *Arch. Surg.,* 116:1391–1398.
5. Schwarten, D. E. (1986): Extracardiac uses for the "steerable" coronary balloon angioplasty systems. *Ann. Radiol.,* 29:120–126.
6. Martin, E. C., Diamond, N. G., and Casarella, W. J. (1980): Percutaneous transluminal angioplasty in non-atherosclerotic disease. *Radiology,* 135:27–33.
7. Cicuto, K. P., McLean, G. K., Oleaga, J. A., et al. (1981): Renal artery stenosis: Anatomic classification for percutaneous transluminal angioplasty. *Am. J. Roentgenol.,* 137:599–601.
8. Katzen, B. T., Chang, J., Lukowsky, G. H., and Abramson, E. G. (1979): Percutaneous transluminal angioplasty for the treatment of renovascular hypertension. *Radiology,* 131:53–58.
9. Tegtmeyer, C. J., Dyer, R., Teates, C. D., et al. (1980): Percutaneous transluminal dilatation of the renal arteries: Techniques and results. Radiology, 135:589–599.
10. Beinart, C., Sos, T. A., Saddekini, et al. (1983): Arterial spasm during renal angioplasty. *Radiology,* 149:97–100.
11. Schwarten, D. E. (1986): Percutaneous transluminal renal angioplasty (Abstr.). *Interventional Radiology, University of Minnesota, July 25–27, 1986, pp. 63–66.*
12. Schwarten, D. E. (1986): Renal angioplasty: Long-term results in 500 patients. *Ann. Radiol. (Paris) (submitted).*
13. Tegtmeyer, C. J., Elson, J., and Glass, T. A. (1982): Percutaneous transluminal angioplasty: The treatment of choice for renovascular hypertension due to fibromuscular dysplasia. *Radiology,* 143:631–637.
14. Casarella, W. J. (1986): Non-coronary angioplasty. *Curr. Probl. Cardiol.,* 11:3.
15. Grim, C. E., Luft, F. C., Yune, H. Y., Klatte, E. C., and Weinberger, M. H. (1981): Percutaneous transluminal dilatation in the treatment of renal vascular hypertension. *Ann. Intern. Med.,* 95:439–442.
16. Tegtmeyer, C. J., Kellum, C. D., and Ayers, C. (1984): Percutaneous transluminal angioplasty of the renal artery: Results and long term follow-up. *Radiology,* 153:77–84.
17. Colapinto, R. F., Stronell, R. D., Harries-Jones, E. P., et al. (1982): Percutaneous transluminal dilatation of the renal artery: Follow-up studies on renovascular hypertension. *Am. J. Roentgenol.,* 139:727–732.
18. Schreiber, M. J., Novick, A. C., and Pohl, M. A. (1984): The natural history of atherosclerotic and fibrous renal artery disease. *Urol. Clin. North Am.,* 11:383–392.
19. Novick, A. C., Pohl, M. A., Schreiber, M. J., et al. (1983): Renal revascularization for preservation of kidney function in patients with atherosclerotic renovascular disease. *J. Urol.,* 129:907.
20. Van Breda, A., Katzen, B. T., and Schwarten, D. E. (1987): Fibrin lysis and percutaneous transluminal angioplasty for the reversal of acute renal failure. *Am. J. Roentgenol. (submitted).*
21. Gruentzig, A., Vetter, W., Meier, B., et al. (1978): Treatment of renovascular hypertension with percutaneous dilatation of a renal artery stenosis. *Lancet,* 1:801–802.

The Kidney in Hypertension, edited by Norman M. Kaplan, Barry M. Brenner, and John H. Laragh. Raven Press, New York © 1987.

Management of Hypertension in the Patient with Renal Insufficiency or Renal Failure

*Richard S. Muther, *Gerald M. Reid, and **William M. Bennett

**Sections of Nephrology/Hypertension, University of Missouri at Kansas City, Research Medical Center, Kansas City, Missouri 64131; **Oregon Health Sciences University, Portland, Oregon 97201*

The management of hypertension in patients with renal disease differs even among experienced clinicians. This chapter outlines one of many approaches to the treatment of hypertension in patients with varying degrees of renal failure and following renal transplantation. Before considering such therapy, it is important to review the rationale for treatment, goals of therapy, and the pathophysiology of hypertension in patients with renal insufficiency.

RATIONALE FOR THERAPY

It is generally accepted that the major reason to treat hypertension in patients with renal disease (as in all hypertensive patients) is to decrease cardiovascular morbidity and mortality (78,79). Cardiovascular events are the major cause of death in patients with renal disease, who as a group have a heightened susceptibility to atherogenesis (46,51). Although the predisposition to atherosclerosis is in part related to the various lipid abnormalities associated with renal dysfunction, hypertension is an equally important risk factor (31,50,80).

Indeed, the effect of hypertension *per se* on atherogenesis probably accounts for the excess mortality documented in hypertensive versus normotensive dialysis patients (5,18,29). Control of hypertension in affected dialysis patients has improved long-term survival (18). Although complications directly related to hypertension are less well documented in patients with milder degrees of renal insufficiency, atherosclerotic changes probably develop during this predialytic period (70). In addition, several recent studies demonstrate improved cardiovascular morbidity with treatment of even mild hypertension, if careful attention is paid to proper drug selection in attempt to avoid lipid and electrolyte abnormalities (34,37,54). Even though these studies excluded patients with renal insufficiency, it seems reasonable to extrapolate the findings to patients with renal parenchymal disease.

Another compelling argument for strict blood pressure control in patients with renal parenchymal disease is the adverse effect of hypertension on the course of such disease. Once a critical level of irreversible renal parenchymal damage is reached, progression to end stage disease appears inevitable, even if the initiating insult has resolved. The mechanism by which hypertension aggravates this progressive renal parenchymal disease is unknown. It is clear from experimental data that progressive renal deterioration is at least in part related to high intraglomerular pressures in remaining functioning nephrons (2,14,26,35). Dietary restriction of protein can reduce intraglomerular pressure in animals with induced forms of progressive nephron loss (14,42), resulting in improved renal outcomes. (55,59). Control of systemic arterial pressure with angiotensin converting enzyme (ACE) inhibitors also lowers intraglomerular pressure and favorably influences the course of experimental renal disease (58). Thus, therapy aimed at specifically lowering intraglomerular pressure may offer particular advantage in treating hypertension in patients with predialytic renal insufficiency.

This body of experimental data provides a scientific rationale for explaining numerous observations on the beneficial effect of blood pressure control in progressive chronic renal disease. The course of diabetic nephropathy is known to be favorably affected by antihypertensive therapy. This holds true not only for well-established disease with proteinuria and reduced glomerular filtration rate (GFR) (60,64), but also for indolent or subclinical diabetic renal disease (63). Accumulating evidence in experimental models (66,67) and early studies in humans (10,12,30,41) are consistent with similar outcomes in other forms of glomerulonephritis and interstitial nephritis.

GOAL OF THERAPY

The optimal level to which blood pressure should be lowered is unknown. Epidemiologic data suggest that the lowest obtainable blood pressures, without causing symptoms, are best for reducing atherogenic risk (49). Even small blood pressure reductions have favorably influenced the course of chronic renal diseases with severe renal insufficiency (10,60). Given these dramatic benefits, an aggressive approach is warranted in patients with moderate to severe azotemia.

One caution should be raised when considering aggressive therapy in these patients. As is frequently seen when treating malignant hypertension, a rapid and significant fall in blood pressure often causes severe worsening of renal function. This probably results from dropping renal perfusion pressure below a critical level due to a fixed preglomerular arterial lesion. In malignant hypertension, this obstructive arteriopathy is at least in part due to acute injury with edema of the vessel wall. As this injury resolves, renal function will usually improve, even though blood pressure is maintained at a low level. In other renal diseases with similar preglomerular changes (scleroderma, vasculitis, chronic nephrosclerosis), the arterial lesion is more chronic and often fixed so that renal function remains significantly impaired despite excellent blood pressure control. In these patients, the clinician may need to compromise, settling for a higher arterial pressure in the interest of improved renal perfusion.

PATHOPHYSIOLOGY

The exact mechanisms responsible for the development of hypertension with renal parenchymal disease are unclear. Nevertheless, several key factors are known to be operative, including (a) extracellular volume expansion, (b) inappropriate activation of the renin-angiotensin system relative to actual volume status, and (c) increased sympathetic nervous system activity. Of these, extracellular volume appears to be most important.

As GFR falls, the kidney excretes salt and water less appropriately. This decreased excretory capacity leads to overexpansion of extracellular and total body sodium, resulting in increased blood pressure (15,17). The relative importance of this mechanism of hypertension appears to roughly parallel the decline in renal function such that the lower the GFR, the more important role volume factors play in the genesis of hypertension (43,44) (Fig. 1).

Although volume is of critical importance, Weidman et al. have clearly demonstrated inappropriate plasma renin activity in patients with hypertension and severe renal insufficiency (9,82,83) (Fig. 2). In certain cases, renin may be oversecreted due to a specific disease. In other instances, renin secretion may not be appropriately suppressed. The resulting stimulation of angiotensin and aldosterone by renin may aggravate sodium retention. Regardless of the mechanism, renin-angiotensin overactivity seems to contribute significantly to the hypertension in some patients with renal parenchymal disease. In addition, progressive nephron loss seen in patients with predialytic renal insufficiency could be accelerated because angiotensin II increases intraglomerular pressure.

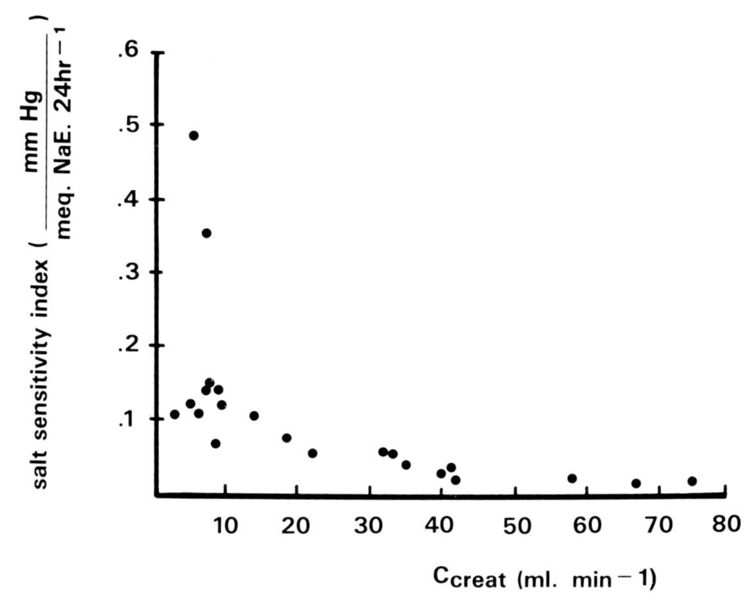

FIG. 1. Relationship between creatinine clearance and salt-sensitivity index in 22 patients. The salt-sensitivity index was calculated from the increase in mean arterial pressure accompanying a certain amount of sodium excretion increase.

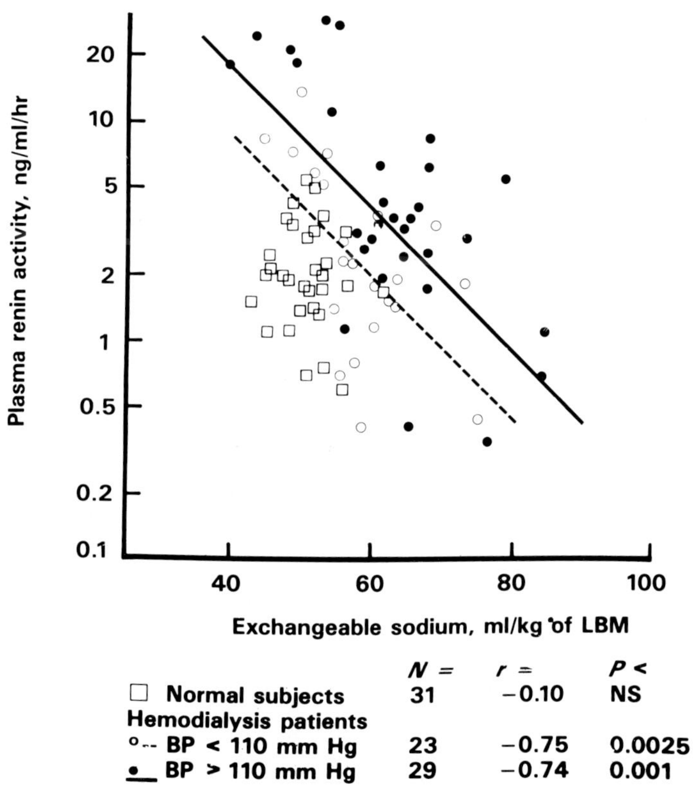

FIG. 2. Relationship between exchangeable sodium and plasma renin activity in normal subjects and hemodialysis patients with normal or elevated blood pressure.

If intraglomerular hypertension is indeed a critical factor in progressive nephron loss, certain antihypertensive agents that lower this pressure may be preferable independently of their systemic antihypertensive effects. In a renal ablation model characterized by arterial hypertension, intraglomerular hypertension, and progressive renal failure, the ACE inhibitor enalapril normalized arterial and glomerular capillary pressure, decreasing proteinuria and glomerular histologic injury (58). When a similar systemic antihypertensive effect was achieved in the same experimental model using a "triple drug" regimen of reserpine, hydralazine, and hydrochlorothiazide, beneficial renal effects were not observed (3). Only when ACE was inhibited did intraglomerular hypertension fall, proteinuria decrease, and glomerular injury decelerate (3). Studies of two other models of hypertension associated with renal injury have yielded similar results (27,68).

If these animal data can be extrapolated to humans, it would appear that antihypertensive agents that specifically lower intraglomerular pressure may have the additional advantage of slowing renal functional deterioration in patients with renal disease over and above the favorable effects of blood pressure reduction in cardiovascular risk factors.

The role of the sympathetic nervous system in the hypertension of renal disease is less clear. Circulating levels of norepinephrine are high (13), and the pressor responsiveness to norepinephrine is increased (46). Sodium retention, by sensitizing the wall of resistance vessels to norepinephrine and angiotensin II or by stimulating norepinephrine release, may contribute to the augmented adrenergic activity (7).

Another potential pathophysiologic factor to explain the hypertension of renal disease is the loss of various vasodepressor substances (kinins, prostaglandins, and others) by the damaged kidney (61). Although this is an intriguing possibility, the fact that nephrectomy normalized blood pressure in 80% of patients with chronic renal failure (24) is against this loss of vasodilator factors as a major contributor to the hypertension of most renal diseases.

Regardless of the mechanism, 80% to 90% of patients with end-stage renal disease present with hypertension (16,23,45). Although hypertension appears more prevalent with glomerular and vascular diseases, a majority of patients with primary tubulointerstitial disease may also be hypertensive (11). There appear to be no significant differences in the pathophysiologic mechanisms to distinguish these patients. Thus a therapeutic strategy for patients with hypertension and renal failure cannot be based on the nature of the original renal disease.

THERAPEUTIC APPROACH

In general, the best guide to antihypertensive drug therapy is the blood pressure response. Nevertheless, Table 1 presents pharmacokinetic parameters and dosing guidelines for the common drugs used to treat hypertension in renal failure.

Predialytic Renal Failure

Because extracellular fluid volume expansion appears to be important pathophysiologically, strategies aimed at volume reduction should be used as initial therapy in patients with hypertension and renal insufficiency (Fig. 3). The importance of volume control can be documented in several studies showing salt sensitivity of blood pressure in chronic renal failure (Fig. 1) and the therapeutic benefit of volume contraction (43,44). Dietary sodium should be restricted to less than 85 mEq (2,000 mg) daily. Because this salt sensitivity appears to increase as GFR falls (43), more severe degrees of sodium restriction (1,000–1,500 mg daily) may be necessary as renal failure progresses.

Other nonpharmacologic treatment modalities do not appear useful in the treatment of hypertension in renal insufficiency. Although dietary calcium supplementation is of benefit in some patients with essential hypertension (56), preliminary experimental evidence suggests it could be harmful in hypertension associated with renal parenchymal injury (28) if serum phosphorus is not controlled (49). Potassium sup-

Table 1. *Drug prescribing in renal failure*

Drug toxicity notes	Elimination and metabolism	Half-life (hr) (normal/ESRD)	Plasma protein binding %	Vol of distrib (liters/kg)	Adjustment for renal failure: Method	GFR (ml/min) >50	GFR (ml/min) 10–50	GFR (ml/min) <10	Supplement for dialysis
Antihypertensive drugs									
In this group blood pressure is best guide to dose and interval									
Adrenergic modulators and blockers									
Clonidine	R	6–23/39–42	20–40	3–6	D	None	None	50–75	No(He)
Rebound hypertension if drug is abruptly withdrawn; tricyclic antidepressants decrease efficacy; potentiate CNS depressant effects of alcohol, sedatives and hypnotics									
Guanabenz	NR	12–14/?	90	10–12	D	None	None	None	?
Guanethidine	R(NR)	Biphasic 48–72; 96–196/?	0	?	I	24	24	24–36[a]	?
Tricyclic antidepressants decrease efficacy; orthostatic hypotension; may decrease renal blood flow									
Guanfacine	H	12–23/15–25[a]	65	4–6.5	D	None	None	None	No(He)
Methyldopa	R(H)	Biphasic/ biphasic 1.4 and/3–6 and 5.8 7/16	<15	0.5	I	6	9–18	12–24	Yes(He, P)
Orthostatic hypotension; retroperitoneal fibrosis; prolonged hypotension due to retained active metabolites; interference with serum creatinine measurement									

(*continued*)

Table 1. *Continued*

Drug toxicity notes	Elimination and metabolism	Half-life (hr) (normal/ESRD)	Plasma protein binding %	Vol of distrib (liters/kg)	Adjustment for renal failure: Method	GFR (ml/min): >50	10–50	<10	Supplement for dialysis
Prazosin	H(R)	2–3/?	97	1.2–1.7	D	None	None	None[b]	No(He,P)
May produce profound hypotension with first dose									
Reserpine	H(NR)	Biphasic:/ 87–320 4.5 and/ 50–170[c]	40	?	D	None	None	Avoid	No(He,P)
Excessive sedation, gastrointestinal bleeding									
Angiotensin converting enzyme inhibitors									
Hypotensive effect magnified by natriuretic agents or sodium depletion hyperkalemia; acute renal dysfunction with bilateral or transplant renal artery stenosis									
Captopril	R(H)	1.9/21–32	25–30	0.7	D	None	75	50	Yes(He)
Rare proteinuria, nephrotic syndrome; dygeusia, granulocytopenia					I	8–12	12–18	24	
Enalapril	H[d]	24–36/40–60	50–60	?	D	100	75–100	50	Yes(He)
Beta-blockers									
Acebutolol	R(H)	8–9/7	25	1.2	D	None	50	30–50[e]	No(He)
Atenolol	R	6–9/15–35	<5	0.7	D	None	50	25	Yes(He)
Significant accumulation in ESRD					I	24	48	96	No(P)
Labetalol	H	3–8/3–8	50	3–10	D	None	None	None	No(He)
Metoprolol	H	2.5–4.5/ 2.5–4.5	12	5–6	D	None	None	None	Yes(He)
Nadolol	R	14–24/45	25–30	2	D	None	50	25[e]	Yes(He)
Pindolol	H(R)	3–4/3–4	40–57	2	D	None	None	None	?

Propranolol Metabolites may accumulate; increases bilirubin by assay interference; less frequent doses in some patients with ESRD; hypoglycemia reported in ESRD	H	3.5–6[f]/2.3[g]	90–96	3–4	D	None	None	None	No(He)
Sotalol	R	5–8[f]/40–50	54	0.7	D	None	30	15–30	Yes(He)
Timolol	H	3–4/4	10	2–4	D	None	None	None	No(He)
Calcium blocking agents Headache, flushing and dizziness in patients with renal disease; may increase serum digoxin levels									
Diltiazem Active metabolites acute renal dysfunction reported	H	2–8/?	80–86	3–5	D	None	None	None	?
Nifedipine Active metabolites edema	H	4–5.5/?	92–98	?	D	None	None	None	No(He)
Verapamil Active metabolites	H	3–7/2.4–4	83–93	3–6	D	None	None	50–75	No(He)
Vasodilators									
Diazoxide Sodium and water retention; 10–30 sec injections to overcome protein binding	R(H)	17–31/>30	790[h]	0.2–0.3	D	None	None	None	Yes(He,P)
Hydralazine May induce lupus nephritis	H(NR)	2–4.5/7–16	87	0.5–0.9	I	8	8	8–16 (fast acetylator) 12–24 (slow acetylator)	No(He,P)
Minoxidil Fluid retention; pericardial effusion	H	2.8–4.2[i]/ Unch	0	2–3	D	None	None	None	Yes(He)

(*continued*)

Table 1. *Continued*

Drug toxicity notes	Elimination and metabolism	Half-life (hr) (normal/ESRD)	Plasma protein binding %	Vol of distrib (liters/kg)	Adjustment for renal failure				Supplement for dialysis
						GFR (ml/min)			
					Method	>50	10–50	<10	
Sodium nitroprusside Toxic metabolite, thiocyanate accumulates producing seizures, coma, hypothyroidism	NR	<10 min/<10 min	0	0.20	D	None	None	None[j]	Yes(He)[j]
Diuretics Natriuretic agents may produce extracellular fluid volume depletion									
Acetazolamide May potentiate acidosis, produce urolithiasis	R	8/?	70–90	0.2	I	6	12	Avoid[k]	?
Amiloride Hyperkalemia with GFR <30 ml/min (diabetics especially susceptible); hyperchloremic metabolic acidosis	R	6/8–144	0–10	5–5.2	D	None	50	Avoid	?
Bumetanide Ototoxic in combination with aminoglycosides; high doses effective in ESRD; muscle cramps, gynecomastia	R(H)	1.2–1.5/1.5	96	0.2–0.5	D	None	None	None	?
Chlorthalidone	R(NR)	44/?	90[l]	3.9	I	24	24	48	?
Ethacrynic Acid Ototoxic in combination with aminoglycosides	H(R)	2–4/?	90	0.1	I	6	6	Avoid[m]	No(He)

Furosemide Ototoxic in combination with aminoglycosides; high doses effective in ESRD	R(H)	0.5–1.1/2-4	95	0.07–0.21[n]	D	None	None	None	No(He)
Indapamide	R	14–18/Unch	76–79	0.3–1.3	D	None	None	None	No(He)
Metolazone High doses useful in renal failure, gynecomastia, impotence	R	4/?	95	1.6	D	None	None	None	No(He)
Spironolactone Hyperkalemia common with GFR <30 ml/min (diabetes especially susceptible)	H(R)[o]	10–35/10–35	98	?	I	6–12	12–24	Avoid	?
Thiazides Prototype chlorothiazide; hyperuricemia	R	1–2/4–6	20–80	?	D	None	None[p]	Avoid	?
Triamterene Folic acid antagonists, urolithiasis; hyperkalemia common with GFR <30 ml/min (diabetics especially susceptible)	H(R)	2–12[q]/10	40–70	2.2–3.7	I	12	12	Avoid	?

[a]Decreased renal clearance matched by increased extrarenal metabolism. [b]May get response to lower dose in ESRD. [c]Plasma $t\frac{1}{2}$ does not reflect extensive tissue uptake; biologic $t\frac{1}{2}$ = 11.5–16 days. [d]Enalaprilat, the active moeity, is formed by hepatic ester hydrolysis. [e]Active metabolites with long $t\frac{1}{2}$ accumulate. [f]Clearance depends on hepatic blood flow; p.o. dose <30 mg extracted by normal liver. [g]Decreased hepatic extraction in ESRD. [h]Decreased protein binding in uremia. [i]Plasma $t\frac{1}{2}$ does not reflect extensive tissue binding, $t\frac{1}{2}$ for blood pressure 12–24 hr. [j]Need to monitor to keep thiocyanate levels <10 mg/dl; $t\frac{1}{2}$ for thiocyanate is 1 week but metabolite is dialyzable. [k]Ineffective. [l]Bound to red blood cells. [m]Ototoxic alone in ESRD. [n]Increased in ESRD. [o]Pharmacologically active metabolites excreted by the kidney. [p]Ineffective. [q]Active metabolites with long $t\frac{1}{2}$.

Abbreviations: ($t\frac{1}{2}$) biologic half-life; (ESRD) end-stage renal disease; (GFR) glomerular filtration rate; (I) interval extension method of dosage adjustment; units are hours between maintenance doses; (D) dose reduction method of dosage adjustment; units are percent of usual maintenance dose; (H) hemodialysis; (P) peritoneal dialysis; (Unch) unchanged; (None) no dosage adjustment necessary; (R) renal; (NR) nonrenal.

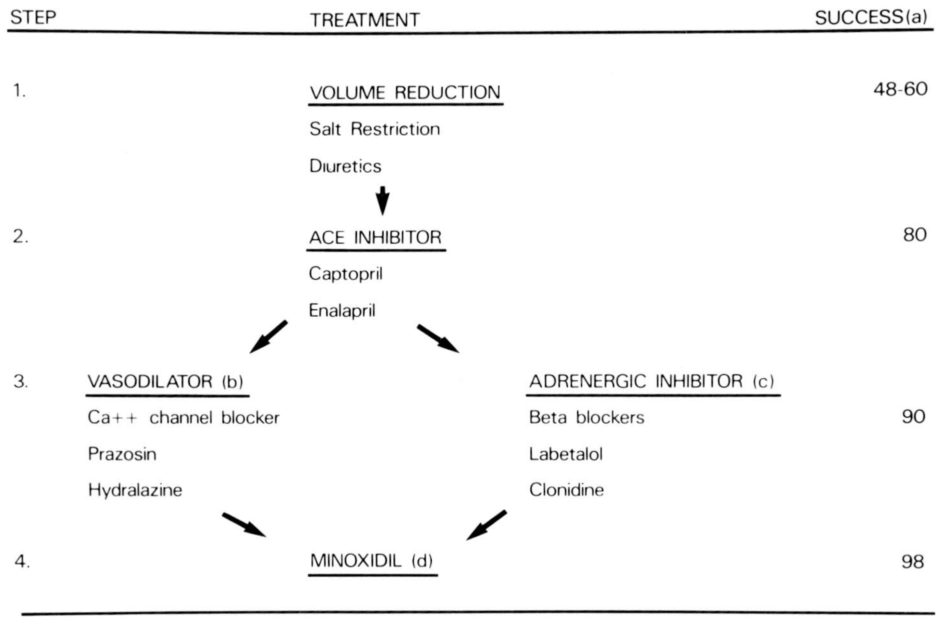

FIG. 3. Approach to antihypertensive therapy in patients with predialytic chronic renal insufficiency (see text). (a) Approximate percentage of patients achieving pressure control. (b) If angiotensin converting enzyme (ACE) inhibitor discontinued. (c) If ACE inhibitor incompletely effective but continued. (d) Generally, other vasodilators and ACE inhibitors can be discontinued.

plementation may also favorably affect blood pressure, but its use in patients with renal insufficiency should be undertaken with extreme caution.

If one does not see an appropriate fall in blood pressure with dietary salt restriction, diuretic therapy should be instituted (6). Thiazide type diuretics are preferred early in the course. Either hydrochlorothiazide 25 mg every 12 hr or chlorthalidone 25 mg daily can be effective. Increasing the dosage above these levels rarely adds benefit and increases the patient's propensity to side effects. If these drugs are not effective in lowering blood pressure, one can switch to metolazone or a more potent loop diuretic. It is generally true, however, that if sodium restriction and thiazides are not effective in normalizing blood pressure, nondiuretic drug therapy will usually be required.

As the GFR approaches 30 ml/min, thiazide diuretics become less effective. Metolazone (5–10 mg q12–24 hr) may work in some patients, but usually a loop diuretic is needed to effectively reduce extracellular fluid volume. Furosemide, bumetamide, and ethacrynic acid are currently available for this purpose. Although ethacrynic acid is the only nonsulfa derivative of the three and can be used in diuretic-associated allergic interstitial nephritis, severe ototoxicity precludes its use when the GFR is <10 ml/min. Because furosemide and bumetamide exert their action on the luminal side of the tubular basement membrane and require tubular secretion, increasing dosages are required as renal function (and tubular secretion) fall. In addition, the half-life is prolonged as the GFR falls. Thus, a furosemide dose of 240 to 400 mg once daily would not be unusual in patients with severe renal impairment.

Because of the reduced GFR and decreased sodium excretory capacity in these patients, hypokalemia is less common than in patients with essential hypertension. When hypokalemia does occur, we favor supplementation with potassium as the chloride or alkali (bicarbonate or citrate) salt. The nonchloride potassium salts are particularly useful when hyperchloremic metabolic acidosis is present. Potassium-sparing diuretics should be avoided altogether or used very carefully as the GFR falls below 30 to 50 ml/min.

Other diuretic side effects are also important to consider in the context of preexisting renal insufficiency. Hyperuricemia can precipitate acute gout, increase adhesiveness of platelets, and potentially further worsen renal function by interstitial deposition of urate. The latter process is surprisingly poorly documented despite the theoretical likelihood of its occurrence. Hyperglycemia is a cause for concern in diabetics. In view of the propensity to atherogenesis in patients with renal disease, thiazide-induced increases in plasma lipids (40,49) may be particularly detrimental. If baseline serum lipids are elevated or values increase significantly on diuretic therapy, one should probably avoid thiazides, emphasize dietary salt restriction, and use other agents for blood pressure control.

If dietary salt restriction and diuretic therapy are insufficient to adequately lower the blood pressure, a trial of an ACE inhibitor (captopril or enalapril) is indicated as the next therapeutic step. Several factors support the use of this class of antihypertensive drugs, including the demonstrated overactivity of the renin-angiogensin system in renal parenchymal hypertension (9,82), the suggestion (albeit preliminary) that these agents may slow progressive nephron loss, and, most importantly, the general acceptance of these agents by the patients (19).

Use of ACE inhibitors in patients with renal insufficiency is not without potential problems. Not the least of these is hyperkalemia due to inhibition of aldosterone-controlled distal tubular potassium secretion (74,86). This is especially true in patients with tubulointerstitial diseases, diabetic nephropathy, or other patients with hyporeninemic hypoaldosteronism, even those with relative preservation of GFR. As the GFR falls to 10 to 15 ml/min (serum creatinine >4 mg/dl), hyperkalemia is much more likely and may limit the general applicability of these agents. Potassium supplements and potassium-sparing diuretics should be stopped when ACE inhibitors are started. Oral potassium can be carefully added later should the need arise. Concomitant use of ACE inhibitors and potassium-sparing diuretics should be avoided. Beta-blockers, which alter potassium distribution across cell membranes, should also be prescribed with caution.

Another problem is that ACE inhibitors are eliminated by the kidneys, leading to the potential for drug accumulation in patients with renal insufficiency. Several studies document that serious toxicity (granulocytopenia, proteinuria) is dose-related and therefore more common when dosages are not adjusted according to renal function. Thus we would recommend a starting dose of 6.25 to 12.5 mg q8 hr for captopril and 2.5 to 5 mg q12 hr or 5 to 10 mg daily for enalapril. Daily dosages should not exceed 100 to 150 mg of captopril or 30 mg of enalapril. As with all antihypertensives, blood pressure is the best guide to dose and interval.

ACE inhibitors may also cause acute renal failure in patients with bilateral renal artery stenosis or renal artery stenosis in a solitary kidney (36). The renal failure is functional, likely due to alterations in glomerular hemodynamics, and for the most part is reversible. Its occurrence is much more frequent in patients simultaneously taking diuretics. If bilateral renal artery stenosis is suspected and the patient is already taking diuretics, ACE inhibitors should be used with extreme caution.

Despite the potential problems with ACE inhibitors in patients with renal disease, they are effective (25,69) and extremely well tolerated by patients. If a decrease in intraglomerular pressure is an important factor in progressive renal deterioration, these agents may preserve renal function over time. In addition, they do not appear to alter the lipid profile. ACE inhibitors are also useful in decreasing nephrotic range proteinuria in diabetics (73) and perhaps other patients with nephrotic syndrome. We therefore feel their careful use as initial nondiuretic drug therapy in patients with reduced renal function is justified.

If a patient's blood pressure is refractory to volume control and ACE inhibition, a third agent must be added or substituted. Both adrenergic inhibitors and vasodilators are effective. Each group offers the clinician several advantages. If one continues ACE inhibitor (vasodilator) therapy, an adrenergic inhibitor rather than an additional vasodilator might offer a theoretical advantage as the next therapeutic step. Centrally acting adrenergic drugs are not without problems, however, as clonidine, methyldopa, and guanabenz may cause excessive sedation and thus aggravate uremic symptomatology. In addition, methyldopa has an active metabolite (methyl-*O*-sulfate) which accumulates in renal failure and causes prolonged hypotension (71). Methyldopa is therefore best avoided if the GFR is <30 ml/min, especially since there are adequate alternatives.

Beta-blockers are effective and usually very well tolerated in patients with renal insufficiency. However, their adverse effect on lipids [increased very low density lipoproteins (VLDL), decreased high density lipoproteins (HDL)] has somewhat tempered our enthusiasm for the long-term use of these agents (40,49). In addition, atenolol, nadolol, and propranolol (or its active metabolites) may all accumulate in severe renal insufficiency. If a beta-blocker is chosen, metoprolol offers the advantage of beta-1 selectivity and a stable half-life, making dosage adjustments unnecessary even with severe degrees of renal failure. The reported adverse effect of beta-blockers on renal blood flow (7) has not been a major clinical problem and by itself does not prevent use of these drugs.

Labetalol, a drug with combined alpha- and beta-blocking effects, can also be used successfully in patients with renal disease. Initial doses of 200 mg every 12 hr can be increased to 400 mg every 12 hr. Because labetalol affects plasma lipids minimally compared to traditional beta-blockers, it serves as a reasonable alternative for long-term antihypertensive therapy. Perhaps the best use of labetalol, however, is parenterally in patients with renal disease and accelerated hypertension (47,84).

Vasodilator therapy is effective in treating sustained hypertension with renal disease, particularly in patients also suffering from cardiac failure. Of the calcium channel blockers, nifedipine is effective (1) and fairly well tolerated, although gastrointestinal upset and fluid retention may aggravate uremic symptoms. Diltiazem is also effective but has active metabolites that may accumulate in renal failure. No effect on plasma lipids has been noted with the calcium blockers. These agents are also advantageous as antianginal agents in appropriate patients.

Prazosin (included as a vasodilator because of its functional effects) is another effective drug that favorably alters the lipid profile (62,76). Some patients have required high dosages (up to 40 mg daily), but generally the dose can be less than 15 mg daily. Hydralazine can be used as a b.i.d. or even daily dose with severe renal failure as the half-life and antihypertensive action is prolonged. With all vasodilating drugs, reflex sympathetic discharge and tachycardia may become a problem.

Basically, the adrenergic inhibitors and vasodilators mentioned are all effective and can be used nearly interchangeably or in combination. The decision on which specific agent to use should therefore be based on the patient's concomitant medical problems, associated conditions, cost, and patient acceptance.

For very resistant or accelerated hypertension, minoxidil or the parenteral agent nitroprusside can be used. Minoxidil, an extremely potent vasodilator, successfully controls blood pressure in most of these individuals (4,8) and has largely been responsible for the declining use of therapeutic nephrectomy for refractory hypertension in renal failure. The drug is well tolerated and has predictable side effects, including hirsutism and fluid retention in most patients. The former is usually well controlled by cosmetic agents but may preclude its use in some women. The fluid retention is usually controllable by an increase in diuretic drugs. Rarely, minoxidil may cause pericardial effusion. Its distinction from uremic pericarditis can sometimes be difficult.

When parenteral therapy is required for accelerated or malignant hypertension, either intravenous labetalol or nitroprusside can be used. Nitroprusside should be used as briefly as possible (usually less than 24–48 hr), as toxic thiocyanate levels may accumulate very rapidly, causing seizures and coma. Thiocyanate levels should be monitored and kept less than 10 mg/dl. Switching patients to oral minoxidil is recommended as early as possible.

Labetalol is effective parenterally as intermittent bolus (20–80 mg) (84) or continuous infusion (2 mg/min) (47). An excellent antihypertensive response is achieved within minutes and may persist for several hours. Labetalol is preferred to nitroprusside if parenteral therapy is required longer than 24–48 hr.

Control of extracellular fluid volume must also be emphasized in patients with accelerated hypertension. They often require transient ultrafiltration dialysis to effectively treat pulmonary edema.

End-Stage Renal Disease

As end-stage disease approaches, the proportion of patients who are hypertensive increases (Fig. 4). Between 75% and 90% of dialysis patients are initially hypertensive (16). In at least 75% of these, the blood pressure can be controlled with limitation of dietary sodium to 60 to 80 mEq daily, control of fluid intake, and aggressive ultrafiltration (39,77,84). In actual practice, achieving this degree of success is often quite difficult. Persistent effort is required by the patient, physician, and dialysis personnel to attain and maintain optimal "dry weight" through dietary adherence and careful attention to fluid removal during dialysis treatments. In general, the practice of "holding" antihypertensive drug therapy before each dialysis treatment is discouraged. Occasionally, however, transient hypotension during hemodialysis may limit fluid removal and achievement of dry weight. In these cases, predialysis antihypertensives can be withheld, but the clinician should frequently reevaluate the long term need for such therapy. A change from acetate to bicarbonate dialysate and a higher sodium concentration in the dialy-

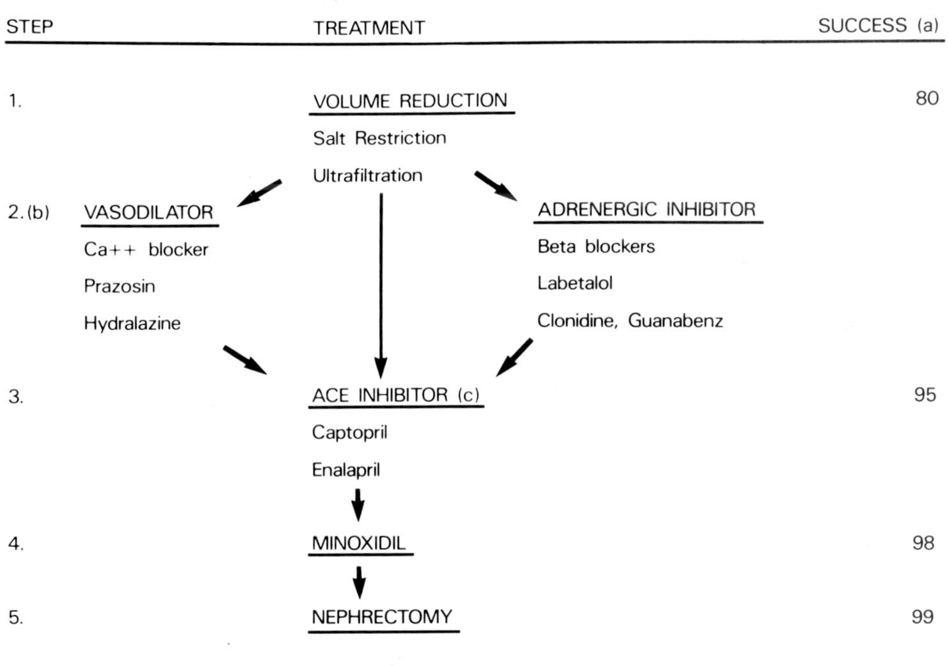

FIG. 4. Approach to antihypertensive therapy in dialysis patients (see text). (a) Approximate percentage of patients achieving blood pressure control. (b) Combined use of vasodilators and adrenergic inhibitors may improve therapy. (c) Alone or in combination with a step 2 drug.

sate may also help avoid the problem of hypotension with ultrafiltration dialysis. The latter solution will likely increase interdialytic weight gain, making "dry weight" and therefore control of hypertension more difficult to achieve.

In the occasional patient in whom hemodialysis-induced hypotension makes achievement of dry weight difficult, changing the treatment modality to chronic ambulatory peritoneal dialysis (CAPD) should be considered. In fact, some authorities have suggested that CAPD is the preferred dialysis modality for severe hypertension complicating dialysis. They argue that the slower yet constant ultrafiltration rate and solute clearance make volume control easier. However, two studies that evaluated antihypertensive therapy on CAPD concluded that blood pressure control was similar to that attained with hemodialysis as long as the same degree of volume control was achieved (48,85).

Hypertensive dialysis patients who fail to respond to volume contraction alone can be separated into two general categories: those that are easily controlled with medication and a more resistant group. In the easily treatable group, vasodilators, low-dose ACE inhibitors, and adrenergic inhibitors are of approximately equal benefit. The clinician can therefore select a drug based largely on the patient's other medical problems, cardiovascular status, drug acceptance, cost, and side effects. Again, because of accelerated atherogenesis, vasodilators or ACE inhibitors are preferable. Diuretics are of little value as long as volume is controlled with dietary salt restriction and ultrafiltration.

Beta-blockers are widely used in this setting, both as primary therapy and adjunctively. These agents are easy to use, generally well accepted, and very effective (52,53). For long-term use, however, their adverse effects on the lipid profile are of concern in this high-risk population. In one prospective crossover study of the treatment of hypertension in 10 hemodialysis patients, propranolol was compared to prazosin (33). VLDL triglyceride increased during propranolol therapy but fell with prazosin. Alternatively, HDL cholesterol decreased during propranolol therapy but increased with prazosin. The overall effect on lipids favored prazosin in lowering this risk factor.

Hypertensive dialysis patients resistant to initial drug therapy usually have significant elevations in circulating renin activity (32,77,82) (Fig. 2). Historically, bilateral nephrectomy was the only effective treatment modality for these patients. Now, nearly all can be controlled with the potent pharmacologic agents available. ACE inhibitors (75,81) can be pushed to maximal dosages (captopril 50 mg q8–12 hr, enalapril 20 mg q 12 hr or 30–40 mg daily). Both drugs are well dialyzed, helping to prevent major drug accumulation but necessitating their administration postdialysis (Table 1).

Minoxidil is an excellent alternative agent (4,65). Although tachycardia and hypertrichosis can be expected, it is extremely effective even in the most resistant cases of hypertension. The significant fluid retention seen in patients with mild to moderate renal insufficiency is much less common in dialysis patients and can be controlled with ultrafiltration. Minoxidil is partially removed by hemodialysis, but its major clearance is hepatic and usual doses can be given to dialysis patients. We suggest starting at 2.5 mg every 8 hr but pushing the dose to 10 mg every 8 hr (Table 1).

Bilateral nephrectomy (45,77,82) and nonsurgical embolization of the kidneys are both highly effective in controlling hypertension. However, the cost is extremely high, as residual renal function and urine volume are lost; anemia and metabolic bone disease may worsen. This procedure should therefore be considered prohibitive except as preparation for renal transplant. If erythropoietin therapy becomes a reality for the anemia of uremia, this option could be reconsidered.

Renal Transplants

Hypertension in recipients of renal transplants has been recently extensively reviewed (23) and will be only briefly discussed here (Fig. 5). The approach must be individualized to the particular clinical characteristics of the patient involved.

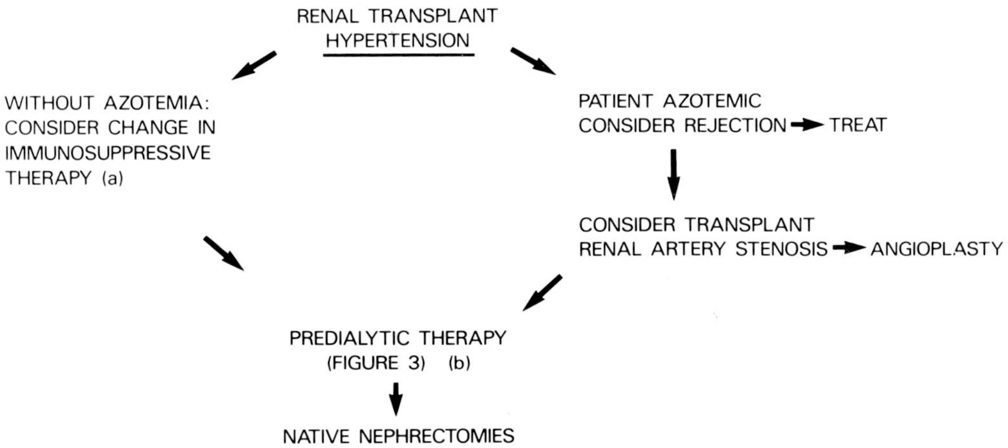

FIG. 5. Approach to hypertension following renal transplantation (see text). (a) If consistent with posttransplant immunologic circumstances, consider reducing cyclosporine dosage, converting to azothioprine, and/or converting to alternate day steroids. (b) If renal dysfunction produced by ACE inhibitors, work up for transplant renal artery stenosis.

When graft dysfunction accompanies hypertension, first consideration must be given to acute rejection. If this diagnosis is made, effective treatment of the rejection episode often will lower the blood pressure. Patients with chronic rejection, recurrence of original renal diseases, or transplant glomerulopathy should be approached in a fashion similar to patients with any parenchymal renal disease, as discussed previously. If hypertension is severe or refractory to therapy, transplant renal artery stenosis must be considered.

In the presence of a well-functioning graft, hypertension is usually mild and easily controlled. For long-term therapy, consideration can be given to conversion to alternate day steroids (21) or conversion from cyclosporine immunosuppression to azathioprine (57). Either of those maneuvers may be helpful in lowering blood pressure.

Certain patients with good graft function have persistent and difficulty to control hypertension. The sudden worsening of blood pressure, new onset of a bruit, or development of azotemia after ACE inhibitor therapy (22,38) all should prompt an investigation for transplant renal artery stenosis. Angioplasty is preferable to surgical revascularization when technically feasible as the therapeutic approach of choice. If transplant stenosis is not present and the patient is more than 1 year posttransplant with good graft function, then native kidney nephrectomy should be strongly considered.

REFERENCES

1. Ambroso, G. C., Como, G., Scalamogna, A. C., Herio, A., Casati, S., and Ponticelli, C. (1985): Treatment of arterial hypertension with nifedipine in patients with chronic renal insufficiency. *Clin. Nephrol.*, 23:41–45.
2. Anderson, S., Meyer, T. W., Rennke, H. G., and Brenner, B. M. (1985): Control of glomerular injury in rats with reduced renal mass. *J. Clin. Invest.*, 76:612–619.
3. Anderson, S., Rennke, H. G., and Brenner, B. M. (1986): In arresting progressive renal disease, all antihypertensive drugs are not created equal (Abstr.). *Kidney Int.*, 29:314.
4. Andreucci, V. E., Usberti, M., Federico, S., Pecoraro, C., Balletta, M., and Meccarrello, S. (1983): Long term follow-up of minoxidil therapy in refractory hypertension. *Clin. Nephrol.*, 19:55–60.
5. Argy, W. P., Chester, A. C., Siemsen, A. S., Rakowski, T. A., and Schreiner, G. E. (1982): Hypertension in two hemodialysis cohorts. *Trans. Am. Soc. Artif. Intern. Organs.*, 28:329–332.
6. Bank, N., Liet, P. D., and Piczon, O. (1978): Use of diuretics in treatment of hypertension secondary to renal disease. *Arch. Intern. Med.*, 138:1524–1529.
7. Bauer, J. H., and Brooks, C. S. (1979): The long term effect of propranolol therapy on renal function. *Am. J. Med.*, 66:405–410.

8. Bennett, W. M., Golper, T. A., Muther, R. S., and McCarron, D. A. (1980): Efficacy of minoxidil in the treatment of severe hypertension in systemic disorders. *J. Cardiovasc. Pharmacol.*, 2:5142–5148.
9. Beretta-Piccoli, C., Weidmann, P., DeChutel, R. D., and Reub, F. C. (1976): Hypertension associated with early stage kidney disease. *Am. J. Med.*, 61:739–747.
10. Bergstrom, J., Alvestrand, A., Bucht, H., and Gutierrez, A. (1986): Progression of chronic renal failure in man is retarded with more frequent clinical follow-ups and better blood pressure control. *Clin. Nephrol.*, 25:1–6.
11. Blythe, W. B., (1985): Natural history of hypertension in renal parenchymal disease. *Am. J. Kidney Dis.*, 5:A50–A56.
12. Branca, G. F., Satta, A., Faedda, R., Soggia, G., Olmeo, N. A., Vacca, R., and Bartoli, E. (1983): Effects of blood pressure controls on the progression of renal insufficiency in chronic renal failure. *Panminerva Med.*, 25:215–218.
13. Brecht, H. M., Ernst, W., and Koch, K. M. (1976): Plasma noradrenaline levels in regular hemodialysis patients. *Proc. Eur. Dial. Transplant. Assoc.*, 12:281–290.
14. Brenner, B. M., Meyer, T. W., and Hostetter, T. H. (1982): Dietary protein intake and the progressive nature of kidney disease: The role of hemodynamically mediated glomerular injury in the pathogenesis of progressive glomerular sclerosis in aging, renal ablation, and intrinsic renal disease. *N. Engl. J. Med.*, 307:652–659.
15. Brod, J., Bahlmann, J., Cachovan, M., Hubrich, W., and Pretschner, P. D. (1982): Mechanisms for the elevation of blood pressure in human renal disease. *Hypertension*, 4:839–844.
16. Brown, J., Dusterdieck, G., Fraser, R., Lever, A. F., Robertson, J. I. S., Tree, M., and Wier, R. J. (1971): Hypertension and chronic renal failure. *Br. Med. Bull.*, 27:128.
17. Cangiano, J. L., Ramirez-Muxo, O., Ramirez-Gonzalez, R., Trevino, A., and Campos, J. A. (1976): Normal renin uremic hypertension. *Arch. Intern. Med.*, 136:17–21.
18. Charra, B., Calemard, E., Cuche, M., and Laurent, G. (1983): Control of hypertension and prolonged survival on maintenance hemodialysis. *Nephron*, 33:96–99.
19. Croog, S. H., Levine, S., Testa, M. A., Brown, B., Bulpitt, C. J., Jenkins, D., Klerman, G. L., and Williams, G. H. (1986): The effects of antihypertensive therapy on the quality of life. *N. Engl. J. Med.*, 314:1657–1664.
20. Curtis, J. J. (1986): Hypertension and kidney transplantation. *Am. J. Kidney Dis.*, 7:181–196.
21. Curtis, J. J., Galla, J. H., and Kotchen, T. A. (1976): Prevalence of hypertension in a renal transplant population on alternate-day steroid therapy. *Clin. Nephrol.*, 5:123–127.
22. Curtis, J. J., Luke, R. G., Whelchel, J. D., Diethelm, A. G., Jones, P., and Dustan, H. P. (1983): Inhibition of angiotensin converting enzyme in renal transplant recipients with hypertension. *N. Engl. J. Med.*, 308:377–381.
23. Darrelson, H., Kornerup, H. J., Olsen, S., and Posberg, V. (1983): Arterial hypertension in chronic glomerulonephritis. An analysis of 310 cases. *Clin. Nephrol.*, 19:284.
24. Del Greco, F., Davies, W. A., Simon, N. M., Huang, C., and Krumlousky, F. A. (1975): Hypertension of chronic renal failure: Role of sodium and the renal pressor system. *Kidney Int.*, 7:5176–5183.
25. Delin, K., Aurell, M., and Herlitz, H. (1984): Captopril in the treatment of hypertension in predialytic end-stage renal disease. *Contrib. Nephrol.*, 41:299–303.
26. Dworkin, L. D., and Feiner, H. D. (1986): Glomerular injury in uninephrectomized spontaneously hypertensive rats, a consequence of glomerular capillary hypertension. *J. Clin. Invest.*, 77:797–809.
27. Dworkin, L. D., Feiner, H. D., and Randazzo, J. (1985): Evidence for hemodynamically mediated glomerular injury despite antihypertensive therapy in rats with desoxycorticosterone-salt hypertension. (Abstr.). *Kidney Int.*, 27:189.
28. Dworkin, L. D., Feiner, H. D., and Randazzo, J. (1986): Increasing dietary calcium augments glomerular capillary hypertension and worsens glomerular injury in rats with desoxycorticosterone-salt hypertension (Abstr.). *Kidney Int.*, 29:244.
29. Eliahou, H. E., Iaina, A., Reisin, E., and Shapira, J. (1977): Probability of survival in hypertensive and nonhypertensive patients on maintenance hemodialysis. *Isr. J. Med. Sci.*, 13:33–38.
30. Fujise, Y., and Miyahara, M. (1975): Comparison of the prognosis of hypertension associated with chronic glomerulonephritis with that of essential hypertension. *Jpn. Circ. J.*, 39:793–798.
31. Green, D., Stone, N. J., and Krumlovsky, F. A. (1983): Atherogenic factors in patients with chronic renal failure. *Prog. Cardiovasc. Dis.*, 26:133–141.
32. Gutkin, M., Levinson, G. E., King, A. S., and Lasker, N. (1969): Plasma renin activity in end-stage kidney disease. *Circulation*, 40:563–574.
33. Harter, H. R., Meltzer, V. N., Tindira, C. A., Naumovich, A. D., and Goldberg, A. P. (1986): Comparison of the effects of prazosin vs. propranolol on plasma lipoprotein lipids in patients receiving hemodialysis. *Am. J. Med.*, 80(*Suppl.* 2A):82–89.
34. Helgelund, A. (1980): Treatment of mild hypertension: A five year controlled drug trial. *Am J. Med.*, 69:725–732.
35. Hostetter, T. H., Olson, J. L., Rennke, H. G., Venkatachalan, M. A., and Brenner, B. M. (1981): Hyperfiltration in remnant nephrons: A potentially adverse response to renal ablation. *Am. J. Physiol.*, 241:F85–F93.
36. Hricik, D. E., Browning, P. J., Kopelman, R., Goorno, W. E., Madias, N. E., and Dzav, V. J. (1983): Captopril induced functional renal insufficiency in patients with bilateral renal artery stenosis or renal artery stenosis in a solitary kidney. *N. Engl. J. Med.*, 308:373–376.
37. Hypertension Detection and Follow-Up Program Cooperative Group (1979): Five year findings of the hypertension detection and follow-up program. *JAMA*, 242:2562–2571.
38. Ibels, L. S., Alfrey, A. C., Haut, L., and Huffer, W. E. (1978): Preservation of function in experimental renal disease by dietary restriction of phosphate. *N. Engl. J. Med.*, 298:122–126.

39. Jacobs, C., Simon, N., Patte, R., Dupuy, C. A., and Sari, R. (1984): Control of blood pressure in patients treated by maintenance hemodialysis. *Contrib. Nephrol.*, 41:128–136.
40. Johnson, B. F. (1982): The emerging problem of plasma lipid changes during antihypertensive therapy. *J. Cardiovasc. Pharmacol.*, 4(*Suppl.* 2):S213–221.
41. Kajiwara, N. (1975): Therapy and prognosis of hypertension in chronic nephritis. *Jpn. Circ. J.*, 39:779–786.
42. Kleinkrecht, C., Salusky, I., Broyer, M., and Gubler, M. C. (1979): Effect of various protein diets on growth, renal function and survival of uremic rats. *Kidney Int.*, 15:534–541.
43. Koomans, H. A., Roos, J. C., Boer, P., Geyskes, G. G., and Dorhout Mees, E. J. (1982): Salt sensitivity of blood pressure in chronic renal failure. *Hypertension,* 4:190–196.
44. Koomans, H. A., Roos, J. C., Dorhout Mees, E. J., and Delaw, I. M. K. (1985): Sodium balance in renal failure. *Hypertension,* 7:714–721.
45. Lazarus, J. M., Hampers, C. C., and Merrill, J. P. (1974): Hypertension in chronic renal failure. Treatment with hemodialysis and nephrectomy. *Arch. Intern. Med.*, 133:1059–1066.
46. Lazarus, J. M., Lowrie, E. G., Hampers, C. L., and Merrill, J. P. (1975): Cardiovascular disease in uremic patients on hemodialysis. *Kidney Int.*, 7(*Suppl.* 2):S167–172.
47. Lebel, M., Langlois, S., Belleau, L. J., and Grose, J. H. (1985): Labetolol infusion in hypertensive emergencies. *Clin. Pharmacol. Ther.*, 6:615–618.
48. Leenen, F. H., Smith, D. L., Khanna, R., and Oreopoulos, D. G. (1983): Changes in left ventricular anatomy and function on CAPD. *Perit. Dial. Bull.* (*Suppl.*), July–Sept:S26–S28.
49. Leren, P., Eide, I., Foss, O. P., Helgeland, A., Hjermann, I., Holme, I., Kjeldsen, S. E., and Lund-Larsen, P. G. (1982): Antihypertensive drugs and blood lipids: The Oslo study. *J. Cardiovasc. Pharmacol.*, 4(*Suppl.* 2):5222–5224.
50. Lew, A. (1973): High blood pressure, other risk factors and longevity: The insurance viewpoint *Am. J. Med.*, 55:281–285.
51. Lindner, A., Charra, B., Sherrard, D. J., and Scribner, B. H. (1974): Accelerated atherosclerosis in prolonged maintenance hemodialysis. *N. Engl. J. Med.*, 290:697–701.
52. Lindner, A., Douglas, S. W., and Adamson, J. W. (1978): Propranolol effects in long term hemodialysis patients with renin-dependent hypertension. *Ann. Intern. Med.*, 88:457–462.
53. Maggiore, Q., Zoccal, C., Monzani, G., and Contini, C. (1978): Chronic hemodynamic effects of propranolol treatment in dialysis-refractory hypertension. *Nephron,* 22:392–398.
54. Management Committee (1980): The Australian therapeutic trial in mild hypertension. *Lancet,* 1:1261–1267.
55. Maschio, G., Oldrizzi, L., Tessitore, N., et al. (1982): Effects of dietary protein and phosphorus restriction on the progression of early renal failure. *Kidney Int.*, 22:371–376.
56. McCarron, D. A., and Morris, C. D. (1985): Blood pressure response to oral calcium in persons with mild to moderate hypertension. *Ann. Intern. Med.*, 103:825–831.
57. Merion, R. M., White, D. J., and Thiro, S. (1984): Cyclosporine: Five years experience in cadaveric renal transplantation. *N. Engl. J. Med.*, 310:699–705.
58. Meyer, T. W., Anderson, S., Rennke, H. G., and Brenner, B. M. (1985): Converting enzyme inhibitor therapy limits progressive glomerular injury in rats with renal insufficiency. *Am. J. Med.*, 79(*Suppl.* 3C):31–36.
59. Mitch, W. E., Walser, M., Steinman, T. I., Hills, S., Zeger, S., and Tungsanga, K. (1984): The effect of a ketoacid-aminoacid supplement to a restricted diet on the progression of chronic renal failure. *N. Engl. J. Med.*, 311:623–629.
60. Mogensen, C. E. (1982): Long term antihypertensive treatment inhibiting progression of diabetic nephropathy. *Br. Med. J.*, 285:685–688.
61. Muirhead, E. E. (1986): Renomedullary system of blood pressure control. *Hypertension,* 8(*Suppl.* I):I38–I46.
62. Neusy, A. J., and Lowenstein, J. (1986): Effects of prazosin, atenolol and thiazide diuretic on plasma lipids in patients with essential hypertension. *Am. J. Med.*, 80(*Suppl.* 2A):94–99.
63. Parving, H. H., Anderson, A. R., Smidt, V. M., Christiansen, J. S., Oxenboll, B., and Swendsen, P. A. (1983): Diabetic nephropathy and arterial hypertension. The effect of antihypertensive treatment. *Diabetes,* 32(*Suppl.* 2):83–87.
64. Parving, H. H., Smidt, V. M., Anderson, A. R., and Swedsen, P. A. (1983): Early aggressive antihypertensive treatment reduces rate of decline in kidney function in diabetic nephropathy. *Lancet,* 1:1175–1178.
65. Pettinger, W. A., and Mitchell, H. C. (1973): Minoxidil—An alternative to nephrectomy for refractory hypertension. *N. Engl. J. Med.*, 289:167–171.
66. Raij, L., Azar, S., and Keane, W. F. (1984): Mesangial immune injury, hypertension, and progressive glomerular damage in Dahl rats. *Kidney Int.*, 26:137–143.
67. Raij, L., Azar, S., and Keane, W. F. (1985): Role of hypertension in progressive glomerular immune injury. *Hypertension,* 7:398–404.
68. Raij, L., Chiou, X. C., Owens, R., and Wrigley, B. (1985): Therapeutic implications of hypertension-induced glomerular injury. *Am. J. Med.*, 79(*Suppi.* 3C):37–41.
69. Reams, G. P., and Baver, J. H. (1986): Effects of enalapril in the treatment of renal parenchymal hypertension (Abstr.). *Kidney Int.*, 29:256.
70. Rostand, S. G., Gretes, J. C., Kirk, K. A., Rutsky, E. A., and Andreoli, T. E. (1979): Ischemic heart disease in patients with uremia undergoing maintenance hemodialysis. *Kidney Int.*, 16:600–611.
71. Saavecka, J. A., Reid, J. L., and Jordan, W. (1975): Plasma concentrations of alpha-methyldopa and sulfate conjugate after oral administration of methyldopa and intravenous administration of methyldopa hydrochloride ethyl ester. *Eur. J. Clin. Pharmacol.*, 8:381.
72. Schohn, O., Weidman, P., Jahn, H., and Beretta-Piccoli, C. (1985): Norepinephrine-related mechanism in hypertension accompanying renal failure. *Kidney Int.*, 28:814–822.

73. Taguma, Y., Kitamoto, Y., Futaki, G., Veda, H., Monma, H., Ishizaki, M., Takahashi, H., Sekino, H., and Sasaki, Y. (1985): Effect of captopril on heavy proteinuria in azotemic diabetics. *N. Engl. J. Med.*, 313:1617–1620.

74. Textor, S. C., Bravo, E. L., Fouad, F. M., and Tarazi, R. C. (1982): Hyperkalemia in azotemic patients during angiotensin converting enzyme inhibition and aldosterone reduction with captopril. *Am. J. Med.*, 73:719–725.

75. Vaughan, E. D., Carey, R. M., Ayers, C. R., and Deach, M. J. (1979): Hemodialysis-resistant hypertension: Control with an orally active inhibitor of angiotensin-converting enzyme. *J. Clin. Endocrinol. Metab.*, 48:869–871.

76. Velasco, M., Hurt, E., Silva, H., Urbina-Quintana, A., Hernandez-Pieretti, O., Feldstein, E., and Camejo, G. B. (1986): Effects of prazosin and propranolol on blood lipids and lipoproteins in hypertensive patients. *Am. J. Med.*, 80(*Suppl.* 2A): 109–113.

77. Vertez, V., Cangiano, J. L., Berman, L. B., and Gould, A. (1969): Hypertension in end-stage renal disease. *N. Engl. J. Med.*, 280:978–981.

78. Veterans Administration Cooperative Study Group (1967): Effects of treatment on morbidity in hypertension: Results in patients with diastolic blood pressure averaging 115 through 129 mm Hg. *JAMA*, 202:1028–1034.

79. Veterans Administration Cooperative Study Group (1970): Effects of treatment on morbidity in hypertension: II Results in patients with diastolic blood pressure averaging 90 through 114 mm Hg. *JAMA*, 213:1143–1152.

80. Vincent, F., Amend, W. J., Abele, J., et al. (1980): The role of hypertension in hemodialysis-associated atherosclerosis. *Am. J. Med.*, 68:363–369.

81. Wauters, J. P., Waeber, B., Brunner, H. R., Guignard, J. P., Tunni, G. A., and Gavras, H. (1981): Uncontrollable hypertension in patients on hemodialysis: Long term treatment with captopril and salt subtraction. *Clin. Nephrol.*, 16:86–92.

82. Weidmann, P., Beretta-Piccoli, C., Steffen, F., Blumberg, A., and Reubi, F. C. (1976): Hypertension in terminal renal failure. *Kidney Int.*, 9:294–301.

83. Weidmann, P., Maxwell, M. H., Lupu, A. N., Levin, A. J., and Massry, S. G. (1971): Plasma renin activity and blood pressure in terminal renal failure. *N. Engl. J. Med.*, 285:757–762.

84. Wilson, D. J., Wallin, J. D., Vlachakis, N. D., Freis, E. D., Vidt, D. G., Michelson, E. L., Langford, H. G., Flamenbaum, W., and Dolund, M. P. (1983): Intravenous labetolol in the treatment of severe hypertension and hypertensive emergencies. *Am. J. Med.*, 75(*Suppl.* 4A):95–101.

85. Young, M. A., Nolph, K. D., Dutton, S., and Prowant, B. (1984): Antihypertensive drug requirements in continuous ambulatory peritoneal dialysis. *Perit. Dial. Bull.*, April–June:85–88.

86. Zavella, M. T., Matte, E., Draibe, S. A., Kater, C. E., and Ajzen, H. (1985): Inadequate aldosterone response to hyperkalemia during angiotensin converting enzyme inhibition in chronic renal failure. *Clin. Pharmacol. Ther.*, 38:613–617.

Subject Index